Orthopedics

Editors

MIKEL SABATER GONZÁLEZ
DANIEL CALVO CARRASCO

VETERINARY CLINICS OF NORTH AMERICA: EXOTIC ANIMAL PRACTICE

www.vetexotic.theclinics.com

Consulting Editor
JÖRG MAYER

May 2019 • Volume 22 • Number 2

ELSEVIER

1600 John F. Kennedy Boulevard • Suite 1800 • Philadelphia, Pennsylvania, 19103-2899
http://www.vetexotic.theclinics.com

VETERINARY CLINICS OF NORTH AMERICA: EXOTIC ANIMAL PRACTICE Volume 22, Number 2
May 2019 ISSN 1094-9194, ISBN-13: 978-0-323-67801-8

Editor: Colleen Dietzler
Developmental Editor: Meredith Madeira

Veterinary Clinics of North America: Exotic Animal Practice (ISSN 1094-9194) is published in January, May, and September by Elsevier, Inc., 360 Park Avenue South, New York, NY 10010-1710. Subscription prices are $284.00 per year for US individuals, $519.00 per year for US institutions, $100.00 per year for US students and residents, $338.00 per year for Canadian individuals, $626.00 per year for Canadian institutions, $352.00 per year for international individuals, $626.00 per year for international institutions and $165.00 per year for Canadian and foreign students/residents. To receive student/resident rate, orders must be accompanied by name of affiliated institution, date of term, and the *signature* of program/residency coordinator on institution letterhead. Orders will be billed at individual rate until proof of status is received. Foreign air speed delivery is included in all *Clinics* subscription prices. All prices are subject to change without notice. **POSTMASTER:** Send address changes to *Veterinary Clinics of North America: Exotic Animal Practice*, Elsevier Health Sciences Division, Subscription Customer Service, 3251 Riverport Lane, Maryland Heights, MO 63043. **Customer Service: Telephone: 1-800-654-2452** (U.S. and Canada); **1-314-447-8871** (outside U.S. and Canada). **Fax: 1-314-447-8029. E-mail: journalscustomerservice-usa@elsevier.com (for print support); journalsonlinesupport-usa@elsevier.com (for online support).**

Reprints. For copies of 100 or more of articles in this publication, please contact the Commercial Reprints Department, Elsevier Inc., 360 Park Avenue South, New York, New York 10010-1710. Tel.: 212-633-3874; Fax: 212-633-3820; E-mail: reprints@elsevier.com.

Veterinary Clinics of North America: Exotic Animal Practice is covered in *MEDLINE/PubMed (Index Medicus)*.

Contributors

CONSULTING EDITOR

JÖRG MAYER, Dr med vet, Msc
Diplomate, American Board of Veterinary Practitioners (Exotic Companion Mammals);
Diplomate, European College of Zoological Medicine (Small Mammals); Diplomate,
American College of Zoological Medicine; Associate Professor of Zoological Medicine,
Department of Small Animal Medicine and Surgery, University of Georgia College of
Veterinary Medicine, Athens, Georgia, USA

EDITORS

MIKEL SABATER GONZÁLEZ, LV, CertZooMed, MRCVS
Diplomate, European College of Zoological Medicine (Avian); Exoticsvet, Valencia, Spain

DANIEL CALVO CARRASCO, LV, CertAVP (ZooMed), MRCVS
Great Western Exotics, Vets Now Swindon, Swindon, United Kingdom; Wildfowl &
Wetlands Trust (WWT), Slimbridge, Gloucestershire, United Kingdom

AUTHORS

**CHIARA ADAMI, DMV, PhD, MRCVS, RCVS, EBVS European Specialist in Veterinary
Anaesthesia and Analgesia**
Diplomate, European College of Anaesthesia and Analgesia; Diplomate, American College
of Anesthesia and Analgesia; Clinical Sciences and Services, Royal Veterinary College,
University of London, Hatfield, United Kingdom

HUGUES BEAUFRÉRE, DVM, PhD
Diplomate, American Board of Veterinary Practitioners (Avian Practice); Diplomate,
European College of Zoological Medicine (Avian); Diplomate, American College of
Zoological Medicine; Department of Clinical Studies, Ontario Veterinary College,
University of Guelph, Guelph, Ontario, Canada

JOÃO BRANDÃO, LMV, MS
Diplomate, European College of Zoological Medicine (Avian); Assistant Professor,
Zoological Medicine, Department of Veterinary Clinical Sciences, Center for Veterinary
Health Sciences, Oklahoma State University, Stillwater, Oklahoma, USA

DANIEL CALVO CARRASCO, LV, CertAVP (ZooMed), MRCVS
Great Western Exotics, Vets Now Swindon, Swindon, United Kingdom; Wildfowl &
Wetlands Trust (WWT), Slimbridge, Gloucestershire, United Kingdom

PETER M. DiGERONIMO, VMD, MSc
Staff Veterinarian, Clinical Exotics and Zoo Medicine, Department of Clinical Science and
Advanced Medicine, School of Veterinary Medicine, University of Pennsylvania,
Philadelphia, Pennsylvania, USA

DARIO D'OVIDIO, DMV, MSc, SPACS, PhD
Diplomate, European College of Zoological Medicine (Small Mammal); Private
practitioner, Arzano, Naples, Italy

MIKEL SABATER GONZÁLEZ, LV, CertZooMed, MRCVS
Diplomate, European College of Zoological Medicine (Avian); Exoticsvet, Valencia, Spain

MINH HUYNH, DVM
Diplomate, European College of Zoological Medicine (Avian); Diplomate, American
College of Zoological Medicine; Centre Hospitalier Vétérinaire Frégis, Arcueil, France

YASUTSUGU MIWA, DVM, PhD
Clinician, Miwa Exotic Animal Hospital, Laboratories of Veterinary Surgery, Graduate
School of Agricultural and Life Sciences, The University of Tokyo, Tokyo, Japan

MICHELLE O'BRIEN, BVetMed, CertZooMed, MRCVS
Diplomate, European College of Zoological Medicine (Zoo Health Management); Wildfowl
& Wetlands Trust, Slimbridge, Gloucestershire, United Kingdom

SARAH PELLETT, BSc (Hons), MA, VetMB, CertAVP (ZM), MRCVS
Diplomate, Zoological Medicine (Reptilian); Animates Veterinary Clinic, Thurlby,
Lincolnshire, United Kingdom

C. IVÁN SERRA, Ldo Vet, PhD
Department of Animal Medicine and Surgery, UCV Veterinary Hospital, Faculty of
Veterinary and Experimental Sciences, Universidad Católica de Valencia San Vicente
Mártir, Valencia, Spain

CARME SOLER, Lda Vet, PhD
Department of Animal Medicine and Surgery, UCV Veterinary Hospital, Faculty of
Veterinary and Experimental Sciences, Universidad Católica de Valencia San Vicente
Mártir, Valencia, Spain

FEDERICO VILAPLANA GROSSO, DVM
Diplomate, European College of Veterinary Diagnostic Imaging; Department of Small
Animal Clinical Sciences, College of Veterinary Medicine, University of Florida,
Gainesville, Florida, USA

Contents

Cartilage and bone are the main skeletal tissues in exotic vertebrates and
are distinguished by their cells and the extracellular matrices they produce.
Differences in cartilage and bone formation and growth exist among small
mammals, birds, and reptiles. A basic knowledge of cartilage and bone
formation, composition, and function in small mammals, birds, and reptiles
commonly kept as pets, and the major differences observed among species, is necessary to correctly evaluate and treat cartilage and bone lesions
in these groups of animals.

Bone strength depends on its structure, its composition, and the forces it is
subjected to. Bone structure varies greatly between species and these differences may have clinical implications in their assessment or treatment.
Fractures occur when the magnitude of the sum of forces affecting it exceeds its ultimate strength. The aim of bone healing is to recover the normal
structure of the bone to maintain its normal function, but the mechanisms of
bone healing differ greatly among species. This article provides a basic
reference for the bone structure of small mammals, birds, and reptiles.

Orthopedic diseases are a common problem in exotic pets. Diagnostic imaging modalities are more accessible and available in exotic animal veterinary medicine; the higher standards of care of the veterinary profession
have progressed toward an increased offer of advanced imaging modalities. The literature on the use of diagnostic imaging modalities in orthopedic disease of exotic pets is scarce. This article discusses when to use the
different diagnostic imaging techniques and reviews the imaging findings
usually found in the most common orthopedic diseases in small mammal,
avian, and reptile exotic pet species using different imaging modalities,
especially radiography and computed tomography.

Orthopedic disorders are a common clinical presentation for the exotic
clinician. Before treating the fracture it is vital to stabilize the patient. Small
exotic mammals are characterized by relatively thinner bones, adding to

the difficulty the small size already represents. A combination of conservative and surgical treatment options are available. The principles of orthopedic surgery and ideas behind the treatment options remain the same as for small mammals, but not all techniques can be directly extrapolated. Historically, the tie-in fixator has been the preferred surgical choice whenever feasible, but further development in bone plates represents a promising advancement.

Osteoarthritis (OA) affects the synovial joint. Animal models commonly used to study the disease and its therapeutic treatment are generally spontaneous or induced. The lack of an animal model representing all types of existing OA requires knowledge about what can be expected from each species and their limitations. The choice of species is crucial, as the selection of the age of individuals at the start of a study, their sex, and nutritional and environmental conditions. A better understanding of the small mammal models used for the study of osteoarthritic pathology may benefit both researcher and clinician dealing with these animals.

In treating avian species with fractures, the clinician must be prepared to think laterally and assess each case individually, taking into account the unique characteristics of the fracture, the temperament of the species and the individual, its lifestyle, and the desired outcome. All this should be considered during the decision making process, which should involve the owner or career of the patient. The clinician should aim for a result as close as possible to the original functional anatomy. The degree of perfection required for postoperative return to normal function is dictated by the species and the lifestyle of the patient.

In most avian species, luxations occur infrequently compared with other orthopedic conditions. A comprehensive review about avian luxations was published 4 years ago. The aim of this article was to review and describe from an orthopedic point of view the different types of luxations and subluxations reported in birds, their surgical treatment, and, whenever possible, the potential limitations and complications related with these procedures.

 Video content accompanies this article at http://www.vetexotic. theclinics.com.

Because the avian skull is the reflection of the wide biodiversity of birds, many anatomic, morphologic, and functional variations are encountered. The main objectives of this article are to review the surgical considerations associated with the functional anatomy of the avian jaw apparatus and its variation among species, and to describe the general medical and surgical management of head traumatic and developmental disorders in birds.

Orthopedics in Reptiles and Amphibians   285

Peter M. DiGeronimo and João Brandão

Musculoskeletal disorders are a common cause for presentation of reptiles and amphibians to the veterinarian. A clinical approach to orthopedic cases starts with a thorough history and review of husbandry, and identification of any underlying or concomitant disease. Medical management is indicated for pathologic fractures. Traumatic fractures may require surgical intervention. Stabilization options include external coaptation and/or external and internal fixation. Special considerations must be given to shell fractures in chelonians. Many techniques used in mammalian practice can be applied to reptiles and amphibians, although some species may require prolonged healing times by comparison.

Locoregional Anesthesia in Exotic Pets   301

Dario d'Ovidio and Chiara Adami

Locoregional techniques are used in exotic pets to improve perioperative analgesia as well as decrease the requirement of systemic analgesics during and after invasive surgeries. This article focuses on the techniques that have been described for exotic mammals, birds, and reptiles, focusing on those that rely on ultrasonographic or nerve stimulator guidance.

Exoskeleton Repair in Invertebrates   315

Sarah Pellett and Michelle O'Brien

This article focuses on exoskeleton repair in invertebrates presented due to physical trauma with impairment of the integument and often with hemolymph loss. Invertebrates, especially the larger-bodied arthropods, can severely damage their exoskeleton if dropped or if they are handled during ecdysis. Clinicians are encouraged to familiarize themselves with the basic first-aid techniques for invertebrate exoskeleton repair. With simple techniques and using items found in most homes, clients can be guided through basic first-aid procedures to prevent fatalities from hemolymph loss until the animal can be properly attended by a clinician.

VETERINARY CLINICS OF NORTH AMERICA: EXOTIC ANIMAL PRACTICE

SERIES OF RELATED INTEREST

Veterinary Clinics of North America: Small Animal Practice
Available at: https://www.vetsmall.theclinics.com/

THE CLINICS ARE NOW AVAILABLE ONLINE!
Access your subscription at:
www.theclinics.com

Preface

Exotic Animal, Zoo, and Wildlife Orthopedics

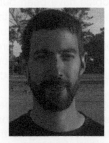 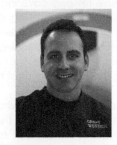

Mikel Sabater González, LV,   Daniel Calvo Carrasco, LV,
CertZooMed, DECZM   CertAVP(ZooMed), MRCVS
(Avian), MRCVS

Editors

Orthopedic disorders are a common reason for presentation in exotics animals. Their optimal management often requires a profound knowledge of the species' anatomy and pathophysiology, and advanced skills not only in surgery but also in related disciplines, such as critical care, diagnostic imaging, or anesthesia.

When we were offered the possibility of compiling this issue about orthopedics in exotic animals, an issue not published by *Veterinary Clinics of North America: Exotic Animal Practice* since 2002, we did not hesitate in accepting the challenge. Since this last issue, significant advances have occurred not only in orthopedics but also in its related disciplines. It has been a pleasure to attempt to compile and review the existent literature while at the same time trying to provide the reader with useful information not previously published.

This issue starts with a review of the similarities and particularities of skeletal bone and cartilage formation, composition, structure, function, and healing in small mammals, birds, and reptiles. Then, the utility of different diagnostic imaging techniques in exotic animal orthopedic cases is discussed before reviewing the medical and surgical management of fractures in small mammals, birds, reptiles, and amphibians. For practical reasons, avian orthopedics was divided in two separated articles: bone orthopedics and articular orthopedics. Apart from this, we considered that selected orthopedic disorders in specific groups of animals deserved a more detailed specific review, which resulted in three supplementary articles. The first one describes osteoarthritis in laboratory animal models with the idea of expanding the reader's knowledge about this and also other articular disorders in small mammals. Articular conditions are commonly seen in the exotic animal daily practice; however, their management has not reached yet the level observed in dogs and cats. This may be sometimes a

Vet Clin Exot Anim 22 (2019) ix–x
https://doi.org/10.1016/j.cvex.2019.02.003
1094-9194/19/© 2019 Published by Elsevier Inc.

consequence of the small size of some patients or due to specific anatomical particularities, but it is frequently the consequence of the limited number of research performed. The second supplementary article reviews the anatomy of the extremely complex avian jaw apparatus and provides a great amount of graphic material never published; at the same time, it reviews the therapeutic options reported for the management of its orthopedic disorders. Orthopedic procedures always require a correct anesthetic and analgesic management of the patient. Because an important number of articles and some comprehensive reviews covering these topics have been published relatively recently, we preferred to focus on describing and promoting the use of locoregional anesthesia in exotic animals undergoing orthopedic procedures, a less commonly reviewed topic. Finally, the increasing number of invertebrates presenting to veterinary clinics, frequently due to traumatic events, justified, in our opinion, a specific article covering the management of their most common orthopedic presentations.

We would like to thank the great team of authors who accompanied us in this challenge for the dedication and commitment reflected in the excellent quality of their contributions. Also, we would like to thank the Elsevier editorial team for giving us the opportunity to compile this issue and supporting us during the whole process.

Mikel Sabater González, LV, CertZooMed, DECZM (Avian), MRCVS
Exoticsvet
Marques de San Juan 23-5
Valencia 46015 Spain

Daniel Calvo Carrasco, LV, CertAVP(ZooMed), MRCVS
Great Western Exotics
Vets-Now Hospital
Swindon, UK

Wildfowl & Wetlands Trust
Slimbridge, UK

23 Webbs Place
Purton SN54FU, UK

E-mail addresses:
exoticsvet@gmail.com (M. Sabater González)
danicalvocarrasco@gmail.com (D. Calvo Carrasco)

Skeletal Cartilage and Bone Formation, Composition, and Function in Small Mammals, Birds, and Reptiles

Mikel Sabater González, LV, CertZooMed, DECZM (Avian), MRCVS

KEYWORDS

* Bone * Cartilage * Composition * Growth * Exotic animals

KEY POINTS

* Living bone is composed of approximately 75% inorganic component (water and minerals) and 25% organic component (extracellular matrix and cells).
* Bone provides the strength and rigidity necessary to support the body and protect vital structures at the same time it plays and important role in maintaining the mineral metabolism and ionic balance of the body.
* In vertebrates, primary cartilage forms the embryonic endoskeletal tissue, which may be replaced by bone except for the hyaline cartilage at the articular surfaces of long bones.
* Secondary cartilage forms between many membrane bones and at sites of muscle, tendon, or ligament insertion onto bone in birds and mammals but it has not been reported in reptiles.
* Differences in cartilage and bone formation and growth exist among small mammals, birds, and reptiles.

INTRODUCTION

Cartilage, bone, enamel, and dentine are the four main skeletal tissues found in vertebrates. Enamel and dentine are included in this list because they arose evolutionarily as skeletal tissues in the exoskeletons of early jawless and toothless vertebrates.[1] These four tissues are distinguished by their cells and the extracellular matrices (ECMs) they produce: osteoblasts and osteocytes form bone; chondroblasts, chondrocytes, and hypertrophic chondrocytes form cartilage; odontoblasts synthesize and deposit dentine matrix; and ameloblasts synthesize and deposit enamel matrix.[1] Chondroid, chondroid bone, chordoid, osteodentin, cementum, and enameloid are considered intermediate skeletal tissues because they share phenotypic and

---

Disclosure Statement: The author has nothing to disclose.
Exoticsvet, Marques de San Juan 23-5, Valencia 46015, Spain
E-mail address: exoticsvet@gmail.com

Vet Clin Exot Anim 22 (2019) 123–134
https://doi.org/10.1016/j.cvex.2019.01.001
1094-9194/19/© 2019 Elsevier Inc. All rights reserved.

vetexotic.theclinics.com

molecular characteristics with more than one main skeletal tissue.[1] Chondroid and chondroid bone are intermediate tissue between bone and cartilage, whereas chordoid is an intermediate tissue between cartilage and notochord, osteodentin and cementum are intermediate tissues between bone and dentine, and enameloid is an intermediate tissue between enamel and dentine.[1]

Cartilage and bone are the main skeletal tissues in exotic vertebrates. A basic knowledge of cartilage and bone formation, composition, and function in small mammals, birds, and reptiles commonly kept as pets, and the major differences observed among these groups of animals, is necessary to correctly evaluate and treat their cartilage and bone lesions. Evolution resulted in the loss of enamel in birds, some reptiles (eg, turtles), and some mammals (eg, armadillos, aardvark, pangolins, anteaters, and baleen whales). The organogenesis, composition, and function of dentine and enamel are not included in this review.[2]

ORGANOGENESIS OF SKELETAL CARTILAGE AND BONE

The skeletogenic mesenchyme of vertebrates derives from two germ layers. The neural crest is the origin of the craniofacial endoskeleton of the head, the visceral arches, and the clavicles, whereas the mesoderm originates the segmented axial skeleton (ie, vertebrae, ribs, and sternum), the appendicular skeleton (ie, limbs and their respective girdles, except for the clavicles), and most of the bones of the cranial vault.[3-5] Being more precise, the segmented axial endoskeleton derives from the sclerotomal portion of the somites, whereas the appendicular skeleton derives from its lateral plate.[5] Variations in the organogenesis of the bones of the cranial vault have been observed in different species (eg, axolotl, chicken, and mouse).[4]

Mesenchymal stem cells are multipotent stem cells able to differentiate into adipocytes, osteoblasts, chondroblasts, and myoblasts.[6] Mesenchymal stem cells lineage "commitment" is regulated by multiple signaling mechanisms, including, but not limited to, transforming growth factor-β/bone morphogenic protein signaling, wingless-type mouse mammary tumor virus (MMTV) integration site signaling, Hedgehogs, Notch, and fibroblast growth factors.[7]

Skeletal Chondrogenesis

Mesenchymal cells committed to form cartilage migrate to areas destined to become cartilage where they produce an ECM rich in hyaluronan and collagen type I and type IIA.[8-10] Then, an increased hyaluronidase activity and the appearance of cell adhesion molecules (neural cadherin and neural cell adhesion molecule) provoke specific cell-cell and cell-matrix interactions that result in the aggregation of mesenchymal cells in precartilaginous nodules, in a process referred as condensation, and initiate the differentiation of mesenchymal derived stem cells (MDSC) into chondroblasts.[7,8,10] At some point, chondroblasts replace the production of collagen type I by collagen types II, IX, and XI; Gla protein; chondroitin sulfate; aggrecan; and link protein.[8] The chondroblasts lose their cytoplasmic processes becoming rounded and differentiate into chondrocytes once they are individually encased by the surrounding matrix in a space called lacuna.[8]

Cartilage grows by two mechanisms. In interstitial growth, chondrocytes trapped within lacunae divide giving rise to an isogenous group of cells (up to eight). These cells produce ECM that separates and encloses each of them individually within a lacuna.[9] The mesenchymal cells surrounding the developing cartilaginous mass give rise to a dense irregular connective tissue sheath, the perichondrium, consisting of an inner chondrogenic layer and an outer fibrous layer.[9] In appositional growth, chondrogenic cells of the perichondrium give rise to chondroblasts that produce ECM. This new cartilage is deposited on the surface of existing cartilage.[9]

Because cartilage is avascular, chondrocytes receive nutrients (including oxygen) by diffusion from blood vessels in the perichondrium.[9] Most chondrocytes continue to divide throughout life, although in some cartilages, such as mammalian articular ones, the number of dividing cells may be less than 1% of the chondrocyte population.[1]

Skeletal Osteogenesis

Skeletal bone formation occurs by replacement of a pre-existing connective tissue. Two processes result in the formation of normal bone tissue:

- Direct ossification or intramembranous ossification refers to the direct conversion of the primitive connective tissue, the mesenchyme, into bone.[5] MDSCs condensate in specific ossification centers of the mesenchyme where they differentiate into osteoblasts that produce osteoid, which becomes mineralized, becoming osteocytes.[1] Simultaneously, the MDSCs around the ossification center divide producing more osteoblasts, which lay down additional bone in their periphery. Primary bone formation continues while the growth rate of the connective tissue separating the nuclei of ossification exceeds the peripheral ossification rate of the nuclei and stops when the two ossification nuclei coalesce and fuse. Bone formed by intramembranous ossification is cancellous.[11] Remodeling of this bone by osteoclasts allows the ordered osteoblastic deposition of compact and cancellous bone.[11] The exoskeleton of vertebrates is formed by membranous ossification.[12]
- Indirect ossification refers to the formation of bone by replacement of another tissue (eg, cartilage, marrow, tendon, or ligament).[13] Endochondral ossification, in which cartilage is replaced by bone, is the most common form of indirect ossification.[13] However, other forms of indirect ossification are observed, such as in tendons and sesamoids.[13]

Although membrane bones are formed by direct ossification, others require a combination of direct and indirect ossification (mainly endochondral).[1] Most membrane bones are part of the exoskeleton, whereas all the bones showing endochondral ossification are endoskeletal.[13] The costoneural plates of the chelonian carapace are an example of membranous ossification derived from the endoskeleton (ribs).[12] In very specific cases, exoskeleton and endoskeleton fuse (eg, in the endochondral bone that replaces Meckel cartilage [endoskeleton] and dermal mandibular bones in hamsters).[13]

Histologically, bone is classified as primary or secondary. Independently of the type of ossification, primary bone presents low mechanic resistance because of the random distribution of collagen fibers (mainly type I), the higher density of cells, and the higher amount of ground substance not completely mineralized. In general, primary bone is replaced by secondary bone except in the sutures of the cranial vault bones, the insertion of tendons, and in dental alveoli (in animals that present them). This bone may be also observed in areas with an accelerated production of bone, such as fracture repairs or some bone tumors. Osteoclasts replace the bone formed by primary ossification by lamellar or secondary bone. Secondary bone is characterized by a lower number of osteocytes located between concentric lamellae surrounding vascular canals (Haver canals) with each lamella presenting collagen fibers parallel oriented separated by organic matrix. This structure combined with the higher degree of mineralization results in the higher mechanical resistance of secondary bone when compared with primary bone.

Postnatally, the skeleton grows intramembranously in membrane bones and at sutural margins of skull bones, and by endochondral or perichondral replacement as in long bones, short bones, vertebrae, and ribs.[13,14] Bone and dentine are often deposited in sufficiently precise layers that age or other aspects of the life history of an individual can be determined with relative accuracy (eg, periosteal growth lines in the mandibles of European hares or concentric osseous annular rings in turtles, snakes, and lizards).[15,16]

The osteogenesis of the flat bones of the cranial vault and long bones is used to illustrate the variability in the formation of different bones and between species.

Osteogenesis of the flat bones of the cranial vault
Neural-crest-derived mesenchymal cells proliferate and condense and form ossification centers following the same initial steps already discussed for skeletal chondrogenesis, except that some of the mesenchymal-derived cells committed to form bone differentiate into osteoblasts instead of differentiating into chondroblasts. Bone morphogenetic proteins from the head epidermis induce the differentiation of mesenchymal-derived cells into osteoblasts.[5] Osteoblasts start synthetizing osteoid, an organic component of the ECM of bone composed of fibers (collagens and elastins) and ground substance.[1] Calcium hydroxyapatite crystals attach to the collagen fibers provoking the progressive mineralization of the ECM in the nucleus of ossification.[1] Osteoblasts surrounded by osteoid become osteocytes. The MDSCs around the ossification center divide producing more osteoblasts that lay down additional bone in their periphery. This bone is cancellous. Mesenchymal-derived cells form parallel compact layers surrounding the cancellous bone, forming the periosteum. The cells of the inner layer of the periosteum are also able to transform into osteoblasts, which deposit osteoid parallel to the existing spicules, forming cortical bone.[5] The two plates of cortical bone fuse with the cancellous bone in between resulting in a flat bone. The interosseous spaces in cancellous bone contain bone marrow.[9] Variations in the organogenesis of these bones, including the moment at which full ossification occurs, have been observed in different species. For example, in mice, the frontal bone derives from the neural crest and the parietal bone derives from the mesoderm, whereas in chickens the rostral aspect of the frontoparietal bone derives from cells originated in the neural crest and its nuchal aspect derives from cells originated in the mesoderm.[4]

Osteogenesis of long bones
During fetal development, a small hyaline cartilage model of the long bone is formed. Mesenchymal-derived cells condense and form the perichondrium along the outer surface of the shaft of the cartilaginous model. Then, the cartilaginous model expands in length by interstitial growth in and near the ends of the model, and in width by appositional growth in the perichondrium. The chondrocytes within the shaft proliferate forming rows parallel to the long axis of the bone and are individually surrounded by a thin layer of ECM.[9] A reciprocal interaction between chondrocytes and the cells of the perichondrium regulates the hypertrophy of the chondrocytes and maturation of the perichondrium.[9] Hypertrophic chondrocytes produce collagen type X, alkaline phosphatase, fibronectin, and matrix metalloproteinase 13, which allow the calcification of the ECM impeding the diffusion of nutrients, which results in the apoptosis of hypertrophic chondrocytes, and facilitates vascular invasion of the perichondrium around the diaphysis.[9] Following this, the osteoprogenitor cells in the perichondrium differentiate   into   osteoblasts,   forming   the   periosteum,   which   grows   by

intramembranous ossification.[9] The degeneration of the calcified cartilage at the center of the cartilaginous template forms a primitive medullary cavity that is invaded by blood vessels, mesenchymal cells, and osteoblasts and osteoclast from the periosteum, forming the primary or diaphyseal center of ossification.[9] Then, osteoclasts remove the dead chondrocytes forming tunnels that, under the influence of VegF, are invaded by blood vessels, which transport osteoblasts that form osteoid on the noncellular calcified cartilaginous matrix, producing cancellous bone.[9,11] Primary ossification of the mesenchyme of a long bone occurs subperiosteally around the shaft and by endochondral replacement of cartilage of the shaft or metaphysis in mammals, important differences in the amount of endochondral ossification or the developmental moment in which it starts, have been observed between species.[1,14,17–22] In mice, periosteal ossification is minimal, and the cartilage is replaced by bone, beginning during embryonic life; therefore, ossification and bone are endochondral. Also, because in avian long bones cartilage is replaced by marrow, which is only replaced by bone after hatching (differences are also observed between altricial and precocial birds), the terms endochondral ossification and endochondral bone may not be completely accurate and therefore, such terms as indirect ossification, perichondral intramembranous ossification, or replacement bone are preferred by some authors.[1,23] In reptiles, the calcification of the diaphysis of long bones is perichondral and occurs in three stages: (1) only peripheral calcification of the mid-diaphyseal region, (2) peripheral calcification in the entire diaphysis accompanied with central calcification in the mid-diaphyseal region, and (3) peripheral and central calcification of the entire diaphysis.[14]

Secondary centers of ossification form in the epiphyses of multiple bones in small mammals, in squamates, in the New Zealand tuatara (*Sphenodon punctatus* [order Rhynchocephalia]), and in the proximal tibiotarsus of birds.[24,25] These centers occur when, in a large number of mammal and avian species, cartilage canals penetrate the epiphyseal cartilage bringing osteogenic cells.[24] However, cartilage canals are not present in all vertebrates. For example, the epiphyses of the mouse, rat, and marsupials (eg, opossums [*Didelphis* spp], terrestrial kangaroos, wallabies and wallaroos [*Macropus* spp], and tree-kangaroos [*Dendrolagus* spp]) lack these canals and therefore, the ossification of secondary centers of ossification occurs directly from the perichondrium.[24,25] Also, cartilage canals have been reported in varanids but not in other lizards.[25] In the epiphyses, the type of ossification varies within species. Periosteal ossification dominates in taxa in which mechanical stresses decrease the importance of secondary centers of ossification (eg, fish, amphibians, and birds), whereas periosteal and endochondral ossification predominates in taxa in which mechanical stress increases the need for secondary centers of ossification (eg, mammals and lizards).[24,25] The New Zealand tuatara presents primitive secondary centers of ossification, but these centers undergo subsequent resorption and replacement by bone when the ossification of the diaphysis extends through the metaphyseal growth zone into the epiphyses.[25] In long bones of turtles and crocodilians, there is a large cartilaginous epiphysis that overlies a growth plate and secondary centers of ossification do not occur.[18,20] In birds, although the tibia and the proximal row of tarsal bones fuse forming the tibiotarsus, the distal tarsal row and the metatarsus fuse forming the tarsometatarsus, and the distal row of carpal bones and the metacarpals fuse forming the carpometacarpus, the only secondary ossification center is in the proximal tibiotarsus.[24]

The time of appearance of these centers during the life of a long bone varies greatly between bones and species.[24] In most species and independently of the type of epiphysial ossification, at some stage, cartilage is restricted to a definitive thin layer in the epiphysial surface that gives rise to the articular cartilage, and to a temporary cartilaginous plate between the diaphysis and the epiphysis in which interstitial growth of cartilage occurs, the epiphysial or growth plate.[9] In the marbled leaf-toed gecko (*Afrogecko porphyreus*), and probably in other very small lizards, the secondary center of ossification is never ossified.[25]

Histologically, the growth plate of mammals is divided into five zones starting from the epiphyseal side of the cartilage: (1) chondrocytic reserve, (2) proliferative, (3) hypertrophic, (4) resorption, and (5) ossification.[5] When the rate of osseous replacement exceeds the mitotic activity within the chondrocytic reserve zone of the growth plate, closure of the plate occurs and the cancellous bone of the metaphysis becomes continuous with the cancellous bone of the epiphysis. In the minimally mineralized humeral and tibial metaphyses of Guinea pigs and mice, many chondrocytes survive and fibrils accumulate within them as they ultrastucturally resemble osteoblasts in a similar process to the metaplastic transformation of secondary cartilage into bone in birds.[26] The closure time of the growth plates of a bone varies between species but also between different bones in the same animal.[9] In mammals, hormonal changes at sexual maturity result in the cessation of growth and fusion of the growth plate, whereas in birds, skeletal maturity occurs at an early age.[11] Although birds lack true epiphyseal (growth) plates, zones of proliferation are evident. This zone is different from the epiphyseal growth plate observed in mammals in three ways: (1) they are wider; (2) they present cells in their zone of hypertrophy not arranged in orderly columns nor are they invaded systematically by vascular channels, which leaves clusters of chondrocytes surrounded by mineralized matrix; and (3) they are vascularized by two sets of vessels (one from the epiphysis and one from the metaphysis) in contrast to the single epiphyseal blood supply in mammals.[11] In lizards with legs, the epiphyseal secondary centers of ossification of long bones consist of several zones of endochondral bone formation: zone of reserve cartilage, zone of multiplication, zone of hypertrophy, zone of calcification, and zone of ossification.[27] In reptiles, apart from the bone growth differences between groups already discussed, determinate growth has been recently confirmed in species that were, at some point, considered to present an indeterminate growth. Degradation of the growth plate cartilage in small-sized species of varanids occurs in adults, whereas it is delayed to senescence in larger species.[28] Osteologic evidence for determinate growth has been reported in the American alligator (*Alligator mississippiensis*).[29]

Factors affecting cartilage and bone growth and mineralization

Bone growth and development is the result of the complex interactions of genetic and environmental factors, including nutrition, hormones, and mechanical stimuli.[30] Cartilage mineralization is species-specific. Mammalian small-cell cartilage normally does not mineralize. Secondary cartilages (those developing from osteochondral progenitor cells) on avian membrane bones mineralize, but Meckel cartilage, a small-cell cartilage, does not.[31] Multiple factors have been reported to affect bone growth in a positive (eg, parathyroid hormones, androgens, tension or compression to a certain level) or a negative way (eg, glucocorticoids, estrogens, or compression after a certain level).[30] Also, cartilage and bone mineralization may be affected by nutritional disorders, such as mineral imbalances (eg, calcium or phosphorus) or vitamin deficiencies or excesses (eg, deficiency or excess of vitamin A; deficiency or excess of vitamin D [rickets/osteomalacia]; and vitamin C deficiency [scurvy] in Guinea pigs [*Cavia porcellus*], in some primates, or in the red-vented bulbul [*Pycnonotus cafer*]).[32,33] In Guinea pigs with or recovering from scurvy, the patterns of circulation and mineralization of condylar, tibial epiphyseal, and tibial articular cartilages are different. Condylar cartilage doubles in width after 26 days but the tibial cartilages show much less change in growth. Recovery is even more rapid, showing a normal condylar width after 3 days of treatment with ascorbic acid.[32]

SKELETAL CARTILAGE COMPOSITION, STRUCTURE, FUNCTION, AND REPAIR

Skeletal cartilage is a supporting and articular skeletal tissue consisting of specialized cells (chondroblasts, chondrocytes, and chondroclasts) separated by pericellular and ECM composed of abundant ground substance rich in glycosaminoglycans (eg, chondroitin sulfate) and proteoglycans (eg, elastin fibers) that, depending on the cartilage type and the species, may mineralize or not (eg, invertebrates).[1] The major extracellular protein of cartilage in small mammals, birds, and reptiles is collagen II.

Based on the types and distribution of fibers, cartilage is classified as hyaline, elastic, or fibrocartilage. Hyaline cartilage contains highly dispersed type II collagen fibers and it is the weakest of the three types of cartilage; elastic cartilage contains type II collagen fibers with elastic fibers scattered throughout the matrix; and fibrocartilage contains dense, coarse type I collagen fibers oriented in the direction of functional stress forces.[9]

In vertebrates, primary cartilage forms the embryonic endoskeletal tissue, which may be replaced by bone except for the hyaline cartilage at the articular surfaces of long bones. Secondary cartilage forms between many membrane bones and at sites of muscle, tendon, or ligament insertion onto bone in birds and mammals but it has not been reported in reptiles.[1,34]

From a mechanical point of view, articular cartilage is a resilient tissue with viscoelastic properties able to resist compressive, shear, and tensile loading stress forces.[35]

Although most chondrocytes continue to divide throughout life, in some cartilages, such as mammalian articular ones, the number of dividing cells may be less than 1% of the chondrocyte population.[1] This reduced rate of division, combined with the avascular and aneural nature of cartilage, explains its limited capacity for intrinsic healing and repair.[13] Nutrition of the cartilage cells occurs by diffusion of nutrients.[13]

SKELETAL BONE COMPOSITION, FUNCTION, AND REMODELING

Bone is a vascular, innervated skeletal tissue only found in vertebrates but not every vertebrate has bone (eg, lampreys and hagfishes).[1] Approximately, bone is composed of 75% inorganic component (water and minerals) and 25% organic component (ECM and cells).[35] The water content of bone is approximately 10% of bone weight.[36] The mineral component of bone consists of calcium hydroxyapatite crystals, which provides strength and rigidity; represents 65% of bone weight; and contains the 99% of calcium, 85% of phosphorus, and 65% of sodium and magnesium of the total corporal reserves.[11,36] The mineral composition varies not only between species, but also within the same individual depending on multiple factors (eg, egg formation in birds or pregnancy and lactation in mammals, or age) and even between different parts of the same bone.[37,38] The organic component represents the remaining 25% of the weight of the bone and consists of cells and ECM. MDSCs are multipotent stromal cells able to differentiate into chondrocytes, myocytes, or adipocytes. Osteoblasts are immature bone cells differentiated from MDSCs. Osteoblasts form a single layer of cells in the surface of bone and, in mature bone, most of them remain inactive and compacted. Active osteoblasts are highly packed cuboidal cells responsible for the synthesis and secretion of osteoid.[1] The composition of osteoid and the function of its more relevant components is summarized in **Table 1**.

Table 1
Composition of osteoid and function of its most relevant components

Osteoid/Bone ECM	Components	Function
Collagens	90% of bone protein.[36] At least 28 types of collagen molecules. Many of them are associated with more than one skeletal tissue. Collagen I (mainly in bone). Collagen II (mainly in cartilage).[1]	Provide structural support to cells.[1] Type I collagen is the major ECM protein associated with mineralization in vertebrates.[1]
Elastins		Provide elasticity to tissues.[1]
Ground substance	Water Proteoglycans: Core protein with one or more GAG attached. Depending on the hexosamine isomer can be: GAGs: Keratan sulfate Heparan sulfate Galactosaminoglycans: Dermatan sulfate Chondroitin sulfate Hyaluronic acid or hyaluronan: Nonsulfate, nonattached to protein GAG.[39] Glycoproteins: Alkaline phosphatase, osteonectin, osteoadherin, thrombospondin, fibronectin, vitronectin, bone sialoprotein (eg, osteopontin), fibrillin, and tetranectin.[40]	The proteoglycans and glycoproteins are highly anionic complexes that have a high ion-binding capacity and participate in the fixation of calcium hydroxyapatite crystals to the collagen fibers.[11] Osteocalcin: Recruits osteoclasts or osteoclast precursors to bone for resorption.[1] It is the only protein unique to bone.[11] Osteopontin: Enhances cell survival and migration but inhibits mineralization.[1] Osteonectin: Expressed as mineralization is initiated; links collagen to hydroxyapatite, serves as a nucleus for mineralization, and regulates the formation and growth of hydroxyapatite crystals.[1] Hyaluronan: Passive space filler and activates and regulates cellular migration, proliferation, and differentiation. Pivotal role in the homeostasis of physiologic events, such as tissue regeneration, wound healing, and tumorigenesis.[41]
	Growth factors and cytokines: Prostaglandin, IGF-1, TGF-β, IL-6.[11]	Growth factors: Control bone cell proliferation, maturation, and metabolism and act as cellular messengers.[11] Cytokines: Activate proteolytic enzymes important for fracture healing and act as cellular messengers.[11]

Abbreviations: GAG, glycosaminoglycan; IGF, insulin-like growth factor; IL, interleukin; TGF, transforming growth factor.

The osteoid rapidly becomes impregnated with hydroxyapatite (mineralized). However, there is always an organic thin layer of unmineralized matrix, the *lamina limitans*, separating the mineralized and nonmineralized parts of the bone matrix.[1] Osteoblasts entrapped within the secreted matrix differentiate to osteocytes through a mechanism not yet completely understood. A suggested explanation is that local damage to bone or local mechanical stress may activate osteocytes making them express osteoblast stimulating factor-1, which stimulates matrix formation and osteoblast differentiation into osteocytes.[42] The osteocytes remain connected by fine cytoplasmic extensions passing through minute interconnecting channels, the canaliculi, that allow the circulation of tissue fluid, nutrients, and metabolites, and rapid communications between osteocytes.[1] Osteocytes are the most common cell population in the bone of adult animals and have two main functions:

- The fine regulation of blood–calcium homeostasis via the resorption and uptake of mineralized matrix in direct response to serum calcium levels and indirectly controlled by hormones secreted by the thyroid and parathyroid glands.[11,42] They also link the action of estrogen on osteoclast resorption by regulating their own apoptosis.[13] Osteocytes resorb perilacunar bone directly through osteocytic osteolysis.[13]
- The functional adaptation of the bone acting as mechanosensors. The modulation of canalicular fluid flow resulting from compression or relaxation of the bone matrix seems a more sensitive mechanism of mechanosignaling in bone than cell deformation because of loading-induced matrix strain.[42] Osteocytes link microdamage and mechanical unloading to osteoclastic bone resorption by regulating their own apoptosis.[13] They also activate osteoclasts to remodel bone matrix and modulate their activity through RANK ligand and secretion of sclerostin.[13]

Osteoblasts are also the main cells regulating bone resorption. The stimulation of osteoblast receptors by systemic bone-resorptive agents provokes the production of matrix-degrading enzymes that contribute to initiate bone resorption, and the summon of osteoclasts to increase bone-resorption.[43]

Osteoclasts are mononucleated or multinucleated giant cells derived from the monocyte-macrophage family.[1,44] During skeletal growth, osteoclasts are actively involved in the resorption of calcified cartilage and modeling of growing bone, whereas they are responsible for bone remodeling in adults.[44] Bone resorption requires solubilization of hydroxyapatite crystals and the suggested mechanism for this process to occur is local acidification. After solubilization of the mineral phase, the organic matrix is degraded, and two major classes of proteolytic enzymes have been studied (lysosomal cysteine proteinases and matrix metalloproteinases). Finally, degradation products are removed from the resorption lacuna. Although *in vitro* studies have shown that an osteoclast can go through more than one resorption cycle, it is unknown if this also occurs *in vivo*. Also, the mechanism that destroys multinucleated osteoclasts *in situ* is not yet completely understood.[44]

From a mechanical point of view, despite its relative light weight, bone presents a high tensile strength and some degree of flexibility.[9] The mineralized structure of bone provides the strength and rigidity necessary to support the body and protect vital structures. However, bone is also a metabolically active tissue, which undergoes replacement and remodeling that allows maintaining the mineral metabolism and ionic balance of the body. Its structure, shape, and composition vary depending on the stress forces supported and metabolic, nutritional, and endocrine factors.[9,13] As demonstrated in rabbit cortical bone, the elastic stiffness and strength of bone increases with age as a result of higher bone mineral density, changes in the relative composition, and alterations in the orientation and remodeling of the collagen fibers and mineral crystals, at the same time their viscoelastic properties decrease.[45] Remodeling may not be continuous as demonstrated by the seasonal remodeling and resorption of the keel bone observed in female blackbirds (*Turdus merula*) only during the breeding season or the diurnal rhythm of remodeling of fracture callus in repairing long bones, which is abolished following hypophysectomy.[13] Also, the rates of remodeling are not constant even within the same bone.[13]

REFERENCES

1. Hall BK. Vertebrate skeletal tissues. In: Hall BK, editor. Bones and cartilage. Developmental and evolutionary skeletal biology. 2nd edition. San Diego (CA): Elsevier Academic press; 2015. p. 3–16.
2. Davit-Béal T, Tucker AS, Sire JY. Loss of teeth and enamel in tetrapods: fossil record, genetic data and morphological adaptations. J Anat 2009;214(4):477–501.
3. Hall BK. Skeletal origins: somitic mesoderm, vertebrae, pectoral and pelvic girdles. In: Hall BK, editor. Bones and cartilage. Developmental and evolutionary skeletal biology. 2nd edition. San Diego (CA): Elsevier Academic press; 2015. p. 261–80.
4. Maddin HC, Piekarski N, Sefton, et al. Homology of the cranial vault in birds: new insights based on embryonic fate-mapping and character analysis. R Soc Open Sci 2016;3(8):160356.
5. Sinowatz F. Musculo-skeletal system. In: Hyttel P, Sinowatz F, Vejlsted M, editors. Essentials of domestic animal embryology. Edinburgh (United Kingdom): Elsevier Health Sciences; 2010. p. 286–316.
6. Hall BK. Stem and progenitor cells in adults. In: Hall BK, editor. Bones and cartilage. Developmental and evolutionary skeletal biology. 2nd edition. San Diego (CA): Elsevier Academic press; 2015. p. 166–77.
7. Assis-Ribas T, Forni MF, Brochado Winnischofer SM, et al. Extracellular matrix dynamics during mesenchymal stem cells differentiation. Dev Biol 2018;437(2): 63–74.
8. Delise AM, Fischer L, Tuan RS. Cellular interactions and signaling in cartilage development. Osteoarthritis Cartilage 2000;8:309–34.
9. McGeady TA, Quinn PJ, FitzPatrick ES, et al. Muscular and skeletal systems. In: McGeady TA, Quinn PJ, FitzPatrick ES, et al, editors. Veterinary embryology. Blackwell publishing.; 2006. p. 184–204.
10. Goldring MB, Tsuchimochi K, Ijiri K. The control of chondrogenesis. J Cell Biochem 2006;97:33–44.
11. Dunning D. Basic mammalian bone anatomy and healing. Vet Clin North Am Exot Anim Pract 2002;5(1):115–28.
12. Hirasawa T, Nagashima H, Kuratani S. The endoskeletal origin of the turtle carapace. Nat Commun 2013;4:2107.
13. Hall BK. Bone. In: Hall BK, editor. Bones and cartilage. Developmental and evolutionary skeletal biology. 2nd edition. San Diego (CA): Elsevier Academic press; 2015. p. 17–42.
14. Mathur JK, Goel SC. Patterns of chondrogenesis and calcification in the developing limb of the lizard. *Calotes versicolor*. J Morphol 1976;149:401–20.
15. Hall BK. Lessons from fossils. In: Hall BK, editor. Bones and cartilage. Developmental and evolutionary skeletal biology. 2nd edition. San Diego (CA): Elsevier Academic press; 2015. p. 98–110.
16. Castanet J, Cheylan M. Les marques de croissance des os et des écailles comme indicateur de l'âge chez *Testudo hermanni* et *Testudo graeca* (Reptilia, Chelonia, Testudinidae). Can J Zool 1979;57:1649–65.

17. Rieppel O. Studies on skeletal formation in reptiles. I. The postembryonic development of the skeleton in *Cyrtodactylus pubisculus* (Reptilia: Gekkonidae). J Zool 1992;227:87–100.
18. Rieppel O. Studies on skeletal formation in reptiles. Patterns of ossification in the skeleton of *Chelydra serpentina* (Reptilia, Testudines). J Zool 1993;231:487–509.
19. Rieppel O. Studies on skeletal formation in reptiles. II. *Chamaeleo hoehnelii* (Squamata: Chamaeleoninae), with comments on the homology of carpal and tarsal bones. Herpetologica 1993;49:66–78.
20. Rieppel O. Studies on skeletal formation in reptiles. V. Patterns of ossification in the skeleton of *Alligator mississippiensis* Daudin (Reptilia, Crocodylia). Zool J Linn Soc 1993;109:301–25.
21. Rieppel O. Studies on skeleton formation in reptiles. Patterns of ossification in the skeleton of *Lacerta agilis exigua* Eichwald (Reptilia, Squamata). J Herpetol 1994; 28(2):145–53.
22. Rieppel O. Studies on skeletal formation in reptiles. I. Patterns of ossification in the limb skeleton of *Gehyra oceanica* (Lesson) and *Lepidodactylus lugubris* (Dumeril & Bibron). Ann Sci Nat Zool Biol Anim 1994;15:83–91.
23. Hall BK. The temporomandibular joint and cranial synchondroses. In: Hall BK, editor. Bones and cartilage. Developmental and evolutionary skeletal biology. 2nd edition. San Diego (CA): Elsevier Academic press; 2015. p. 511–28.
24. Hall BK. Vertebrate cartilages. In: Hall BK, editor. Bones and cartilage. Developmental and evolutionary skeletal biology. 2nd edition. San Diego (CA): Elsevier Academic press; 2015. p. 43–59.
25. Haines RW. The evolution of epiphyses and of endochondral bone. Biol Rev Cambr Philos Soc 1942;17:267–92.
26. Hall BK. Dedifferentiation of chondrocytes and endochondral ossification. In: Hall BK, editor. Bones and cartilage. Developmental and evolutionary skeletal biology. 2nd edition. San Diego (CA): Elsevier Academic press; 2015. p. 199–218.
27. Jacobson ER. Overview of reptile biology, anatomy, and histology. In: Jacobson ER, editor. Infectious diseases and pathology of reptiles. Color atlas and text. CRC Press. Taylor & Francis Group; 2007. p. 1–130.
28. Frýdlová P, Nutilová V, Dudák J, et al. Patterns of growth in monitor lizards (Varanidae) as revealed by computed tomography of femoral growth plates. Zoomorphology 2016;136(1):95–106.
29. Woodward HN, Horner JR, Farlow JO. Osteohistological evidence for determinate growth in the American alligator. J Herpetol 2011;45(3):339–42.
30. Gkiatas I, Lykissas M, Kostas-Agnantis I, et al. Factors affecting bone growth. Am J Orthop 2015;44(2):61–7.
31. Hall BK. Invertebrate cartilages, notochordal cartilage and cartilage origins. In: Hall BK, editor. Bones and cartilage. Developmental and evolutionary skeletal biology. 2nd edition. San Diego (CA): Elsevier Academic press; 2015. p. 60–78.
32. Hall BK. Dedifferentiation and stem cells: regeneration of urodele limbs and mammalian fingertips In: Hall BK, editor. Bones and cartilage. Developmental and evolutionary skeletal biology. 2nd edition. San Diego (CA): Elsevier Academic press; 2015. p. 219–37.
33. Roy RN, Guha BC. Production of experimental scurvy in a bird species. Nature 1958;182(4650):1689–90.
34. Irwin CR, Ferguson MWJ. Fracture repair of reptilian dermal bones: can reptiles form secondary cartilage? J Anat 1986;146:53–64.

35. Hayes WC, Mockros LF. Viscoelastic properties of human articular cartilage. J Appl Physiol 1971;31(4):562–8.
36. Martin RB, Burr DB, Sharkey NA, et al. Skeletal biology. In: Martin RB, Burr DB, Sharkey NA, et al, editors. Skeletal tissue mechanics. 2nd edition. Springer; 2015. p. 35–93.
37. Biltz RM, Pellegrino ED. The chemical anatomy of bone. I. A comparative study of bone composition in sixteen vertebrates. Bone 1969;51(3):456–66.
38. Weidman SM, Rogers HJ. Studies on the skeletal tissues; the degree of calcification of selected mammalian bones. Biochem J 1950;47(4):493–7.
39. Lamoureax F, Baud'huin M, Duplomb L, et al. Proteoglycans: key partners in bone cell biology. Bioessays 2007;29:758–71.
40. Robey PG, Fedarko NS, Hefferan TE, et al. Structure and molecular regulation of bone matrix proteins. J Bone Miner Res 1993;8(2):483–7.
41. Astachov L, Vago R, Aviv M, et al. Hyaluronan and mesenchymal stem cells: from germ layer to cartilage and bone. Biosci 2011;16:261–76.
42. Nijweide PJ, Burger EH, Feyen JH. Cells of bone: proliferation, differentiation, and hormonal regulation. Physiol Rev 1986;66(4):855–86.
43. Tully TN. Basic avian bone growth and healing. Vet Clin North Am Exot Anim Pract 2002;5(1):23–30.
44. Väänänen K. Mechanism of osteoclast mediated bone resorption: rationale for design of new therapeutics. Adv Drug Deliv Rev 2005;57(7):957–71.
45. Isaksson H, Malkiewicz M, Nowak R, et al. Rabbit cortical bone tissue increases its elastic stiffness but becomes less viscoelastic with age. Bone 2010;47:1030–8.

Skeletal Bone Structure and Repair in Small Mammals, Birds, and Reptiles

Mikel Sabater González, LV, CertZooMed, DECZM (Avian), MRCVS

KEYWORDS

• Bone • Structure • Repair • Fracture • Exotic animals

KEY POINTS

• The structure and composition of normal bone provide it with the maximum resistance to mechanical stresses while maintaining the least bone mass.
• Bone structure varies significantly between species.
• The aim of bone healing is to recover the normal structure of the bone to maintain its normal function.
• Similarities but also important differences also exist in the mechanisms of bone healing in exotic animal species.

INTRODUCTION

The structure and composition of each individual bone provides the maximum resistance to mechanical stresses while maintaining the least bone mass. Bone structure varies greatly between species and these differences may have clinical implications when assessing a bone.

During normal function, bones are subjected to different forces or combinations of forces. Bone strength does not only vary according to its structure and composition but also according to load orientation. Fractures occur when the magnitude of the sum of forces the bone is subjected to (axial compression or tension, shearing, torsion, or bending) exceeds the ultimate strength of the bone. The aim of bone healing is to recover its normal structure to maintain its normal function, but different healing mechanisms have been descried in small mammal, avian, and reptile species.

Skeletal Bone Structure

In general terms, the structure and composition of individual bones provide the maximum resistance to mechanical stresses while maintaining the least bone mass.[1] Bone undergoes changes in its composition, structure, and functional

Disclosure: The author has nothing to disclose.
Exoticsvet, Marques de San Juan 23-5, Valencia 46015, Spain
E-mail address: exoticsvet@gmail.com

properties during growth and maturation to maintain its functions. The elastic stiffness and strength increase as a result of higher bone mineral density, changes in the relative composition, as well as alterations in the orientation and remodeling of the collagen fibers and mineral crystals.[2] In addition, bone development and structure are also influenced by other biological and environmental factors.

Bone structure can be described at different levels ranging from nanostructure to macrostructure. From a macrostructural point of view, bone tissue can be divided into cortical (also referred to as compact bone) and cancellous (also known as trabecular or spongy bone).

The articular surface of a bone forming a synovial joint is covered by a layer of hyaline cartilage with 3 main functions: absorption of stress, distribution of mechanical loads, and resistance to deformation.[1]

The periosteum is the connective tissue layer covering the nonarticular cortical bone and consists of an external layer composed of dense fibrous connective tissue that allows the insertion of muscles, tendons, and ligaments, and an internal layer with osteogenic cells responsible for bone growth in width, remodeling, and fracture repair.[1] The periosteum also has nerves and blood vessels (discussed later).

Cortical bone tissue forms mainly the outer surface of long bones and short bones except for the articular surface, and the outer and inner layer (lamina externa and interna) of the skull vault bones.[3] The osteon, also referred as the haversian system, consists of a neurovascular canal (the haversian canal) surrounded by concentric layers of bone (the lamellae). Osteons are considered the basic structural element of mineralized cortical bone.[4] Osteons can be primary or secondary. A primary osteon has a central canal containing 2 or more blood vessels and lacks a delimiting cement line or interstitial lamellae. A secondary osteon has a larger canal containing a single central blood vessel, is limited externally by a cement line, and is wedged between interstitial lamellae (remnants of old osteons partially resorbed during bone remodeling). The lamellae located near the surface of the bone are arranged parallel to its surface.[2] The time required to form an osteon and its lifespan vary between species. Also, the rate of osteon mineralization is not uniform; 70% of mineralization occurs within 1 to 2 days of deposition of osteoid, and the remaining 30% may take many months.[2] Furthermore, variations such as areas of bone lacking primary or secondary osteons, acellular or avascular areas, and necrotic areas have been reported not only in different species but also within the same individual.[2]

Cancellous bone consists of a network of fine, irregular plates covered by endosteum (trabeculae) separated by intercommunicating spaces filled with bone marrow and hematopoietic cells. In general terms, cancellous bone occupies the epiphyses of long bones, and constitutes most of the vertebrae, the ribs, short bones, and flat bones. However, variations in the distribution of cancellous bone have been reported between species. For example, cancellous bone is scarce or nonexistent in certain flat bones of the skull and pelvis in mammals and birds.[1] Furthermore, bones of the skull, vertebrae, pelvis, sternum, ribs, the humerus, and sometimes the femur in several birds have minimal cancellous bone because of their pneumatic nature.[1]

The bone marrow may be partially or totally responsible for hematopoiesis depending on the species and age of the individual. Active bone marrow consists of a supportive reticulin framework and a system of interconnected blood sinusoids that drains toward the central vein.[1] Three types of multipotent stem cells (endothelial, mesenchymal, and hematopoietic) can be found in the bone marrow.

The endosteum is a thin connective tissue layer that lines the inner surface of the bone tissue that forms the medullary cavity of long bones. It contains osteogenic cells that are responsible for growth, remodeling, and repair of bone fractures.[1]

Bone vascularization varies between species and bones. The blood supply to healthy bone comprises the nutrient artery, the proximal and distal metaphyseal arteries, and the periosteal arterioles.[5] The nutrient artery penetrates the diaphyseal bone through the nutrient foramen, traverses the cortical bone, and reaches the medullary cavity where it bifurcates into ascending and descending branches.[5] These branches divide into arterioles that enter, depending on the species and the part of the bone, the primary vascular canals, the primary osteons, and/or the secondary osteons. However, avascular areas have been reported in the bones of some species (discussed later). Osteons run longitudinally along the cortical bone and are connected between them, with the endosteum and with the periosteum, by the Volkmann canals.[1] This vascular system supplies the 2 inner thirds of the cortical diaphysis.[5] In addition, the branches of the nutrient artery also arborize and enter the sinusoids of the medullary cavity.[5] The medullary arterioles at the extremes of the medullary cavity anastomose with the metaphyseal arteries.[5] The metaphyseal arteries do not provide a substantial contribution to the afferent vascular system in healthy bone but are able to assume cortical bone supply if damage to the nutrient artery occurs.[5] In immature animals, the periosteal arterial blood supply is well developed and runs longitudinally within the periosteum to supply all aspects of the long bone, except the joint surfaces, allowing appositional bone growth.[5] In mature animals, these arterioles atrophy and contact the bone surface only at fascial or ligamentous attachments, where they supply the remaining third (outer) of the cortex. Terminal branches of the periosteal arterioles anastomose with those of the medullary system.[5]

The blood drainage of the cortex and medullary cavity occurs separately. Cortical venous blood flows toward the periosteum, where it is drained into periosteal venules that coalesce into larger periosteal veins before entering the systemic circulation.[5] Medullary venous blood is drained into sinusoids that coalesce into a central venous sinus that forms the nutrient vein, which exits the cortex through the nutrient foramen before reaching the systemic circulation.[5]

Lymphatic ducts are present in the periosteum and within the medullary cavity of mammals.[1] However, further studies are warranted in reptiles and birds.

Sensory neurons innervate the periosteum and medullary cavity of bones.[6] In humans, it has been shown that these neurons have a morphology and a molecular phenotype related to nociception.[6] Also, myelinated and nonmyelinated nerve fibers have been observed in the bone marrow of different mammal species.[7] Further studies on the innervation of bone tissues are warranted in other mammals, reptiles, and birds.

SMALL MAMMALS

Differences in the rate of development and resulting bone structure have been extensively described in mammals.[8–12] Multiple studies concluded that secondary osteons (secondary haversian systems) scale allometrically in the long bones of mammalian species, supporting the hypothesis that the osteon resorption area may be limited by bone's local resistance to avoid fracture in smaller mammalian species but needs to maintain osteocyte viability in larger species.[13–15] The distribution and intensity of bone formation and resorption are largely determined by genetic factors but can be altered by mechanical stress or metabolic requirements. The formation of secondary osteons in the rat can be experimentally induced by feeding a high-calcium diet after feeding a calcium-free diet during pregnancy and suckling, and by mechanical stress.[14] Ovariectomy in rats initiates an endosteal cortical bone resorption but has no effect on the periosteal bone formation. In contrast, orchidectomy accelerates endosteal bone resorption and reduces periosteal bone formation. Estrogen administration in ovariectomized and intact rats reduces the rate of periosteal bone formation.[16] Larger and weaker femurs have been reported in rabbit 16 weeks after ovariectomy.[17] The ferret has also been suggested as an animal model for evaluating the effects of estrogen depletion in a remodeling skeleton.[18]

In rodents, different bone structural patterns have been reported. Mice and hamsters present vascular simple lamellar bone structure with simple remodeling. However, in mice, periosteal ossification is minimal, and the cartilage is replaced by bone, beginning during embryonic life; therefore, ossification and bone are endochondral.[19] Also, bone length growth is stopped by 6 months of age.[14] Dzungarian hamsters present delayed bone development compared with mice.[14] Rats present a more complicated bone structure than mice and hamsters. At 3 months old, the cortical bone is no longer composed of poor vascular simple lamellar bone.[14] In rats 4 to 6 months old, the diaphysis of the femur presents nonvascular bone tissue.[20] Epiphyseal growth plates may still be open until the age of 12 to 24 months, depending on the bone.[21] Older rats have pronounced bone modeling throughout life, which results in mostly fine-fibered lamellar bone, no cortical remodeling (although a few scattered osteon-line structures have been reported), and cancellous bone remodeling.[10,14,21,22] Rats have hemopoietic marrow at most skeletal sites throughout life.[21] Guinea pigs present osteons at 6 months of age.[14] An interesting rodent feature is the conversion of the interpubic cartilage into a flaccid ligament, accompanied by some resorption of the medial edges of the pelvic bones during pregnancy.[23]

Rabbits have faster skeletal change and bone turnover, and significant intracortical haversian remodeling compared with other species, such as primates and some rodents.[24] In rabbits, the basic microstructure of the femur is primary vascular longitudinal bone tissue.[3] In addition, primary vascular radial bone tissue, irregular haversian bone, and/or dense haversian bone tissue can be observed in the middle part of substantia compacta, whereas dense haversian bone tissue can be found in younger tissue areas at 5 to 7 months of age.[14,20] Rabbit cortical bone tissue increases its elastic stiffness but becomes less viscoelastic with age, which indicates significant structural and functional maturation of the bone matrix during growth of the rabbit.[2]

Ferrets reach skeletal maturity between 4 and 7 months of age as shown by closure of the growth plate and maturation of trabeculae from thin rods to thick rods and plates.[18] The long bone of the ferret shows extensive osteon remodeling in the cortical bone and a heavy trabeculation in the medullary canal.[10,18]

In immature mammals, the medullary cavities of most bones contain active bone marrow, which is responsible for hematopoiesis. The stroma contains hematopoietic supporting tissues and mesenchymal stem cells able to differentiate into osteoblasts, chondrocytes, and adipocytes.[25] Hematopoiesis occurs within the reticulin framework and only mature or almost mature blood cells, containing the membrane proteins required to attach and pass the blood vessel endothelium (eg, aquaporins or glycophorin), can be released into the general circulation. Hematopoietic cells can move in the opposite direction, allowing their recruitment from systemic circulation. In adult mammals, active marrow is restricted to the metaphysis and the medullary cavities of the diaphysis are filled with inactive marrow, which is largely composed of fat.[1]

BIRDS

The description of bone structure in birds is limited to a few articles. In general terms, the avian cortex consists of a narrow layer of slowly formed lamellar bone encircling a densely vascularized, rapidly formed, fibrolamellar bone in which primary osteons are arranged in longitudinal, radial, circular, and oblique orientations.[26] The rate of bone deposition and bone microstructure in birds may be affected by nutritional and environmental conditions. In quails, food deprivation induced lower bone deposition, whereas asymmetrical mechanical loads induced different bone deposition rates.[27] In 2-year-old laying hens, prolonged exercise restriction combined with heavy calcium demands resulted in major structural and mechanical effects.[28] Lines of arrested growth have been observed in the outer cortical layer of many birds.[29]

Avian bones present a great variability in their macrostructure and microstructure because of divergent adaptations resulting from the forces they experience. Most of the avian cortical bone retains its primary structure and is not remodeled throughout life to the extent observed in some mammals.[26] In pigeons, cortical bone consists of lamellar bone with few haversian systems. The minimal uptake of fluorescent labeling observed in the periosteal and endosteal layers of these birds indicate low levels of remodeling, which may contribute to its brittle nature.[30] Penguins have a very thick cortical bone in which 3 different zones have been identified.[31] The haversian systems in penguins are located in its inner zone, and between its inner and middle zones.[31] The study of 168 long bones from wings and legs of 22 bird species revealed that the humerus, ulna, and femur generally show torsion-resisting features, such as higher degree of laminarity, whereas other bones (radius, carpometacarpus, tibiotarsus, tarsometatarsus, and foot phalanx) instead show bending/axial load-resisting structural properties.[32] The same conclusion was achieved by a different study that investigated the degree of laminarity (the proportion of circular vascular canals) and the occurrence of secondary osteons in 3 avian species using different primary flight modes: the double-crested cormorant (a continuous flapper), the brown pelican (a static soarer), and the Laysan albatross (a dynamic soarer).[26] Secondary osteons were longitudinally oriented along the endosteal surface in the humeri of cormorants and albatross, and in the carpometacarpi of cormorants, albatross, and pelicans.[26] The torsional and axial compressive properties of the tibiotarsus have been also studied in red-tailed hawks.[33] Apart from interspecies and intraspecies structural variations, these also may occur within a single bone. The hardness of the humerus varies along its length, being the greatest in its diaphysis. This variation may be caused by adaptive remodeling in response to the stresses of flight, or by the bone's midshaft being older and more mineralized than its ends.[34]

Cancellous bone is mainly found in the epiphyses of long bones and in the vertebrae.[35] In some species, the bones of the skull, vertebrae, pelvic girdle, clavicle, sternum/keel, ribs, the humerus, and sometimes the femur or the tibiotarsus have minimal cancellous bone owing to their pneumatic nature. In those species in which the presence of pneumatic bones (vertebral or appendicular) has not been yet completely confirmed in spite of presenting pneumatic foramens at least in their vertebrae (eg, penguins or loons) or birds with reduced bone pneumatization (eg, grebes or ducks), spongy bone may be also observed within the diaphysis of long bones.[31,36–39] The pneumatic regions of some bones (eg, avian skull) may be difficult to distinguish from soft tissue by diagnostic imaging algorithms. The cortices of pneumatic bones are thinner walled and denser than marrow-filled ones but present a lower bending strength.[34,36] According to a study in passerines, bats, and rodents, passerines present the highest density of the cranium, humerus, and femur followed by bats and rodents, suggesting an adaptation for maximizing bone strength and stiffness while minimizing bone mass and volume.[40] To provide better skeletal support and redistribute stress forces, soaring and gliding birds present reinforcing structures such as struts and ridges not observed in flightless birds.[34] Contrarily, diving birds have marrow-filled bones, which are more resistant to impact (eg, against water) and prevent excess buoyancy while diving.[34] In penguins, the long bones are not pneumatic and consist of a hard and thick cortical bone and a small amount of spongy bone containing bone marrow in the center of the bone shaft.[31] Immature birds have more active marrow cavities with increased vascularization and hematopoietic capacity than mature birds.[1] Angiographic studies of immature pigeons have revealed that the intramedullary blood supply of the humerus bones is similar to that of nonpneumatic bones.[1] Avian erythropoiesis occurs within the lumen of the vascular sinusoids in the bone marrow instead of in the reticulin framework as happens in mammals.[1,41] Another characteristic feature of avian bone marrow is that avian heterophils derive from hematopoietic multipotent cells in the extravascular spaces of the bone marrow, whereas mammalian neutrophils develop from precursor cells within the vascular spaces.[41]

Apart from cortical and cancellous bone, a third type of bone exclusive to birds, the medullary bone, may be observed. Medullary bone is formed in response to the activity of gonadal steroids and represents a calcium reservoir found in females during the breeding period, in females with ovarian or oviductal disorders (eg, neoplasia), or in males presenting hormonal disorders such as Sertoli cell tumors.[35,42,43] Despite medullary bone formation occurring regardless of the vitamin D levels of the bird, full mineralization requires adequate vitamin D_3 levels.[44] Approximately 30% to 40% of eggshell calcium is derived from the medullary bone. Medullary bone is formed by the ingrowth of bony spicules from the endosteum into the medullary cavity of well-vascularized long bones, leaving spaces occupied by blood sinuses and red marrow.[45] In medullary bone, haversian systems have not been observed, the collagen fibers and the hydroxyapatite crystals are not oriented, and there is less collagen but more chondroitin sulfate or a different state of polymerization than in cortical bone.[45,46] Medullary bone formation starts 2 weeks before the start of laying in the hen. During the ovulation-oviposition cycle, the medullary bone undergoes alternating phases of growth (when the uptake of calcium and phosphate is enough for normal ossification of the eggshell) and regression (when it is insufficient).[35] The presence of medullary bone (polyostotic hyperostosis) must be considered when interpreting bone density using diagnostic imaging (eg, radiography or computed tomography).

REPTILES

Detailed comparative studies have described the structure of several reptile bones.[47,48] In this article and for descriptive purposes, the groups described by Enlow[49] are used.

Chelonians and Crocodilians

The cortices of the bones in young individuals present a single lamina containing many primary canals.[49] Very limited amounts of plexiform bone, bone with a regularly arranged three-dimensional plexus of primary vascular canals, is observed in young crocodilians.[49] In adults, the cortex is composed of circumferentially arranged, broad laminae each containing a row of primary vascular canals resulting from accumulated periods of growth.[49] On histology, the layers of cortical bone are referred to as growth rings, which are separated by lines of arrested growth (LAGs), and overall represent the intermittent skeletal growth (eg, hibernation).[49] In the metaphyses, the cancellous trabeculae in the medulla are invaded by newly formed endosteal cortical bone, which converts it to compacted cortical bone. Therefore, the cortex of the metaphysis near the epiphyseal cartilage of most long bones is thin and largely composed of endosteal bone. Haversian systems are restricted to localized areas in the corticomedullary transition zone, where the fibrous component of muscle or tendon anchorages into the cortex, allowing the continuous reattachment of the muscle or tendons on resorptive periosteal surfaces during bone lengthening. The central medullary cavity may be small or absent depending on the amounts of cancellous bone showing minimal to no remodeling that surrounds it.[47,49] The amount of cortical and cancellous bone varies not only within species but also within different bones in the same individual or even within a single bone. The radius of the Mediterranean spur-thighed tortoise (*Testudo graeca*) has extensive cancellous bone, whereas it shows thick cortical bone and no cancellous bone in the red-footed tortoise (*Chelonoidis carbonarius*) and the greater padloper (*Homopus femoralis*). *H femoralis* shows the same structural pattern in the tibia, whereas other terrestrial tortoises (eg, the Hermann's tortoise [*Testudo hermanni*], the Mediterranean spur-thighed tortoise, the radiated tortoise [*Astrochelys radiata*], and the red-footed tortoise) show variable development of cancellous bone.[47] The long bones of marine chelonians (eg, the leatherback sea turtle [*Dermochelys coriacea*] or the green sea turtle [*Chelonia mydas*]) tend to present larger amounts of cancellous bone and minimal to absent cortical bone.[50,51] The long bones of turtles and crocodilians present a large cartilaginous epiphysis overlying the growth plate.[52]

Lizards and Snakes

Squamate periosteal bone basically consists of parallel-fibered or lamellar bone with LAGs.[50] However, nonlamellar tissue, lamellar tissue, or circumferential layered combinations of both may be observed depending on the part of the bone and the species.[49] Growth rings in long bones of some lizards may be less evident than in turtles.[49] In most species, cortical bone of periosteal origin is nonvascular.[49] Scarce radially oriented simple vascular canals may be observed in large species (eg, *Python* sp, *Eunectes* sp, or large species of *Varanus*).[50] Diaphyseal vascular canals in the femur and tibia, and less frequently in the fibula, have been observed in large species of varanids.[53,54] The medullary canal consists of cancellous bone and vascular spaces surrounded by endosteal deposits of lamellar bone.[50,52] However, the extension of cancellous bone into the mid-diaphysis of long bones is limited in lizards.[49] In the metaphysis, compacted cancellous bone is formed when the endosteal cortical bone deposits bone in the canals of the cancellous bone of the medulla.[49] Also, some isolated vascular vessels may be encountered in these canals.[49] The reduced extension of cancellous bone and the lack of cortical canals prevents diaphyseal bone remodeling.[49] The epiphyses of long bones in lizards with legs present secondary centers of ossification consisting of several zones of endochondral bone formation (zone of reserve cartilage, zone of multiplication, zone of hypertrophy, zone of calcification, and zone of ossification), which results in an extensive number of cancellous trabeculae that, after being invaded by bone, become compact cortical bone.[52] Vertebrae also present growth plates.[52] Cartilage canals in the epiphyses of lizards have been reported in some *Varanus* spp, *Agama* spp, and in some *Chamaeleo* spp.[48]

Vertebrae consist of cortical and cancellous bone, and often contain marrow.[52] In healthy snakes, remodeling of vertebral bone is seen as irregularly arranged cement or reversal lines resulting in a mosaic appearance.[52]

The New Zealand tuatara, *Sphenodon punctatus* (order Rhynchocephalia), presents primitive secondary centers of ossification, but these centers undergo subsequent resorption and replacement by bone when the ossification of the diaphysis extends through the metaphyseal growth zone into the epiphyses.[48]

Bone Marrow

Bone marrow is present in the vertebrae, ribs, the pelvis, and certain skull bones of all reptiles and in some of the long bones of those presenting extremities.[55] The major blood-forming organ in most lizards and crocodilians is the bone marrow.[52,56] In turtles, the spleen and bone marrow equally produce red cells.[52] Exceptions have been reported, such as in the regal horned lizard (*Phrynosoma solare*), in which the spleen assumes this role, or in the European pond turtle (*Emys orbicularis*), in which bone marrow hematopoiesis has only been observed in 1-year-old individuals but not in younger ones.[57,58] In the Iberian wall lizard (*Podarcis hispanica*), hematopoiesis occurs in the bone marrow, whereas erythropoiesis takes place in the lumen of blood vessels, and granulopoiesis is extravascular.[57]

Osteocytic Necrosis

Extensively distributed or localized small foci of necrotic osteocytes may be observed within the cortical bone of reptiles. Osteocytic necrosis may be a consequence of the sparse distribution or total absence of vascular canals in certain kinds of bone, or the occlusion of canals with ectopic mineral deposits. The mid-diaphyses of long bones are more prone to osteocytic necrosis because they present broader cortices and, therefore, the deeper zones of their cortical plates are farther from the vessels in the inner and outer surfaces.[49]

BONE FRACTURE HEALING

During normal function, bones are subjected to different forces (eg, axial compression or tension, shearing, torsion, or bending) or combinations of them. Bone strength depends on load orientation and its structure and composition. A fracture occurs when the magnitude of the sum of these forces exceeds the ultimate strength of the bone.[59] The aim of bone healing is to recover the normal structure of the bone to maintain its normal function. Using the mechanisms of bone healing in small mammals as a reference, the main variations observed in birds and reptiles are discussed here.

Bone Healing in Small Mammals

Primary bone healing

Primary fracture healing (direct) occurs when there is less than 2% of interfragmentary strain environment and less than a 1-mm interfragmentary gap, and results in the direct formation of cortical bone across the fracture line and no evidence of callus formation.[1,59] Primary healing usually occurs only when the fracture fragments are reduced anatomically and stabilized and when the fragments are placed under interfragmentary compression.[1]

Depending on the distance between fragments, primary healing may be classified as contact healing or gap healing. Contact healing occurs when the interfragmentary space is less than 0.01 mm and consists of the formation of new cortical bone directly across the fracture line (parallel to the long axis of the bone), which undergoes immediate haversian remodeling.[1] Gap healing occurs in interfragmentary spaces greater than 0.01 mm but smaller than 1 mm. Endosteal and periosteal cells deposit cortical bone perpendicular to the long axis of the bone, which is later remodeled by haversian systems into the correct longitudinal orientation.[1]

Clinically, primary bone healing is always a combination of gap and contact healing because fracture reduction with no interfragmentary space along the fracture is almost impossible because of fixation tissue limitations and the plastic deformation of the fracture surfaces that occurs during the initial fracture.[59]

Secondary bone healing

Secondary bone healing (indirect) occurs when the interfragmentary strain is between 2% and 10%. Bone healing is a dynamic process with 3 phases (reactive, reparative, and remodeling). More than 1 phase normally occurs at the same time within the fracture site.

The fracture of the bone normally is associated with a rupture of the medullary and periosteal blood vessels that results in their vasoconstriction to control the hemorrhage. Within the following hours, the extravascular cells form a hematoma between and around the fracture ends.[60] Inflammatory cells, first neutrophils/heterophils and later macrophages, arrive at the hematoma. Macrophages release inflammatory mediators (eg, cytokines, including tumor necrosis factor-alpha and interleukins), which recruit inflammatory cells; promote angiogenesis; stimulate differentiation of osteoblasts and osteoclasts; and are able, at least in vitro, to induce osteogenic differentiation of mesenchymal stem cells.[60] The hematoma becomes acidotic and hypoxic, which causes the death of the cells and the replication and aggregation of fibroblasts between the blood vessels, resulting in the formation of granulation tissue (the first tissue able to provide some stability to the fracture site).[1]

During the reparative phase, pluripotent mesenchymal-derived cells arising from the endosteum, periosteum, or surrounding soft tissues, or recruited from remote hematopoietic sites, proliferate and differentiate into osteogenic cells.[59,60] The periosteal cells close to the fracture gap and the fibroblasts within the granulation site differentiate into chondroblasts, which form a soft callus of hyaline cartilage inside and around the fracture site. At the same time, intramembranous ossification occurs subperiosteally directly adjacent to the distal and proximal ends of the fracture, generating a hard callus of cancellous bone.[60] In animal models (mouse, rat, and rabbit), the peak of soft callus formation and hard callus formation occur around 7 to 9 days and 14 days postfracture, respectively.[60] The gradual shift in the pH toward the neutral or alkalotic range allows alkaline phosphatase function and callus mineralization.[1] Calcified cartilage, progressively replaced by cancellous bone through endochondral ossification, and cancellous bone grow until they fill the space in a semirigid structure known as the fracture callus and are able to allow weight bearing.[1,60]

In addition, remodeling, a process in which the cancellous is reabsorbed by osteoclasts and cortical bone is deposited by osteoblasts, starts as early as 3 to 4 weeks postfracture in animal models and may continue for years.[60] The resulting bone may be even stronger than the initial one. This type of healing is observed in less stable forms of fracture fixation (eg, comminute fractures; fractures treated with intramedullary pins, cerclages, external coaptation; and in nontreated fractures), which in most cases result in malunion of the fracture fragments.[1,60]

Many growth factors (eg, platelet-derived growth factor, insulinlike growth factor 1, transforming growth factor β, bone morphogenetic proteins, and fibroblast growth factor) have been shown to influence bone healing.[1]

Bone Healing in Birds

The number of studies investigating avian bone healing after fracture is still very limited.

Avian fracture callus derives from the periosteum and the endosteum. According to a histomorphometric and angiographic analysis of bone healing in the humerus of pigeons, quantitatively, the periosteal surface forms the largest amount of callus but the endosteal surface was also active.[46] Also, reformation of the intramedullary circulation may not be imperative for osseous union in the humerus of pigeons.[46]

The rate of fracture healing seems to depend on the amount of displacement, the integrity of the blood supply, the presence of infection, and the degree of motion at the fracture.[61] Manually created and nonstabilized fractures of the humerus or antebrachium in pigeons presented both endosteal and periosteal callus consisting of cancellous bone cartilage and fibrous connective tissue after 9 days. After 16 and 21 days, the amount of cancellous bone in the callus increased and cartilage and connective tissue decreased. After 6 and 12 weeks, the callus of well-aligned fractures continued to mature and started developing the components of normal bone, whereas unstable, poorly aligned fractures barely changed between 4 and 12 weeks.[62] A different study in pigeons reported radiographic evidence of a mineralized external callus 5 weeks after internal fixation of ulnar or radius fracture and 8 weeks after internal fixation in pigeons, whereas the endosteal callus was observed after 3 weeks. In ulnar and radius fractures in which the ulna was stabilized with a Kirschner pin, the radius (mainly primary cortical union) healed faster than the stabilized ulna (cancellous bone union). Internal fixation of both bones resulted in fracture healing after 4 weeks and in the start of bone remodeling.[63]

In cage layers, medullary bone formation results in cessation of remodeling of structural bone.[64] Also, birds receiving estrogen therapy show bones with higher content of calcium and higher degrees of calcification in young bone than in older preexisting diaphyseal bone.[43]

Bone Healing in Reptiles

Information about fracture healing in reptiles is limited. Most of the information available derives from single case reports or case series. Controlled experiments to study reptile fracture processes are extremely scarce. According to a study that compared femoral fracture repair in the common lizard (*Zootoca vivipara*) and the rat, several differences were observed.[65] In both the lizards and the rat, cartilage was formed in the periosteum and at the site of the original hematoma. This cartilage was later progressively eroded and replaced by endochondral bone. In the lizard, erosion began under the subperiosteal shell of new bone formed across the fracture gap, and not along linear invasion fronts on each side as occurred in the rat. Cartilage resorption was less organized and slower in the lizards than in the rats. Also, the uneroded cartilage of lizards appeared to become transformed directly into bone.[65] A different experimental study concluded that reptile dermal bones are not able to form secondary cartilage, and that osteoblasts repair the broken bone directly with new bone.[66] Also, it has been reported that lizards are able to regenerate a variable mass of cartilaginous and fibrocartilaginous tissues after damage, fracture, or amputation.[67,68] The persistence of stem cells in the epiphyseal growing centers of the studied bones (eg, femur and tibia), and also the persistence of few progenitor cells able to reactivate in the growth plate and the articular cartilage, were suggested as the mechanisms of epiphyseal cartilage regeneration.[67]

REFERENCES

1. Dunning D. Basic mammalian bone anatomy and healing. Vet Clin North Am Exot Anim Pract 2002;5(1):115–28.
2. Isaksson H, Malkiewicz M, Nowak R, et al. Rabbit cortical bone tissue increases its elastic stiffness but becomes less viscoelastic with age. Bone 2010;47: 1030–8.
3. Martiniaková M, Grosskopf B, Omelka R, et al. Histological study of compact bone tissue in some mammals: a method for species determination. Int J Osteoarchael 2007;17:82–90.
4. Hall BK. Bone. In: Hall BK, editor. Bones and cartilage. Developmental and evolutionary skeletal biology. 2nd edition. San Diego (CA): Elsevier Academic Press; 2015. p. 17–42.

5. Remedios A. Bone and bone healing. Vet Clin North Am Small Anim Pract 1999; 29(5):1029–44.
6. Nencini S, Ivanusic JJ. The physiology of bone pain. How much do we really know? Front Physiol 2016;26(7):157.
7. Calvo W. The innervation of the bone marrow in laboratory animals. Am J Anat 1968;123:315–28.
8. Enlow DH, Brown D, Brown HC. A comparative histological study of fossil and recent bone tissues. Part III. Mammalian bone tissues. Texas J Sci 1958;10: 187–230.
9. Jowsey J. Studies of Haversian systems in man and some animals. J Anat 1966; 100(4):857–64.
10. Singh IJ, Tonna EA, Gandel CP. A comparative histological study of mammalian bone. J Morphol 1974;144(4):421–37.
11. Mulhern DM, Ubelaker DH. Differences in osteon banding between human and nonhuman bone. J Forensic Sci 2001;46(2):220–2.
12. Wang X, Mabrey JD, Agrawal M. An interspecies comparison of bone fracture properties. Biomed Mater Eng 1998;8:1–9.
13. Felder AA, Phillips C, Cornish H, et al. Secondary osteons scale allometrically in mammalian humerus and femur. R Soc Open Sci 2017;4(11):170431.
14. Hörner K, Loeffler K, Holtzmann M. Vergleich der histologischen Struktur der Kompacta der langen Röhrenknochen bei Maus, Hamster, Ratte, Meerschweinchen, Kaninchen, Katze und Hund während der Altersentwicklung. Anat Histol Embryol 1997;26:289–95.
15. Bagi CM, Berryman E, Moalli MR. Comparative bone anatomy of commonly used laboratory animals: implications for drug discovery. Comp Med 2011;61(1): 76–85.
16. Danielsen CC, Moselkide L, Svenstrup B. Cortical bone mass, composition, and mechanical properties in female rats in relation to age, long-term ovariectomy, and estrogen substitution. Calcif Tissue Int 1993;52:26–33.
17. Sevil F, Kara ME. The effects of ovariectomy on bone mineral density, geometrical, and biochemical characteristics in the rabbit femur. Vet Comp Orthop Traumatol 2010;1:31–6.
18. Mackey MS, Stevens DC, Ebert DL, et al. The ferret as a small animal model with BMU-based remodeling for skeletal research. Bone 1995;17(4):181S–96S.
19. Hall BK. Vertebrate skeletal tissues. In: Hall BK, editor. Bones and cartilage. Developmental and evolutionary skeletal biology. 2nd edition. San Diego (CA): Elsevier Academic Press; 2015. p. 3–16.
20. Martiniakova M, Grosskopf B, Omelka R, et al. Differences among species in compact bone tissue microstructure of mammalian skeleton: Use of a discriminant function analysis for species identification. J Forensic Sci 2006;51(6): 1235–9.
21. Moselkide L. Assessing bone quality – Animal models in preclinical osteoporosis research. Bone 1995;17(4):343S–52S.
22. Lieuschner MAK. Biomechanical considerations of animal models used in tissue engineering of bone. Biomaterials 2004;25:1697–714.
23. Hall BK. Vertebrate cartilages. In: Hall BK, editor. Bones and cartilage. Developmental and evolutionary skeletal biology. 2nd edition. San Diego (CA): Elsevier Academic Press; 2015. p. 43–59.
24. Pearce AI, Richards RG, Milz S, et al. Animal models for implant biomaterial research in bone: A review. Eur Cell Mater 2007;13:1–10.

25. Krebsbach PH, Kuznetsov SA, Bianco P, et al. Bone marrow stromal cells: characterization and clinical application. Crit Rev Oral Biol Med 1999;10(2):165–81.
26. Simons ELR, O'Connor PM. Bone laminarity in the avian forelimb skeleton and its relationship to flight mode: Testing functional interpretations. Anat Rec (Hoboken) 2012;295:386–96.
27. Starck JM, Chinsamy A. Bone microstructure and developmental plasticity in birds and other dinosaurs. J Morphol 2002;254:232–46.
28. Shipov A, Sharir A, Zelzer E, et al. The influence of severe prolonged exercise restriction on the mechanical and structural properties of bone in an avian model. Vet J 2010;183:153–60.
29. Ponton F, Elzanowski A, Castanet J, et al. Variation of the outer circumferential layer in the limb bones of birds. Acta Ornithol 2004;39(2):137–40.
30. West PG, Rowland GR, Budsberg SC, et al. Histomorphometric and angiographic analysis of the humerus in pigeons. Am J Vet Res 1996;57:982–6.
31. Mesiter W. Histological structure of the long bones of penguins. Anat Rec 1962; 13:377–87.
32. Margerie E, Sánchez S, Cubo J, et al. Torsional resistance as a principal component of the structural design of long bones: comparative multivariate evidence in bird. Anat Rec A Discov Mol Cell Evol Biol 2005;282A:49–66.
33. Kerrigan SM, Kapatkin AS, Garcia TC, et al. Torsional and axial compressive properties of tibiotarsal bones of red-tailed hawks (Buteo jamaicensis). Am J Vet Res 2018;79(4):388–96.
34. Sullivan TN, Wang B, Espinosa H, et al. Extreme lightweight structures: avian feathers and bones. Mater Today 2017;20(7):377–91.
35. König HE, Maierl J, Weissengruber G, et al. Introduction. In: König HE, Korbel R, Liebich HG, editors. Avian anatomy. Textbook and colour atlas. 2nd edition. 5m. Sheffield (United Kingdom): Taylor Francis; 2016. p. 1–23.
36. Cubo J, Casinos A. Incidence and mechanical significance of pneumatization in the long bones of birds. Zoo J Lin Soc 2000;130:449–510.
37. Apostolaki NE, Rayfield EJ, Barrett PM. Osteological and soft-tissue evidence for pneumatization in the cervical column of the ostrich (Struthio camelus) and observations on the vertebral columns of non-volant semi-volant and semi-aquatic birds. PLoS One 2015;10(12):e0143834.
38. O'Connor PM. Evolution of archosaurian body plans: skeletal adaptations of an air-sac-based breathing apparatus in birds and other archosaurs. J Exp Zool A Ecol Genet Physiol 2009;331(8):629–46.
39. Gutzwiller SC, Su A, O'Connor PM. Postcranial pneumaticity and bone structure in two clades of neognath birds. Anat Rec 2013;296(6):867–76.
40. Dumont ER. Bone density and the lightweight skeletons of birds. Proc Biol Sci 2010;277:2193–8.
41. Fudge AM. Avian cytodiagnosis. In: Fudge AM, editor. Laboratory medicine: avian and exotic pets. Philadelphia: WB Saunders; 2000. p. 124–32.
42. Larsen S, Carpenter JW, Goggin J, et al. What's your diagnosis. J Avian Med Surg 2001;15(3):226–31.
43. Ascenzi A, François C, Bocciarelli DS. On the bone induced by estrogens in birds. J Ultrastruct Res 1963;8:491–505.
44. Dacke CG. The parathyroids, calcitonin, and vitamin D. In: Whittow G, editor. Sturkie's avian physiology. 5th edition. San Diego (CA): Academic Press; 1999. p. 473–89.
45. King AS, McLelland M. Skeletomuscular system. In: King AS, McLelland M, editors. Birds: their structure and function. Eastbourne (United Kingdom): Baillière Tindall; 1984. p. 9–22.

46. West PG, Rowland GR, Budsberg SC, et al. Histomorphometric and angiographic analysis of bone healing in the humerus of pigeons. Am J Vet Res 1996;57:1010–5.
47. Laurin M, Canoville A, Germain D. Bone microanatomy and lifestyle: a descriptive approach. Comptes Rendus Paleovol 2011;10:381–402.
48. Haines RW. The evolution of epiphyses and of endochondral bone. Biol Rev Camb Philos Soc 1942;17:267–92.
49. Enlow DH. The bone of reptiles. In: Gans C, Bellairs A d'A, editors. Biology of the Reptilia: 1A. London: Academic Press; 1969. p. 45–80.
50. Houssaye A. Bone histology of aquatic reptiles: what does it tell us about secondary adaptation to an aquatic life? Biol J Lin Soc 2013;108:3–21.
51. Kriloff A, Germain D, Canoville A, et al. Evolution of bone microanatomy of the tetrapod tibia and its use in palaeobiological inference. J Evol Biol 2008;21:807–26.
52. Jacobson ER. Overview of reptile biology, anatomy, and histology. In: Jacobson ER, editor. : Infectious diseases and pathology of reptiles. Color atlas and text. Boca Ratón (FL): CRC Press. Taylor & Francis Group; 2007. p. 1–130.
53. De Buffrenil V, Houssaye A, Böhme W. Bone vascular supply in monitor lizards (Squamata: Varanidae): influence of size, growth, and phylogeny. J Morphol 2008;269:533–43.
54. Haines RW. Epiphyses and sesamoids. In: Gans C, Bellairs A d'A, editors. Biology of the Reptilia: 1A. London: Academic Press; 1969. p. 81–115.
55. Garner MM. Overview of biopsy and necropsy techniques. In: Mader DR, editor. Reptile medicine and surgery. 2nd edition. St Louis (MO): Saunders Elsevier; 2005. p. 560–90.
56. Finger JW, Isberg SR. A review of innate immune functions in crocodilians. CAB Reviews 2012;7(67):1–11.
57. Zapata A, Leceta J, Villena A. Reptilian bone marrow. An ultrastructural study in the Spanish lizard, *Lacerta hispanica*. J Morphol 1981;168:137–49.
58. Vasse J, Beaupain D. Erythropoiesis and haemoglobin ontogeny in the turtle *Emys orbicularis* L. J Embryol Exp Morphol 1981;62:129–38.
59. Cross AR. Fracture biology and biomechanicals. In: Tobias KM, Johnston SA, editors. Veterinary surgery small animal. St. Louis (MO): Elsevier Saunders; 2012. p. 1966–82.
60. Marsell R, Einhorn TA. The biology of fracture healing. Injury 2011;42(6):551–5.
61. Gandal CP. Anesthetic and surgical techniques. In: Petrak ML, editor. Diseases of cage and aviary birds. Philadelphia: Lea & Febiger; 1982. p. 304–28.
62. Montali RJ, Bush M. Avian fracture repair, radiographic and histologic correlation. Proceedings of the Annual Conference of the American Association of Zoo Veterinarians. San Diego, CA, November 2–6, 1975.
63. Newton CD, Zeitlin S. Avian fracture healing. J Am Vet Med Assoc 1977;170: 620–5.
64. Whitehead CC, Flemming RH. Osteoporosis in cage layers. Poult Sci 2000;79(7): 1033–41.
65. Pritchard JJ, Ruzicka AJ. Comparison of fracture repair in the frog, lizard and rat. J Anat 1950;84(3):236–61.
66. Irwin CR, Ferguson MWJ. Fracture repair of reptilian dermal bones: can reptiles form secondary cartilage? J Anat 1986;146:53–64.
67. Alibardi L. Proliferating cells in knee epiphyses of lizards allow for somatic growth and regeneration after damage. J Funct Morphol Kinesiol 2017;2:23.
68. Lozito TP, Tuan RS. Lizard tail regeneration as an instructive model of enhanced healing capabilities in an adult amniote. Connect Tissue Res 2017;58(2):145–54.

Orthopedic Diagnostic Imaging in Exotic Pets

Federico Vilaplana Grosso, DVM, DECVDI

KEYWORDS

- Radiography • CT • Ultrasound • MRI • Trauma • Fracture
- Metabolic bone disease • Osteomyelitis

KEY POINTS

- Orthopedic disorders in exotic pets are common due to trauma, infection, and metabolic bone disease.
- Knowledge regarding the anatomic, physiologic, and pathophysiologic characteristics of the exotic pet species is crucial when interpreting diagnostic imaging examinations.
- Computed tomography is increasingly used in exotic pet medicine due to public awareness, higher standards of care demand, and the increased availability in small animal practice.

INTRODUCTION

Orthopedic disorders are a common problem in exotic pets. Nevertheless, there are many different species kept as pets, each with a variety of orthopedic conditions with different implications in their health, diagnosis, and treatment options. Therefore, knowledge regarding the anatomic, physiologic, and pathophysiologic characteristics of these exotic pet species is crucial when interpreting diagnostic imaging examinations.

Exotic animals are acquiring popularity, and the number of exotic pets presented to the veterinary practices has significantly increased in recent times, becoming a large percentage of the clientele in many veterinary hospitals and clinics.

On the other hand, nowadays there are diagnostic and therapeutic options available that were not accessible few years ago. Public awareness has translated into an increased expectation of targeted and competent diagnostic testing for pet animals. An increasing number of clients are willing to provide higher standards of medical care regardless of the cost involved on diagnostics and treatment.

There are many species of exotic pet birds, small mammals, and reptiles with major differences in anatomy. In interpreting diagnostic imaging studies in exotic pets,

Disclosure Statement: The author has nothing to disclose.
Department of Small Animal Clinical Sciences, College of Veterinary Medicine, University of Florida, 2015 Southwest 16th Avenue, PO Box 100116, Gainesville, FL 32610-0116, USA
E-mail address: fvilaplanagrosso@ufl.edu

thorough knowledge of the different species anatomy is paramount, but the literature about it is scarce. Fortunately, the number of publications describing the radiographic, tomographic, or MRI anatomy of different exotic pet species and breeds is increasing over the last years.[1–17] The bilateral and symmetric musculoskeletal anatomy may be used for interpreting an imaging examination by means of comparing with the contralateral part of the body or producing contralateral limb radiographs.

DIAGNOSTIC IMAGING MODALITIES

Radiography has been traditionally used as the first diagnostic imaging modality in veterinary care. However, over the past years, other imaging modalities, such as ultrasonography (US) and advanced cross-sectional techniques (eg, computed tomography [CT] and MRI), are becoming more available and accessible. The use of advanced imaging techniques is increasingly used in exotic animal patients as the availability of the advanced imaging equipment becomes readily available in small and exotic animal practice. Radiography and CT are frequently used for the diagnosis of orthopedic diseases as well as for surgical planning and follow-up. US and MRI can be used for assessment of orthopedic diseases affecting soft tissue structures, such as muscles, ligaments, tendons, and joints. For the evaluation of the central nervous system in traumatized or neurologic patients, MRI is the modality of choice. Nuclear scintigraphy (NS) is less frequently used and scarcely available. In musculoskeletal diseases, NS provides information about regions of increased bone metabolism and may be used to determine decreased perfusion of soft tissues after an injury.

Radiography

Radiography is the most common imaging modality used because of its availability and low cost. Similarly, radiography is a very good modality for assessment of bony structures, making it ideal for the evaluation of skeletal diseases. In small exotic pets, this modality allows fast and whole-body radiographic assessment using one single exposure. Quick and whole-body evaluations are an advantage for patients who may present severely ill or in shock after a traumatic incident. In these cases, the use of whole-body radiography is a valuable tool for a rapid health assessment, and for investigation of the underlying cause and extent of the disease. Therefore, a quick diagnosis, prognosis, and detection of life-threatening conditions may be provided, allowing a prompt action in cases that require lifesaving treatment. After stabilization of the patient, collimated orthogonal radiographs of the affected area should be performed for an optimal assessment.

Nowadays, most practices are using digital radiography (DR) instead of conventional radiography. The advantages of DR over analog radiography are numerous. The main advantage of DR as compared with analog radiography is that it provides a wide range of exposures for an acceptable image quality, which means that even being less accurate with the specific exposure technique of the radiograph, the image quality will probably be acceptable and will allow greater flexibility than in the case of analog radiography. Therefore, this will help to reduce the number of retakes because of overexposure and underexposure. DR also permits image postprocessing, such as modification of the brightness and contrast of the image (window width and leveling) and consequently allows an optimal examination of all anatomic areas.[18] Other postprocessing manipulations include image sharpening, edge enhancement and smoothing, image subtraction, and contrast inversion, among others.

In many occasions, the small size of the patients may be a compromising factor because of the limited spatial resolution of the DR systems. These patients may benefit from being examined with analog radiography (eg, high-detail radiographic film or mammography) because of the increased spatial resolution. However, a very precise exposure technique is required.

Horizontal beam radiography is frequently used in exotic pets because it allows easier positioning and sometimes decreases or eliminates the need of restraint. Decreased restraint and manipulation is especially important in patients affected with metabolic bone disease (MBD), where restraint and manipulation may induce pathologic fractures. In addition, horizontally directed radiographic beams are useful when assessing gravity-dependent (fluid, sediment, and mineral) and non-gravity-dependent (gas) structures (**Fig. 1**).

Ultrasonography

US is a noninvasive imaging modality that allows a good evaluation of soft tissues and fluid-filled structures and does not produce any ionizing radiation. In exotic pets affected with orthopedic disorders, US is useful for the assessment of soft tissue swellings, muscles, tendons, and joints.

Another advantage of US is that it provides guidance during the aspiration of fluids or masses, and US-guided biopsies (**Fig. 2**). Fine needle aspirates (FNA) can be very helpful to distinguish between infectious, inflammatory, and neoplastic causes. US can also be used to guide locoregional anesthesia (ie, nerve blocks) or therapy delivering (eg, ethanol ablation), among others.

The use of color and power Doppler US is useful when assessing blood flow of a certain organ or a lesion, ischemia, or the degree of vascularization of a mass. At the same time, use of color and power Doppler US can be used to assess the amount of hemorrhage after performing FNAs or biopsies.

Computed Tomography

CT has become more available and economically affordable, and consequently, its use in exotic pets is exponentially increasing over the last several years. On some occasions, general anesthesia may be required; however, modern multidetector CT machines allow the scanning of large anatomic areas in a very short time. Because of this increased scanning velocity, many patients can be scanned under sedation or

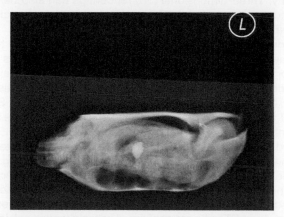

Fig. 1. Horizontal beam radiograph of a tortoise that was attacked by a dog, demonstrating the presence of free gas in the celomic cavity. (*Courtesy of* Federico Vilaplana Grosso and the Diagnostic Imaging Service, College of Veterinary Medicine, University of Florida.)

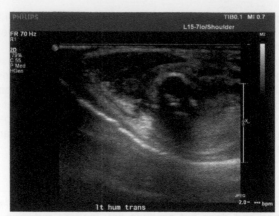

Fig. 2. Transverse ultrasonographic image of the humerus of a marmoset with a pathologic fracture. Multiple small bone fragments are seen as well as a collection of hypoechoic fluid. The examination was performed to obtain FNAs. (*Courtesy of* Federico Vilaplana Grosso and the Diagnostic Imaging Service, College of Veterinary Medicine, University of Florida.)

conscious with the help of commercial physical restraint devices (eg, VetMouseTrap) or self-made restraint devices.[19]

CT has many advantages compared with radiography. The major advantage over DR is the ability to visualize the internal anatomy without superimposition of the adjacent or external structures. This lack of superimposition is very advantageous when evaluating exotic pets, especially for the skull, or in chelonians, where the superimposition of the shell may mask underlying lesions. One study revealed a higher sensitivity of CT when compared with radiography in the detection of fractures and luxations in chelonians.[20]

CT has a higher contrast resolution than radiography, distinguishing between different types of soft tissues and fluids. In addition, the great spatial resolution of CT can help detect subtle fractures that may not be seen with other imaging modalities.

Multiplanar reconstructions (eg, dorsal and sagittal) can be reformatted after acquiring the transverse scan of the patient. Multiplanar reconstructions allow the clinician to appreciate the disease, because it is oriented relative to the surrounding anatomy. Three-dimensional (3D) renderings can also be performed. 3D reconstructions can be very helpful for surgical planning, especially in complicated fractures (**Fig. 3**).

Intravenous iodinated contrast media can be administered during the examination to enhance tissues and vessel visualization. Soft tissue structures with abnormal vascularization or increased vessel permeability due to disease manifest abnormal patterns of enhancement, allowing their differentiation from normal tissues.

Similarly to US, CT-guided FNAs and biopsies can be performed.[21] Some of the disadvantages of CT are the use of ionizing radiation, the higher cost, the lesser availability, and the potential requirement of general anesthesia.

Microcomputed tomography (μ-CT) is becoming more popular in exotic animal practice. Originally, this type of CT was designed for laboratory animals (eg, small rodents), but due to the very high resolution, it may be used in small exotic species.[22] Scanning and operation principles of μ-CT are similar to those of standard CT. Some advantages of μ-CT over standard CT are the much smaller size and the lack of need of lead shielding of the CT room (ie, μ-CT units are configured within a leaded shield structure). The main disadvantage of μ-CT is the limited range of species that can fit in the gantry. Depending on the manufacturer, μ-CT can accommodate patients up to 15 kg.[23]

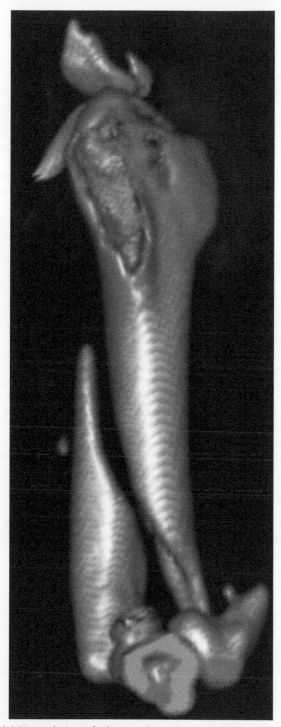

Fig. 3. Craniocaudal 3D rendering of a humeral intercondylar fracture of an eclectus parrot. (*Courtesy of* Federico Vilaplana Grosso and the Diagnostic Imaging Service, College of Veterinary Medicine, University of Florida.)

MRI

MRI is an excellent imaging modality for the investigation of the musculoskeletal and central nervous systems. This modality is considered noninvasive because it does not use ionizing radiation for generating images. MRI has a superior contrast resolution when compared with CT, allowing a better depiction of soft tissue structures.

Same as CT, MRI has the advantage of avoiding the superimposition of structures. However, unlike CT, the different scan planes need to be acquired separately and cannot be reconstructed, therefore increasing the time of the examination. Other factors that may increase the time of the examination are the type of sequence used, the sequence planes, and the overall number of sequences.

The major disadvantages of MRI are the lower availability, the higher cost, and the long scan times that often require the use of general anesthesia. General anesthesia is the main limiting factor. In very small patients, inhalational general anesthesia cannot be performed for MRI examinations due to limiting factors, such as the anesthetic circuit dead spaces and the fact that a ventilator cannot be used inside the MRI room.

Nuclear Scintigraphy

NS is rarely used in exotic animal orthopedic disorders. The main reason is the lack of availability when compared with other imaging modalities. In NS, a radioactive substance, such as 99m technetium methylene diphosphonate, is injected intravenously in the patient. Then, the radiopharmaceutical is localized in areas of increased bone metabolism, where it will emit radiation that can be measured and imaged with a gamma camera. Bone scintigraphy allows whole-body examination but requires heavy sedation or anesthesia to avoid motion while the images are being acquired.

Some indications of musculoskeletal NS in exotic pets are the evaluation of fractures that may not be seen with radiography, polyostotic infectious osteomyelitis, occult lameness, bone and soft tissue viability after a traumatic injury, and neoplastic bone disease (**Fig. 4**).

NS has been previously used to assess ischemia and necrosis of the extremities of a ferret and for evaluation of multifocal infections and plastron necrosis in a Horsfield tortoise.[24,25]

RESTRAINT OF EXOTIC PETS FOR IMAGING

Manual, physical, and chemical restraint can be used in exotic pets. The use of restraints will depend on the species and size of the patient, the behavior, the degree of illness, and the elected imaging modality.

Manual Restraint

Manual restraint may be used in radiography and US in relatively calm birds, small mammals, and reptiles. It is important to take into consideration the human exposure to ionizing radiation during manual restraint in radiographic examinations.

Physical Restraint

Physical restraint with acrylic devices or devices made of other radiolucent material, such as plastic, or cardboard can also be used in radiography and sometimes in CT, especially in critical patients, where the use of sedation or anesthesia might be discouraged. Acrylic tubes, boxes, and plates are routinely used for immobilization of exotic animals for radiography. Ancillary devices for physical restraint and positioning include rope, roll gauze, adhesive tape, towels, sand bags, wedge foam, and Velcro, among others. A large number of specialized radiographic positioning

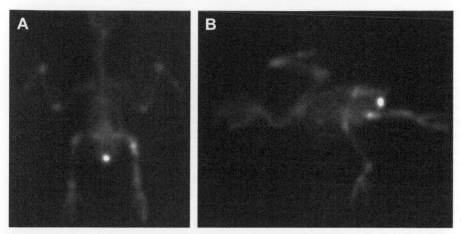

Fig. 4. Ventrodorsal (*A*) and laterolateral (*B*) scintigraphic images of an African gray parrot with a transverse middiaphyseal fracture of the right tibiotarsal bone after being attacked by a cat. NS was performed to investigate soft tissue and bone viability. Decreased radio-pharmaceutical uptake is noted, suggestive of ischemia. (*Courtesy of* Federico Vilaplana Grosso and the Diagnostic Imaging Service, College of Veterinary Medicine, University of Florida.)

aids are also commercially available for the use in small animals (eg, VetMouseTrap, Bird Board).[19,26]

Chemical Restraint

Chemical restraint is generally required in large, powerful, highly stressed or fractious animals, in venomous animals, or in individuals with injuries that can be exacerbated with struggling. Sedation may be achieved with injectable drugs or intranasal drugs, and general anesthesia with injectable or inhalational drugs. Patient monitoring is required whenever a patient is under sedation or anesthesia. Oxygen should be supplied during the examination in critically ill, traumatized, sedated, or anesthetized patients.

For radiographic studies, rabbits and ferrets can be physically restrained with techniques similar to those used with cats. Physical or chemical restraint will be required for small-sized mammals and fractious or stressed individuals.[27] Birds can be physically restrained with tape or commercial restraint devices. Otherwise, chemical restraint is used. Most lizards, tortoises, and turtles can be examined without any restraint or with the help of positioning aids, such as foam rubber block, where the patient can be placed on top. The restraint of a snake can be challenging. Manual restraint or placement of the snake in an acrylic tube is the most common form of restraint. Snakes may be alternatively placed in a bag during radiographic examination, but they tend to curl, making the image difficult to interpret. In such cases, the use of external metallic markers placed on the snake at the level of the potential abnormality may be helpful.

When using CT and MRI, the use of general anesthesia is most of the time required to avoid motion artifacts that will degrade the image quality and make the examination suboptimal. The use of general anesthesia is even more important in the case of MRI because longer examination times are often needed. However, in exceptional cases, CT examinations can be performed with no or light sedation, especially in critical patients.[28]

FRACTURES OF THE APPENDICULAR SKELETON IN EXOTIC PETS
Fracture Classification

Fractures are defined as a disruption in the continuity of the bone. In exotic pets, fractures are classified in the same way as in other species. Fractures may be classified according to the following: 1. Anatomic location; 2. possible communication with the skin (ie, open or closed); 3. fracture configuration (ie, simple, double, multiple, comminuted, or segmental); 4. direction of the fracture line (ie, transverse, oblique, spiral, longitudinal, or irregular); 5. extent of the bone damage (ie, complete or incomplete, such as greenstick fractures and fissures); 6. relative displacement of the bone fragments (ie, avulsion fracture, impacted fracture, compression fracture, and depression fracture); 7. communication with the joint (ie, articular or not articular); 8. fractures of healthy or diseased bone (ie, traumatic or pathologic); 9. age of the fracture (ie, acute or chronic) (**Fig. 5**); and 10. involvement of the physis (ie, Salter Harris fractures types I to VI) (**Fig. 6**).

When the fracture segments are displaced, the distal fracture segment is used to describe the displacement relative to the proximal fracture segment.

Fracture and Bone Healing in Exotic Species

Numerous factors affect the time taken for a fracture to heal (eg, species, nutritional status, presence of underlying MBD, type of bone, fracture configuration, stability of the fracture, age of the patient, vascular supply, method of treatment, presence of systemic diseases, if the fracture was traumatic or pathologic, and presence of complications such as osteomyelitis).

As compared with mammal species, birds have a different bone-healing response in fracture repair.[29–31] For further reading about bone healing in exotic species, please see Mikel Sabater González's article, "Skeletal bone structure and repair in small mammals, birds and reptiles," in this issue.

Avian bones may clinically heal faster than mammalian bones.[30] A simple closed fracture in a healthy individual may clinically heal and be stable by 3 weeks. Radiographic union often lags behind clinical union, requiring approximately 4 to 6 weeks for the development of the radiographically visible osseous callus.

Reptile species are considered slow bone healers. Between the different species of reptiles, snakes often produce a more prominent periosteal reaction than chelonians and lizards.

In reptile and avian species, fracture fibrous union may occur; this means that during the healing process, fibrous tissue would be present at the level of the fracture leading to visualization of a persistent radiolucent line in later follow-ups. Therefore, because of the particular bone-healing process in these species, radiographic evidence of complete bone healing is expected at a later time than in small mammals, being frequently up to 12 to 16 weeks after the injury.[32] In small mammals, fracture healing is generally expected by 4 weeks in young individuals, 6 to 8 weeks in young adults, and around 12 weeks in aged adults. However, specific healing times will also depend on the previously described factors. If complications are suspected or the patient presents clinical complaints related to the fracture, radiographic examination is indicated before the anticipated time of clinical union. When the expected time of clinical union exceeds 6 to 8 weeks, radiographic examination at a halfway stage can be recommended to give assurance of a correct healing. In birds and reptiles, radiographic assessment can be made first at 3 weeks after surgery and then every 2 to 3 weeks until radiographic evidence of union is present.

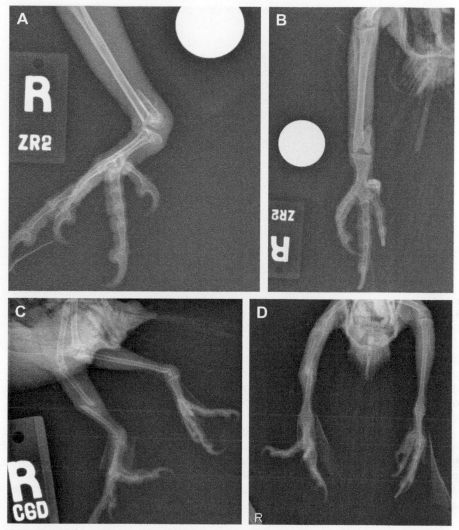

Fig. 5. Mediolateral (*A*) and caudocranial (*B*) radiographs of an Amazon parrot with an acute oblique distal diaphyseal tibiotarsal fracture. Mediolateral (*C*) and caudocranial (*D*) radiographs of a lovebird with a chronic middiaphyseal tibiotarsal fracture. Note the sharp and well-defined fracture margins in (*A*) and (*B*), as compared with the smooth and ill-defined margins in (*C*) and (*D*). (*Courtesy of* Federico Vilaplana Grosso and the Diagnostic Imaging Service, College of Veterinary Medicine, University of Florida.)

Complications

The most common complications in fracture healing are infection (ie, osteomyelitis), sequestration, delayed union, nonunion, and malunion.

Osteomyelitis

Osteomyelitis associated with a fracture may be the result of contamination occurring at the time of the fracture, such as in an open fracture (**Fig. 7**), or due to intraoperative contamination. Fractures may be related to traumatic injuries, such as bites or nail

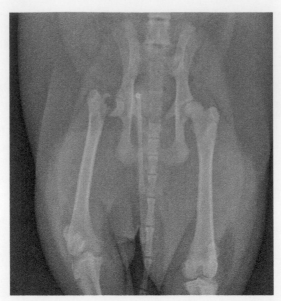

Fig. 6. Ventrodorsal radiograph of a raccoon with a Salter Harris type I fracture of the right femoral head, after falling from a closet. (*Courtesy of* Federico Vilaplana Grosso and the Diagnostic Imaging Service, College of Veterinary Medicine, University of Florida.)

punctures provoked by other animals. In these cases, osteomyelitis might be expected. Severe soft tissue injury may also create an adequate environment for pathogen growing and predisposed bone infection.[33] Although all ballistic fractures are open, the likelihood of osteomyelitis to occur is reduced, because of the heat related to this type of trauma.

In birds, fractures that involve the pneumatic bones are at a greater risk of osteomyelitis, and in very rare cases, secondary extension into the air sacs and, consequently, inducing air sacculitis. As the avian species does not generate much periosteal reaction during fracture healing, the same happens with osteomyelitis, and osteolysis together with soft tissue swelling will be the predominant radiographic abnormality.

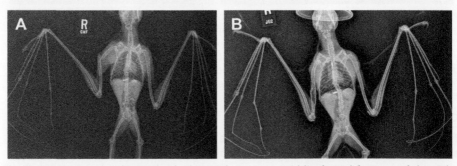

Fig. 7. Ventrodorsal radiograph of a bat with an open middiaphyseal fracture of the right humerus (*A*). An external fixator was placed but removed 2 months later due to osteomyelitis (*B*). Note the heterogeneous bone opacity with mixed pattern of osteolysis and the ill-defined and irregular periosteal reaction. (*Courtesy of* Federico Vilaplana Grosso and the Diagnostic Imaging Service, College of Veterinary Medicine, University of Florida.)

In reptiles, osteomyelitis also yields a predominant lytic reaction with little periosteal proliferation.

In small mammals, from approximately 7 to 10 days after infection of a fracture, a small and ill-defined periosteal proliferation may be detected. If the infection progresses, signs of an aggressive bone lesion will be noted, including extensive lysis and marked irregular periosteal reaction. If surgical implants were used, ill-defined radiolucency around the implants and endosteal sclerosis can be noted as a sign of osteomyelitis.

Radiography is very useful in the detection of osteomyelitis, although radiographic changes will be noted at least 1 to 2 weeks after infection and even later in birds and reptiles. In cases of suspected of early infection, US may show changes, such as fluid collections, before the patient develops radiographic changes. US also allows sampling for cytologic analysis and culture.

Sequestration

Sequestration can occur in combination with osteomyelitis. A sequestrum is an avascular, nonviable fragment of bone that may serve as a focus of infection that will not be eliminated without removing this fragment. A sequestrum is recognized radiographically as a sharply marginated sclerotic bone fragment surrounded by, or separated from, the rest of the bone by a radiolucent region called involucrum. If a draining tract originates from the involucrum and communicates with the skin, it means that a cloaca is present. Sequestration is particularly relevant in birds that have comminuted fractures, in which the bone fragments may lose the blood supply. For the assessment of draining tracts, radiographic or CT contrast studies (ie, sinusograms and fistulograms) can be performed. Administration of nonionic iodinated contrast media through the draining tract is done with a catheter or a cannula. This procedure may confirm or rule out communication between the draining tract with and osseous or articular structures.

Delayed union and nonunion

Delayed union and nonunion are common in exotic pets. With delayed union, a subjectively longer than expected time to heal for the type and location of the fracture occurs, although little evidence of bone healing is present. Some reasons for delayed union are limb disuse, instability, poor fracture reduction, poor vascular irrigation, poor nutrition, MBD, old age, infection, presence of a sequestrum, or undetected underlying pathologic condition, such as a tumor. Usually given enough time and in the absence of instability or other complications, a delayed union fracture should heal. If not, the fracture will progress to nonunion, at which point it is considered that complete healing will not occur. Nonunion is defined as a fracture that has not healed and has no evidence of progression on later follow-ups. Determination of nonunion is also subjective, and no specific time is strictly defined. In avian and reptile species, nonunion may be considered after 16 weeks, and after 12 weeks in small mammals, especially when there is no evidence of radiographic healing in sequential radiographs.

In nonunion cases, intervention to improve the stabilization and application of bone grafting may be used to increase the chance of a successful union. Otherwise, amputation of the limb may be required.

Malunion fractures

Malunion fractures are healed but have abnormal anatomic alignment. In exotic pets, especially in small-sized animals, malunion fractures are mainly related to lack of initial reduction and stabilization or because of poor reduction or instability, which is more frequent when external coaptation is applied. This type of complication can produce bone shortening, angulation or rotation of the limb, development of joint pain, or cosmetic deformity (**Fig. 8**). Severe malunion fractures may require surgical correction[34] (**Fig. 9**).

ORTHOPEDIC DISEASES IN EXOTIC PETS
Traumatic Injuries of the Appendicular and Axial Skeleton

Orthopedic trauma is very frequent in exotic pet species. In small mammals, it often results from household accidents such as falls, injury from a falling object, a closing door, or a human stepping on the pet. Other types of traumatic injuries may happen in the cage, in which fractures most frequently occur when a limb becomes entrapped in a rodent wheel or a wire cage or toy. In cities with tall buildings, high-rise syndrome can occur, especially in ferrets, with injuries similar to those described in cats. Injuries are also the result of the attack by other animals.

After a traumatic event, whole-body radiographs are indicated to detect life-threatening conditions, as well as fractures of the axial and appendicular skeleton, in a fast manner. After stabilization of the patient, collimated radiographs of the affected area should be acquired.

Most of the traumatic fractures in small mammals occur in the long bones. When fractures occur distal to the elbow and stifle, they are usually open because of the small amount of soft tissues covering the bone. The femur is the most commonly fractured bone in ferrets.[35] In rabbits, fractures of the limbs occur more frequently in the femur, tibia, radius, and ulna[17] (**Fig. 10**). The most common fractured bone in Guinea pigs is the femur.[17]

The most common traumatic fracture in chinchillas is the tibial fracture, presumably because their tibia is longer than the femur and because of their very thin fibula.[36] A frequent reason for this type of fracture includes catching their limb in its cage or grabbing the animal by its hind limb.[37] Tibial fractures tend to be short spiral or transverse. Nonunion can result with tibial fractures in chinchillas because of their thin and fragile bone structures as well as their active behavior. Bones in rabbits and chinchillas are thin and fragile. For this reason, surgical repair can be difficult, and complications

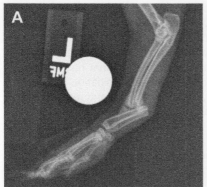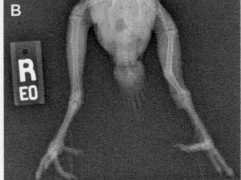

Fig. 8. Mediolateral radiograph of a rabbit with a chronic distal diaphyseal radioulnar fracture with malalignment and extensive osseous callus (*A*). If this fracture was not corrected, it would progress into a malunion fracture. Ventrodorsal radiograph of an aracari with a malunion fracture of the left tibiotarsal bone (*B*). (*Courtesy of* Federico Vilaplana Grosso and the Diagnostic Imaging Service, College of Veterinary Medicine, University of Florida.)

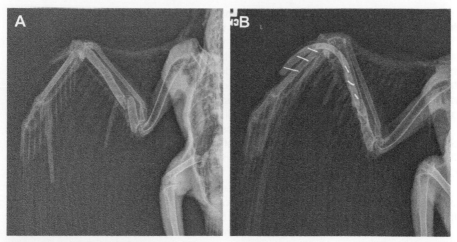

Fig. 9. Ventrodorsal radiograph of a blue and gold macaw with proximal diaphyseal radio-ulnar malunion fracture and carpal fractures (*A*). Ventrodorsal radiograph of the same macaw after surgical correction of the radioulnar malunion and carpal arthrodesis (*B*). (*Courtesy of* Federico Vilaplana Grosso and the Diagnostic Imaging Service, College of Veterinary Medicine, University of Florida.)

are common. These complications include bone-pin loosening, infection, nonunion, necrosis of the distal limb, and self-mutilation.

In captive birds, diaphyseal fractures to the pelvic limbs are the most common traumatic injury.[29] However, in wild birds, thoracic limb and thoracic girdle fractures are more common. Fractures of the shoulder girdle may be difficult to assess radiographically because of superimposition. Consequently, fractures of the scapula, coracoids, and clavicle are often underdiagnosed. A specific oblique radiographic view has been recently reported for the assessment of fractures of the thoracic girdle in raptors.[38] This radiographic view can also be used in other bird species. Thoracic girdle fractures are easily assessable with CT.

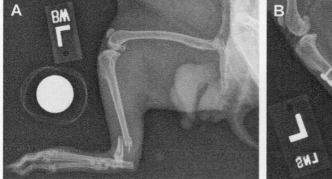
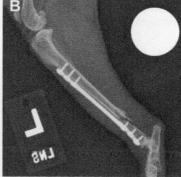

Fig. 10. Mediolateral radiograph of a rabbit with a comminuted distal diaphyseal tibial fracture (*A*). Immediate postoperative mediolateral radiograph after reduction of the fracture with internal osteosynthesis (*B*). (*Courtesy of* Federico Vilaplana Grosso and the Diagnostic Imaging Service, College of Veterinary Medicine, University of Florida.)

In adult reptiles, fractures are most commonly traumatic, whereas in young reptiles, fractures are usually pathologic secondary to fibrous osteodystrophy (**Fig. 11**).

Assessment of fractures in chelonians is very limited because of the external shell and their propensity to retract their head, tail, and appendages into the shell. Shell fractures usually occur because of a fall, dog bite, or vehicular accident. If external trauma to the shell is seen, radiography, and, even better, CT, are indicated to determine the extent of the internal damage, fractures, and luxations. 3D reconstructions are very useful for surgical planning of shell fractures (**Fig. 12**).

In chelonians, the vertebral column is closely connected to the shell, which means that in case of shell trauma, the vertebral column may also be affected. Vertebral fractures carry a very bad prognosis in chelonians, and for this reason, their detection with CT is very important (**Fig. 13**).

Vertebral fractures are also regularly diagnosed in lizards and snakes, generally pathologic secondary to fibrous osteodystrophy or osteomyelitis. However, traumatic fractures may occur, especially if attacked by another animal (**Fig. 14**).

Traumatic spinal fractures in small mammals are generally due to crush injuries (**Fig. 15**). In rabbits, the most common reason of acute posterior paralysis is vertebral fracture or luxation.[39] Fractures are more common than luxations, and the most frequent site for them to occur is the lumbosacral junction (L7).[39] This type of traumatic injury often results from improper handling or restraint (eg, a startled rabbit that jumps from a table or chair), but can also happen in caged rabbits that are frightened.[39,40] The spinal injury generally occurs when the muscled hind limbs are hyperextended and causes hyperextension of the vertebral column, which may result in disc damage, luxations, and fractures with subsequent spinal cord compression, paresis, or paralysis.[39]

In birds, cranial impact against a window is frequent. This type of trauma can produce vertebral fractures that usually happen cranial to the fused synsacrum (ie, between the notarium and synsacrum, usually at the level of L3 but varies among the species).[29] For that reason, thorough examination of the vertebral region immediately cranial to the synsacrum should be performed in avian patients with suspected vertebral trauma. These fractures will be easier to recognize with CT because it avoids the superimposition of structures.

For evaluation of spinal fractures and luxations, radiography is an excellent imaging modality; however, for less clearly visible lesions, such as subluxations or small nondisplaced fractures, CT is a better modality. When assessing for compressive myelopathy, myelography, CT-myelography, and MRI are indicated. With MRI, no need of intrathecal injection of nonionic iodinated contrast media is required, being therefore

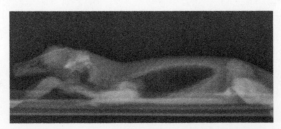

Fig. 11. Laterolateral radiograph of a gecko with a pathologic bilateral mandibular fracture. Note the severe generalized osteopenia because of nutritional secondary hyperparathyroidism and fibrous osteodystrophy. (*Courtesy of* Federico Vilaplana Grosso and the Diagnostic Imaging Service, College of Veterinary Medicine, University of Florida.)

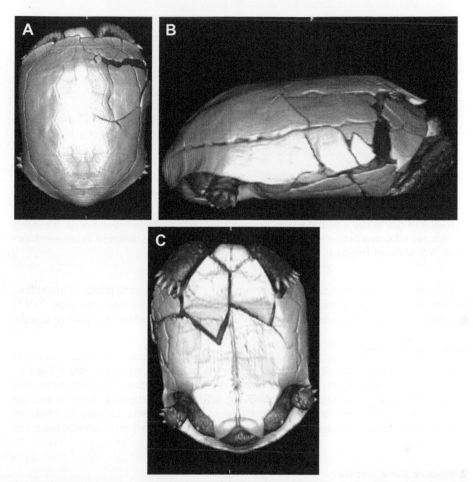

Fig. 12. Dorsal (*A*), lateral (*B*), and ventral (*C*) 3D reconstructions of a tortoise with multiple carapacial and plastral fractures after being hit by a car. (*Courtesy of* Federico Vilaplana Grosso and the Diagnostic Imaging Service, College of Veterinary Medicine, University of Florida.)

less invasive. Also, it may aid in the detection of spinal cord disorders, such as spinal contusions, edema, myelomalacia, or hemorrhage.

Skull fractures generally occur secondary to severe trauma. This type of fractures is difficult to assess in exotic pets because of their reduced size. In birds, cranial fractures are frequently a diagnostic challenge because of the fine cortical bone, the numerous air sac extensions, and the complexity of the avian jaw apparatus.[2] For additional information about avian skull orthopedics, please refer Minh Huynh and colleagues' article, "Avian skull orthopedics", in this issue. In general, CT can be performed to fully assess the severity of the injury. Mandibular and maxillary fractures can occur in association with dental disease.[17]

Elbow luxations are a common condition in ferrets and can occur spontaneously or secondary to a traumatic insult.[35] Elbow luxations are also frequent in rabbits and traumatic in nature.[41,42] Craniodorsal coxofemoral luxation is also a common orthopedic condition in rabbits and may be iatrogenic, traumatic, or congenital.

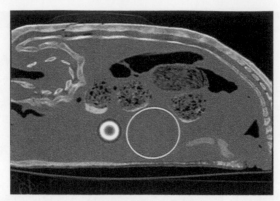

Fig. 13. Sagittal CT image of a tortoise with a carapacial and vertebral fracture. Note the presence of gas in the epidural space. Several mineralized eggs are also noted. (*Courtesy of* Federico Vilaplana Grosso and the Diagnostic Imaging Service, College of Veterinary Medicine, University of Florida.)

In birds, luxations seem to be more prevalent in the coxofemoral joints, in the stifles, and involving the digits; however, luxations of other joints have been reported.[29,43,44] Luxations are uncommon in reptiles and mainly affect the coxofemoral joint of lizards.

Pathologic Fractures

Pathologic fractures are spontaneous fractures that occur without evident trauma, because of weakening of the bone by an underlying disease. In exotic pets, this type of fracture is usually due to underlying MBD or osteomyelitis. Bone neoplasia is a less frequent cause of pathologic fractures. In cage birds, pathologic fractures secondary to MBD have been described to be more common than traumatic fractures or infection.[29]

Metabolic Bone Disease

One of the most common osseous diseases in exotic pets is *fibrous osteodystrophy*. Exotic species seem to be quite susceptible to nutritional secondary hyperparathyroidism. Nutritional deficiencies (eg, calcium or vitamin D3) due to feeding an improper

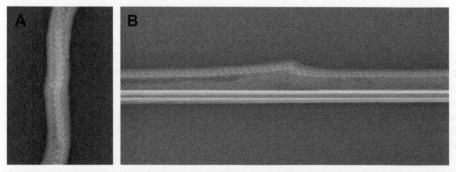

Fig. 14. Dorsoventral (*A*) and laterolateral (*B*) radiographs of a pet snake with a luxated vertebral fracture after being attacked by a dog. (*Courtesy of* Federico Vilaplana Grosso and the Diagnostic Imaging Service, College of Veterinary Medicine, University of Florida.)

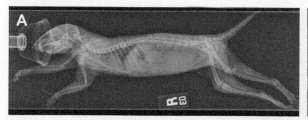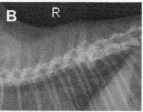

Fig. 15. Laterolateral whole-body radiograph of a squirrel with hind limb paraparesis. A chronic compressive thoracic vertebral fracture with dorsal subluxation is noted (A). Collimated view of the vertebral fracture (B). (*Courtesy of* Federico Vilaplana Grosso and the Diagnostic Imaging Service, College of Veterinary Medicine, University of Florida.)

diet will cause calcium/phosphorus imbalances that result in secondary hyperparathyroidism and fibrous osteodystrophy.

Renal secondary hyperparathyroidism can also occur because of chronic kidney disease or renal dysplasia. In small mammals, it happens more frequently in older rabbits that are infected with *Encephalitozoon cuniculi*.[17] In reptiles, renal secondary hyperparathyroidism may occur secondary to visceral gout. Animals affected with renal secondary hyperparathyroidism may present pathologic mandibular fractures, although the opacity of the long bones may appear normal.[32]

The most obvious radiographic feature of this disease is osteopenia. Radiographically, osteopenia is characterized by a severe decrease in bone opacity compared with the soft tissues, thinning of the cortices, and coarse bone trabeculation. Radiography is relatively insensitive for bone loss, because approximately 30% to 60% of the bone must be lost before being radiographically evident.[45] Frequently, the pattern of demineralization is irregular and may mimic aggressive bone lesions with a patchy pattern of demineralization, especially in the long bones **(Fig. 16)**.

The bones of animals diagnosed with MBD are very fragile and predisposed to pathologic, folding, and incomplete fractures. The handling, restraint, and positioning of these patients has to be very careful because of their fragile body condition **(Fig. 17)**.

Guinea pigs are the only small mammal that is genetically susceptible to vitamin C deficiency. *Hypovitaminosis C* in Guinea pigs will present clinical complaints, such as poor wound healing, weakness, or diarrhea, and can show radiographic evidence of bone and/or joint disease. Radiographic changes include enlargement of the epiphyses of long bones and costochondral junctions of the ribs, and there may be an increase in soft tissue opacity in the joints. Pathologic fractures may occur.[37]

Articular gout is a common cause of lameness in reptiles and birds, such as parakeets and small psittacines. Gout in birds is thought to result from chronic kidney disease or high dietary levels of proteins.[43] In reptiles, gout develops secondary to renal disease and hyperuricemia. Radiographic findings of gout are subchondral bone lysis and periarticular new bone formation.[46]

Orthopedic Diseases Secondary to Infection

Osteomyelitis and septic arthritis may result from open fractures, penetrating wounds, hematogenous spread, extension from a soft tissue infection (eg, pododermatitis, cellulitis, or abscess), or may be iatrogenic. In birds, it can also happen because of extension of an air sac infection to the pneumatized bones.

In early stages of osteomyelitis, radiographic changes may not be readily apparent. Later in the course of the disease, soft tissue swelling, osteolysis, and aggressive periosteal reactions are often seen. Fungal osteomyelitis may cause a marked periosteal

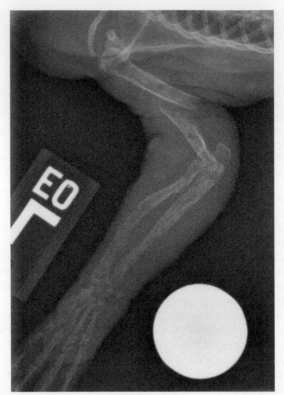

Fig. 16. Mediolateral radiograph of a capuchin monkey with severe osteopenia secondary to fibrous osteodystrophy with multiple pathologic fractures. This was confirmed with histopathology. (*Courtesy of* Federico Vilaplana Grosso and the Diagnostic Imaging Service, College of Veterinary Medicine, University of Florida.)

reaction and increased opacity of the medullary cavity of the bone due to granuloma formation (**Fig. 18**). In the case of acute septic arthritis, the only radiographic finding may be soft tissue swelling. As the infection progresses, lytic changes to the cartilage and subchondral bone (ie, erosive arthritis) as well as ill-defined periarticular new bone formation may be seen.

Posttraumatic osteomyelitis is a potential complication of fractures in ferrets, rabbits, and small rodents and occurs secondary to inciting trauma to the joint and/or bones, bone avascularity, or wound contamination with secondary postoperative infection.[35,47]

Radiographic examination is indicated in ulcerative pododermatitis (ie, bumblefoot), because in chronic or severe cases, osteomyelitis may be present. Septic arthritis is most commonly seen in the intertarsal joints of cage birds.

Avian tuberculosis (*Mycobacterium* spp) may result in focal areas of increased medullary opacity and periosteal proliferation, affecting principally the long bones and causing lameness.[29,43]

Degenerative Diseases

Degenerative joint disease

Degenerative joint disease may occur because of prior trauma or age-related degeneration (**Fig. 19**). Age-related osteoarthritis is commonly seen in exotic pets, affecting

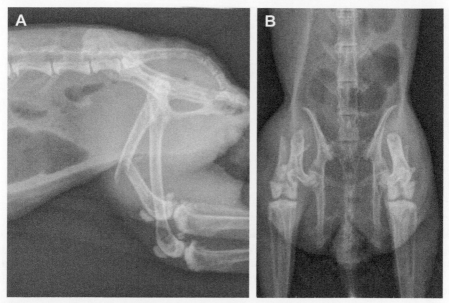

Fig. 17. Laterolateral radiograph of a rabbit with renal secondary hyperparathyroidism and pathologic fracture of the left femur (*A*). Ventrodorsal view of the same rabbit showing an additional pathologic fracture of the right femur that occurred during the examination (*B*). (*Courtesy of* Federico Vilaplana Grosso and the Diagnostic Imaging Service, College of Veterinary Medicine, University of Florida.)

principally the stifle, coxofemoral, and shoulder joints, and is usually bilateral. Degenerative joint disease is often underdiagnosed in certain exotic pet species, such as rodents, and it is frequently an incidental finding. Spontaneous cartilage degeneration has been reported in Guinea pigs, resulting in degenerative changes and arthritis of the stifle joint[37] (**Fig. 20**). Radiographic findings include periarticular osteophytes, enthesophytes, subchondral bone sclerosis and lysis, joint space narrowing, and periarticular dystrophic mineralization. Periarticular mineralized bodies and linear dystrophic mineralization of entheses and muscles are commonly seen in rodents and usually lack of clinical significance.[48]

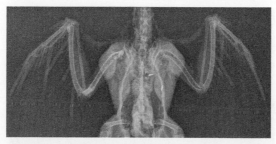

Fig. 18. Ventrodorsal radiograph of a macaw with fungal osteomyelitis of the right humerus. Note the patchy multifocal intramedullary increased opacity and distal periosteal reaction. (*Courtesy of* Federico Vilaplana Grosso and the Diagnostic Imaging Service, College of Veterinary Medicine, University of Florida.)

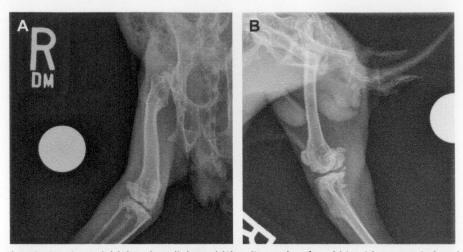

Fig. 19. Craniocaudal (*A*) and mediolateral (*B*) radiographs of a rabbit with trauma-induced marked coxofemoral and stifle degenerative joint disease. (*Courtesy of* Federico Vilaplana Grosso and the Diagnostic Imaging Service, College of Veterinary Medicine, University of Florida.)

Degenerative intervertebral disc disease

Degenerative intervertebral disc disease has been reported in hedgehogs.[49] In a series of 4 cases, radiographic findings included spondylosis deformans, intervertebral disc space narrowing, and intervertebral disc mineralization.[50] Degenerative intervertebral disc disease is common in older pet rabbits (**Fig. 21**). Radiographic findings are similar to those encountered in other species (eg, dog), such as spur-shaped or bridging new bone formation ventrally to adjacent endplates, endplate sclerosis, or intervertebral disc space narrowing.

Neoplasia *Osteosarcomas* have been diagnosed in small mammals, reptiles, and birds affecting the appendicular and axial skeleton, but overall, bone tumors are rare in exotic pets.[29,51–53] In rabbits, it seems that osteosarcomas more commonly affect the skull. Bone neoplasia in exotic pets is usually characterized by osteolysis with minimal periosteal change; however, osteoblastic neoplasia with marked periosteal reaction may occur. Soft tissue neoplasia may involve the bone and be a cause of lameness. The most frequent radiographic findings are bone lysis and reactive periosteal reaction.

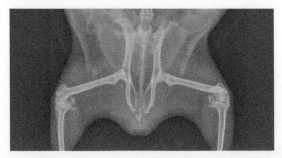

Fig. 20. Ventrodorsal radiograph of a Guinea pig with severe bilateral stifle degenerative joint disease. (*Courtesy of* Federico Vilaplana Grosso and the Diagnostic Imaging Service, College of Veterinary Medicine, University of Florida.)

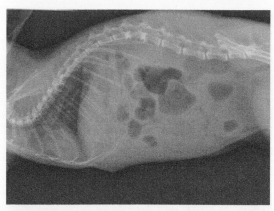

Fig. 21. Laterolateral radiograph of a rabbit with degenerative intervertebral disc disease. Note the narrowing of the intervertebral disc spaces L1-L3 with associated endplate sclerosis and mild spondylosis deformans. (*Courtesy of* Federico Vilaplana Grosso and the Diagnostic Imaging Service, College of Veterinary Medicine, University of Florida.)

Chordomas are the most common type of musculoskeletal neoplasia reported in ferrets. Cervical chordomas may induce osteolytic reaction of the vertebrae and can develop compressive myelopathy and compression of the adjacent tissues[54] (**Fig. 22**).

Also, in ferrets, lymphoma, invasive histiocytic sarcoma, and plasma cell neoplasia can cause osteolytic lesions with associated spinal cord compression.[55,56] Metastatic bone disease is rare in exotic species.

Miscellaneous *Polyostotic hyperostosis* is seen seasonally in reproductively active female birds because of the storage of calcium salts before the beginning of the egg laying and usually happens in the ulna and tibia. Radiographically, polyostotic hyperostosis is characterized by a diffuse, uniform, or patchy increase in the opacity of the medullary cavity of nonpneumatic bones, such as the femur, tibiotarsus, radius, and ulna.[43] Polyostotic hyperostosis can also occur in female birds with oviductal neoplasia or male birds with Sertoli cell tumors.[57]

Spine curvature disorders (eg, scoliosis, lordosis, and kyphosis) *and angular limb deformities* (eg, tibiotarsal valgus or splayed legs) are commonly seen exotic species, probably secondary to MBD (with concomitant folding fractures) and malunion

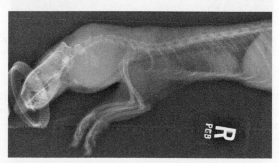

Fig. 22. Laterolateral radiograph of a ferret with a cervical chordomas. A large soft tissue opaque mass with associated amorphous dystrophic mineralization is seen. (*Courtesy of* Federico Vilaplana Grosso and the Diagnostic Imaging Service, College of Veterinary Medicine, University of Florida.)

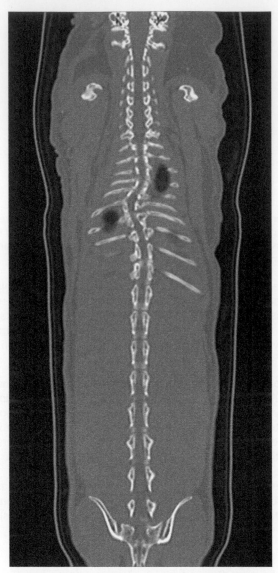

Fig. 23. Dorsal CT reconstruction of a rabbit showing scoliosis. (*Courtesy of* Federico Vila-plana Grosso and the Diagnostic Imaging Service, College of Veterinary Medicine, University of Florida.)

fractures. Scoliosis is the most usual spine curvature malformation and in most cases is difficult to determine the underlying cause (**Fig. 23**). Congenital causes are also possible but less frequent. In reptiles, improper incubation temperatures during embryogenesis may lead to these abnormalities.[46]

REFERENCES

1. Pees M, Kiefer I, Ludewig E, et al. Computed tomography of the lungs of Indian pythons (*Python molurus*). Am J Vet Res 2007;68:428–34.

2. Paul-Murphy JR, Koblik PD, Stein G, et al. Psittacine skull radiography: Anatomy, radiographic technique, and patient application. Vet Radiol Ultrasound 1990;31: 218–24.

3. Smith BJ, Smith SA, Spaulding KA, et al. The normal xeroradiographic and radiographic anatomy of the cockatiel (*Nymphzcus hollandz*). Vet Radiol Ultrasound 1990;31:226–34.

4. Smith BJ, Smith SA, Flammer K, et al. The normal xeroradiographic and radiographic anatomy of the orange-winged amazon parrot (*Amazona amazonica amazonica*). Vet Radiol Ultrasound 1990;31(3):114–24.

5. Ahranjani BA, Shojaei B, Tootian Z, et al. Anatomical, radiographical and computed tomographic study of the limbs skeleton of the Euphrates soft shell turtle (*Rafetus euphraticus*). Vet Res Forum 2016;2:117–24.

6. Banzato T, Selleri P, Veladiano IA, et al. Comparative evaluation of the cadaveric and computed tomographic features of the coelomic cavity in the green iguana (*Iguana iguana*), black-and-white tegu (*Tupinambis merianae*) and bearded dragon (*Pogona vitticeps*). Anat Histol Embryol 2013;42:453–60.

7. BanzatoT, Selleri P, Veladiano IA, et al. Comparative evaluation of the cadaveric, radiographic and computed tomographic anatomy of the heads of green iguana (*Iguana iguana*), common tegu (*Tupinambis merianae*) and bearded dragon (*Pogona vitticeps*). BMC Vet Res 2012;8:53.

8. Veladiano IA, Banzato T, Bellini L, et al. Computed tomographic anatomy of the heads of blue-and-gold macaws (*Ara ararauna*), African grey parrots (*Psittacus erithacus*), and monk parakeets (*Myiopsitta monachus*). Am J Vet Res 2016;77: 1346–56.

9. Müllhaupt D, Wenger S, Kircher P, et al. Computed tomography of the thorax in rabbits: a prospective study in ten clinically healthy New Zealand white rabbits. Acta Vet Scand 2017;59:72.

10. Zotti A, Banzato T, Cozzi B. Cross-sectional anatomy of the rabbit neck and trunk: comparison of computed tomography and cadaver anatomy. Res Vet Sci 2009; 87:171–6.

11. Banzato T, Russo E, Di Tomma A, et al. Evaluation of radiographic, computed tomographic and cadaveric anatomy of the head of boa constrictors. Am J Vet Res 2011;72:1592–9.

12. Veladiano IA, Banzato T, Bellini L, et al. Normal computed tomographic features and reference values for the coelomic cavity in pet parrots. BMC Vet Res 2016; 12:182.

13. King AM, Cranfield F, Hall J, et al. Radiographic anatomy of the rabbit skull with particular reference to the tympanic bulla and temporomandibular joint Part 1: Lateral and long axis rotational angles. Vet J 2010;186:232–43.

14. King AM, Cranfield F, Hall J, et al. Radiographic anatomy of the rabbit skull with particular reference to the tympanic bulla and temporomandibular joint. Part 2: ventral and dorsal rotational angles. Vet J 2010;186:242–51.

15. Hashemi M, Javadi S, Hadian M, et al. Radiological investigations of the hedgehog (*Erinaceus concolor*) appendicular skeleton. J Zoo Wildl Med 2009;40:1–7.

16. Smith SA, Smith BJ. Radiographic evaluation of general avian anatomy. In: Smith SA, Smith BJ, editors. Atlas of avian radiographic anatomy. Philadelphia: WB Saunders; 1992. p. 5–18.

17. Krautwald-Junghanns ME, Pees M, Reese S, et al. Diagnostic imaging of exotic pets. Hannover (Germany): Schlutersche; 2009.

18. Lo WY, Puchalski SM. Digital image processing. Vet Radiol Ultrasound 2008;49: 42–7.

19. Oliveira CR, Ranallo FN, Pijanowski GJ, et al. The VetMousetrap: a device for computed tomographic imaging of the thorax of awake cats. Vet Radiol Ultrasound 2011;52:41–52.

20. Abou-Madi N, Scrivani PV, Kollias GV, et al. Diagnosis of skeletal injuries in chelonians using computed tomography. J Zoo Wildl Med 2004;35:226–31.

21. Di Girolamo N, Selleri P, Nardini G, et al. Computed tomography-guided bone biopsies for evaluation of proliferative vertebral lesions in two boa constrictors (*Boa constrictor imperator*). J Zoo Wildl Med 2014;45:973–8.

22. De Rycke LM, Boone MN, Van Caelenberg AI, et al. Micro-computed tomography of the head and dentition in cadavers of clinically normal rabbits. Am J Vet Res 2012;73:227–32.

23. Capello V. Diagnostic imaging of dental disease in pet rabbits and rodents. Vet Clin North Am Exot Anim Pract 2016;19:757–82.

24. Goggin JM, Hoskinson JJ, Carpenter JW, et al. Scintigraphic assessment of distal extremity perfusion in 17 patients. Vet Radiol Ultrasound 1997;38:211–20.

25. Hernandez-Divers SJ, Strunk A, Frank PM, et al. Scintigraphic imaging of a Horsfields Tortoise (*Testudo horsfieldi*) with multifocal bacterial and fungal infections, and plastron necrosis. Proceedings of the Association of Reptilian and amphibians veterinarians 2002;103–4.

26. Silverman S, Tell LA. Radiology equipment and positioning techniques. In: Radiology of birds. St. Louis (MO): Saunders Elsevier; 2010. p. 1–15.

27. Sirois M, Anthony E, Mauragis D. Radiography of avian and exotic animals. In: Handbook of radiographic positioning for veterinary technicians. New York: Delmar Cengage Learning; 2010. p. 181–223.

28. DeCourcy K, Hostnik ET, Lorbach J, et al. Unsedated computed tomography for diagnosis of pelvic canal obstruction in a leopard gecko (*Eublepharis macularius*). J Zoo Wildl Med 2016;47:1073–6.

29. McMillan MC. Imaging techniques. In: Ritchie BW, Harrison GJ, Harrison LR, editors. Avian medicine: principles and application. FL: Wingers Publishing; 1994. p. 246–326.

30. Bush M, Montali RJ, Novak GR, et al. The healing of the avian fractures: a histologic xeroradiopgrahic study. J Am Anim Hosp Assoc 1976;12:768–76.

31. Silverman S, Janssen DL. Diagnostic imaging. In: Mader DR, editor. Reptile medicine and surgery. Philadelphia: WB Saunders; 1996. p. 258–64.

32. Williams J. Orthopedic radiography in exotic animal practice. Vet Clin North Am Exot Anim Pract 2002;5:1–22.

33. Henry GA. Fracture healing and complications. In: Thrall D, editor. Textbook of veterinary diagnostic radiology. 6th edition. MO: Saunders Elsevier; 2013. p. 283–306.

34. Meij BP, Hazewinkel HAW, Westerhof I, et al. Treatment of fractures and angular limb deformities of the tibiotarsus in birds by type II external skeletal fixation. J Avian Med Surg 1996;10:153–62.

35. Ritzman KT, Knapp D. Ferret orthopedics. Vet Clin North Am Exot Anim Pract 2002;5:129–55.

36. Cevik-Demirkan A, Ozdemir V, Turkmenoglu I, et al. Anatomy of the hind limb skeleton of the chinchilla (*Chinchilla lanigera*). Acta Vet Brno 2007;76:501–7.

37. Schaeffer DO, Donnelly TM. Disease problems of Guinea pigs and chinchillas. In: Hillyer EV, Quesenberry KE, editors. Ferrets, rabbits, and rodents: clinical medicine and surgery. Philadelphia: WB Saunders; 1997. p. 260–79.

38. Visser M, Hespel AM, de Swarte M, et al. Use of a caudoventral craniodorsal oblique radiographic view made at 45° to the frontal plane to evaluate the pectoral girdle in raptors. J Am Vet Med Assoc 2015;247(9):1037–41.
39. Keeble E. Common neurological and musculoskeletal problems in rabbits. Practitioner 2006;28:212–8.
40. Oglesbee B. Vertebral fracture or luxation. In: Oglesbee BL, editor. The 5-minute veterinary consult: ferret and rabbit. Ames (IA): Blackwell Publishing; 2006. p. 381.
41. Ertelt J, Maierl J, Kaiser A, et al. Anatomical and pathophysiological features and treatment of elbow luxation in rabbits. Tierarztl Prax Ausg K Kleintiere Heimtiere 2010;38:201–10.
42. Calvo Carrasco D, Minier K, Shimizu N, et al. Surgical management of a traumatic elbow luxation with circumferential suture prostheses in a rabbit (Oryctolagus cuniculus). J Exot Pet Med 2018;27:38–42.
43. Quesenberry K. Disorders of the musculoskeletal system. In: Altman RB, Clubb SL, Dorrestein GM, et al, editors. Avian medicine and surgery. Philadelphia: WB Saunders; 1997. p. 523–39.
44. Azmanis PN, Wernick MB, Hatt JM. Avian luxations: occurrence, diagnosis and treatment. Vet Q 2014;34(1):11–21.
45. Dennis R, Kirberger RM, Barr F, et al. Skeletal system: general. In: Handbook of small animal radiology and ultrasound. 2nd edition. New York: Churchill Livingstone Elsevier; 2010. p. 1–37.
46. Raiti P. Non-invasive imaging. In: Girling SJ, Raiti P, editors. BSAVA manual of reptiles. 2nd edition. Gloucester (United Kingdom): Quedgeley; 2004. p. 87–102.
47. Kapatkin A. Orthopedics in small mammals. In: Hillyer EV, Quesenberry KE, editors. Ferrets, rabbits, and rodents: clinical medicine and surgery. Philadelphia: WB Saunders; 1997. p. 346–57.
48. Drees R. Rabbits and rodents. In: Schwarz T, Saunders, editors. J. Veterinary computed tomography. Chichester (United Kingdom): Wiley-Blackwell; 2011. p. 509–16.
49. Raymond JT, White MR. Necropsy and histopathologic findings in 14 African hedgehogs (Atelerix albiventris): a retrospective study. J Zoo Wildl Med 1999; 30:273–7.
50. Raymond JT, Aguilar R, Dunker F, et al. Intervertebral disc disease in African hedgehogs (Atelerix albiventris): four cases. J Exot Pet Med 2009;18:220–3.
51. Weiss ATA, Müller K. Spinal osteolytic osteosarcoma in a pet rabbit. Vet Rec 2011;168(10):266.
52. Ishikawa M, Kondo H, Onuma M, et al. Osteoblastic osteosarcoma in a rabbit. Comp Med 2012;62(2):124–6.
53. Cowan ML, Monks DJ, Raidal SR. Osteosarcoma in a woma python (Aspidites ramsayi). Aust Vet J 2011;89(12):520–3.
54. Geoffrey W, Bennett A, Gregory D, et al. Thoracic vertebral chordoma in a domestic ferret (Mustela putorius furo). J Zoo Wildl Med 2000;31(1):107–11.
55. Warschau M, Hoffmann M, Dziallas P, et al. Invasive histiocytic sarcoma of the lumbar spine in a ferret (Mustela putorius furo). J Small Anim Pract 2017;58: 115–8.
56. Suran JN, Wyre NR. Imaging findings in 14 domestic ferrets (Mustela putorius furo) with lymphoma. Vet Radiol Ultrasound 2013;54(5):522–31.
57. Stauber E, Papageorges M, Sande R, et al. Polyostotic hyperostosis associated with oviductal tumor in a cockatiel. J Am Vet Med Assoc 1990;196(6):939–40.

Exotic Mammal Orthopedics

Yasutsugu Miwa, DVM, PhD[a,b],
Daniel Calvo Carrasco, LV, CertAVP (ZooMed), MRCVS[c,d],*

KEYWORDS

- Orthopedics • Exotic • Small mammal • Rabbit • Ferret • Fracture • Bone plate
- Luxation

KEY POINTS

- A complete full examination and a complete understanding of the ongoing pathologic processes of the patient are required as part of the treatment decision-making process.
- Supportive care should include fluid therapy, analgesia, supplemental feeding, and prokinetics in herbivore species.
- Physiologic and anatomic particularities, as well as the orthopedic pathologic characteristics, must be considered when elaborating a treatment plan.
- Conservative management is a valid option but should be used adequately and its limitations understood.
- Tie-in fixators are currently one of the preferred options because of their versatility, light weight, and are relative ease of use.

INTRODUCTION

The commonly used term "exotic mammal" is widely understood as those mammals, other than dogs and cats, kept as pets. The more common exotic small mammal pet species include rodents, rabbits, and ferrets, which, despite the consistency of the different skeletal elements across Mammalia, significantly vary in size and, even in the largest species, skeletal strength, bone density, thickness of cortical bone, and muscle strength. Some species, such as squirrels, sugar gliders, and chinchillas, have a very different locomotion, a factor to be considered when planning their orthopedic treatment. Equally, many of them are prey species who present a low stress tolerance compared with dogs and cats and which may manifest as self-mutilation of the surgical site, even when careful postoperative care is provided.

Disclosure Statement: The authors have nothing to disclose.
[a] Miwa Exotic Animal Hospital, 1-25-5 Komagome, Toshima-ku, Tokyo 170-0003A, Japan; [b] Laboratories of Veterinary Surgery, Graduate School of Agricultural and Life Sciences, The University of Tokyo, 1-1-1 Yayoi, Bunkyo-ku, Tokyo 113-8657, Japan; [c] Great Western Exotics, Vets Now Swindon, Swindon, UK; [d] Wildfowl & Wetlands Trust (WWT), Newgrounds Ln, Gloucestershire, England, Gloucester GL2 7BT, United Kingdom
* Corresponding author. Wildfowl &Wetlands Trust (WWT), Newgrounds Ln, Gloucestershire, England, Gloucester GL2 7BT, United Kingdom.
E-mail address: danicalvocarrasco@gmail.com

The principles of fracture management in exotic small mammals are similar to those established for dogs and cats; however, many aspects such as anatomy, tolerance to stress, postoperative care, and the level of overall understanding of the species from both veterinary surgeons and owners significantly differ from those of dogs and cats.[1] In addition, scientific information about the orthopedic treatment of small exotic mammals is limited to few case reports and a scarce number of clinical studies.[2–16] In the other hand, rodents and rabbits are commonly used as experimental models for human studies, although the utility of these for the clinician can greatly vary, given that their main purpose was humans rather than the species in question.

Treating orthopedic diseases in small exotic mammals may be challenging. To obtain a successful outcome, it is important to follow the principles of orthopedic surgery described for other species such as dogs and cats while being flexible and able to adapt to each specific case. Other things to consider include the cost of treatment, ease of application, availability of surgical equipment, the surgeon's experience, and the patient's character, among others.

This article discusses orthopedic conditions, including fracture and luxation management, in exotic small mammals, focusing on those treatment options that differ with respect to dogs and cats.

FRACTURES IN SMALL EXOTIC MAMMALS (CAUSE, LESION, AND OTHER SPECIFIC FEATURES)

One of the most common causes of fractures in dogs and cats are road traffic accidents. The incidence rate of this type of injury seems to have decreased in recent years, particularly in urban areas, where dogs and cats are increasingly kept indoors. In exotic small mammals, fractures are seen relatively often despite most of these animals being kept exclusively indoors. In exotic small mammals, other causes of traumatic fractures include being trapped by wire cages and wheels and stepped on or sat on by the owner; falls from heights are common causes of traumatic fractures in hamsters and chinchillas, or being dropped by the owner in rabbits and fennec foxes. Overall the origin of these pathologies remains mostly traumatic, often the result of improper handling and restraint or suboptimal husbandry conditions. Primary pathologic fractures do not seem as common as in other exotic pet species such as reptiles and birds, but in the author's (D.C.C.) opinion is not unlikely that metabolic bone disease, either by low calcium intake and/or low ultraviolet B exposure, is to some degree an (often underconsidered) underlying predisposing factor.

A 13-year summary of the types of orthopedic trauma in small mammals presented to the teaching hospital of a Veterinary School in the United States presented the rabbit as the most common species treated for orthopedic injuries (67.5%), followed by chinchillas (13%).[17] This result seems to correlate with the cases seen in one exotic referral practice in the United Kingdom, according to the experience of one of the authors (D.C.C.), but not with the cases seen in first opinion or general practice. Orthopedic conditions caused by trauma occur frequently in certain species of rodents, but may not be seen in referral hospitals of Western countries because further specialized treatment is often declined owing to cost limitations. By contrast, the hamster is the most common presented species to exotic referral practices because of fractures in Japan, followed by chinchillas and sugar gliders, whereas fractures in guinea pigs, hedgehogs, and ferrets are not as commonly seen (Y.M.).

Different factors may predispose different species to be presented to the exotic practice. Hamsters are popular pets among children, leading them to suffer a high number of accidental injuries. Rabbits are a common pet worldwide (the third most commonly kept pet in the United Kingdom, around 1 million in 2018), possess relatively thin cortices and strong muscles, particularly in the hind limbs, and present a locomotion based on hopping rather than walking.[15,18,19] Chinchillas have relatively long and thin hind limbs and present a range of activity that includes the vertical plane (tall enclosures) in addition to the horizontal plane. Contrarily, Guinea pigs and hedgehogs have short limbs and lack the ability to jump.

A retrospective study in rabbits reported accidental falls as the most common cause of fracture, causing nearly half of the fractures, followed by 36.3% being a direct consequence of human error, including mishandling and injuries that occurred under veterinary care.[20]

In the authors' experience, most fractures in exotic small mammals occur in the long bones of the limbs and particularly involve the pelvic limbs. Sasai and colleagues[16] reported the tibia as the most common site for fractures in rabbits, followed by the femur and the radius. Additionally the distal aspect of the limbs such as metacarpal bone, talus, and phalanges were also common fracture sites in rabbits. These distal areas, especially the tibia, were not only common lesions but also prone to open-wound fractures because of the small soft-tissue coverage.

Apart from traumatic fractures, pathologic fractures caused by metabolic bone disease (particularly relevant in sugar gliders), iatrogenic fractures of rabbits under hospital care, and primary neoplasia or metastatic tumors, such as metastasis of uterine tumors in rabbits, are occasionally seen.

Based on the authors' experience, most small exotic mammals attended to are herbivorous and their cortex is relatively thin and light in comparison with dog cortex and is prone to shatter, as seen in rabbits.

In addition, rodents are prone to self-trauma at the affected area, and most are prey species that tend to hide signs of illness, which often results in a delayed detection of the fracture by the owner, resulting in severe infections of open-wound fractures.

FEATURES OF RABBIT BONE AND ITS FRACTURE

Management of long bone fractures in rabbits and other small mammals is challenging because of their particular anatomy and composition of their bony tissues when compared with dogs and cats. The rabbit skeleton constitutes only 7% of the total body weight, which is a much smaller contribution to the whole body mass than the one observed in dogs or cats (**Fig. 1**) where it represents around 12% of the body weight.[15,19] The ratio of the thickness cortex/bone is 26% in the Chihuahua (a dog breed of a similar size) and 12% in rabbits (see **Fig. 1**). In addition, the full length of the femur is around 15 mm longer in rabbits than in Chihuahuas (**Fig. 2**). Rabbit bones also possess a lower density and a higher mineral composition, which makes them brittle. The already mentioned features combined with their relatively large muscles are a potential explanation for the higher predisposition to fractures when compared with dogs and cats.

Although rabbits have a greater risk for spinal injuries than dogs and cats, the features mentioned earlier increase the chances of accidental iatrogenic damage to the long bone, resulting in further damage while being manipulated.[19] According to Sasai and colleagues[16] limb fractures were the most common and accounted for 63.6% of all fractures, especially distal bones such as the tibia, the ulna, and the radius. This research showed a higher ratio of hind limb fractures compared with forelimb (1:2).

Rabbits have a higher ratio of segmental (or comminuted) fractures compared with dogs, not only regarding high-energy traumatic events but also low-energy impacts.

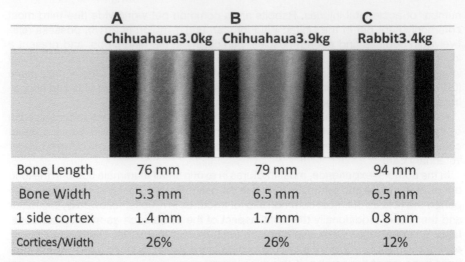

	A Chihuahaua3.0kg	B Chihuahaua3.9kg	C Rabbit3.4kg
Bone Length	76 mm	79 mm	94 mm
Bone Width	5.3 mm	6.5 mm	6.5 mm
1 side cortex	1.4 mm	1.7 mm	0.8 mm
Cortices/Width	26%	26%	12%

Fig. 1. Comparison of the thickness of femoral bone in dogs and rabbits of similar body. The cortex/bone diameter is 26% in Chihuahua (*A, B*) and 12% in rabbits (*C*). (*Courtesy of* Muneki Honnami, DVM, PhD, Tokyo, Japan.)

The fact that rabbit bones shatter very easily makes the surgical approach particularly challenging because the possibility of the occurrence of macroscopically invisible fissures in each bone fragment complicates the procedure.

Owing to the sizable power-to-weight ratio, secondary fractures need to be included on the list of postsurgical complications. Moreover, rabbits are prone to postoperative infections and rapid development of osteomyelitis, which significantly aggravates the prognosis.[21–23] Various experimental studies on efficacy of implant placement have been reported in rabbits used as experimental models.[24] Generally even the smallest implants applied in orthopedics of cats and dogs are too large and heavy to use in rabbits.[15] However, some successful reports of long bone fracture repair in rabbits have been published in recent years. External skeletal fixation (ESF) is preferred to the other methods thanks to the versatility in construct, minimal disruption of the vascularity, and low cost of the equipment.[10,21]

DIAGNOSIS
Initial Care and Physical Examination

The basic diagnostic workup for diagnosis in exotic small mammals is similar to those of dogs and cats. Although the fracture may appear to be the most dramatic consequence of the injury, a complete assessment of the animal should be performed.

At first, the injured animal should be considered a traumatic patient (as the primary cause of fractures is trauma); therefore shock, potential bleeding, any concomitant fractures, and any thoracic and/or abdominal lesions must be addressed and treated immediately before a full orthopedic evaluation is considered. In most cases, fractures are not life threatening except for a few conditions that directly affect the central nervous system or respiratory system. A thorough physical examination and appropriate initial treatment of metabolic compromise and/or shock should be the priority, and further diagnostics such as radiographs should only be carried out once stabilized.

Despite a single fracture perhaps being obvious, the clinician must rule out the presence of other fractures or concomitant injuries (**Fig. 3**). On physical examination,

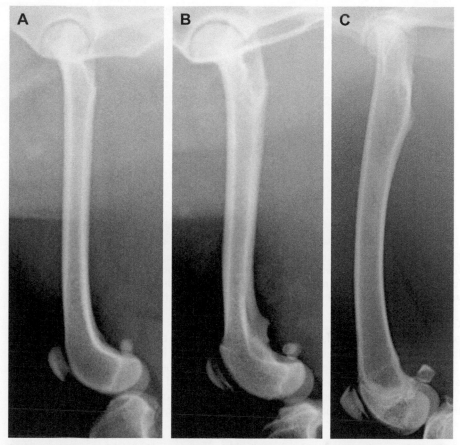

Fig. 2. Comparison of the femoral bone in dogs and rabbits. Radiographs represented femoral bones of a Chihuahua with body weight 3 kg (*A*), a Chihuahua with body weight 3.9 kg (*B*), and a rabbit with body weight 3.4 kg (*C*). The rabbit femur is more elongated and presents thinner cortices compared with the femur of dogs of a similar body weight. (*Courtesy of* Muneki Honnami, DVM, PhD, Tokyo, Japan.)

checking the fracture site for instability, soft-tissue damage, and active hemorrhage is important, and special care is required in locating any skin wounds at the fracture site, which could reveal the existence of a contaminated or open fracture (**Fig. 4**). The tibial bone is the most commonly contaminated bone because of its relatively small amount of surrounding soft tissue (**Fig. 5**).

Radiographs

Following the complete physical examination, orthogonal radiographs of the whole body should be taken to determine whether other injuries or fractures are present that may have been initially overseen on physical examination. In general, whole-body survey radiographs are not considered as an ideal diagnostic technique, although they may be useful to reveal significant abnormalities before the animal can be safely restrained for isolated radiographic examination of affected bones.[25] Analgesics or sedative agents may be needed to facilitate obtaining the radiographs.

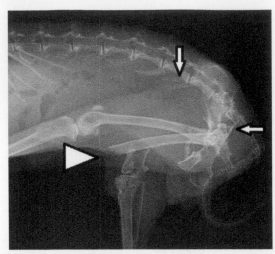

Fig. 3. Lateral radiograph of a rabbit with a suspected leg injury following trauma. The femoral fracture (*arrowhead*) is easily seen, but the clinician must ensure not to miss other lesions by focusing in the more obvious radiographic findings (*arrows*; fractures of pelvic and transverse process of vertebra). (*Courtesy of* Yasutsugu Miwa, DVM, PhD, Tokyo, Japan.)

Good-quality, diagnostic, properly positioned orthogonal radiographs (eg, limb; laterolateral and craniocaudal views that include the joints proximal and distal to the fracture site) are essential to evaluate the fracture.

In some cases, pathologic fractures related to bone tumors or metastatic tumors are suspected based on radiographic findings (**Figs. 6** and **7**).

Micro–computed tomography (CT) is another useful diagnostic method to evaluate the detailed conditions such as fissures and fragments of affected bone in small exotic

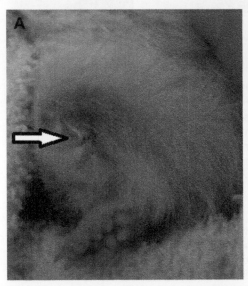
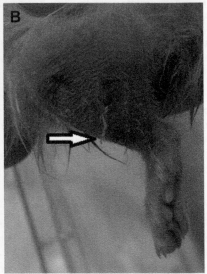

Fig. 4. Open fracture in Syrian hamster. Open-wound fracture (*arrows*) is occasionally unclear (*A*), so hair clipping (*B*) and close examination are recommended to avoid missing open-wound fractures. (*Courtesy of* Yasutsugu Miwa, DVM, PhD, Tokyo, Japan.)

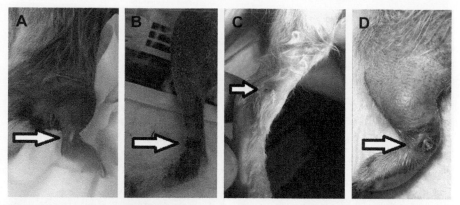

Fig. 5. Open-wound fractures in small exotic mammals. (*A*) Djungarian hamster, (*B*) chinchilla, (*C*) guinea pig, (*D*) Richardson's ground squirrel. Open-wound fractures (*arrows*) are common in small exotic mammals (*A–D*). The tibial bone is the most common location because of the relatively small amount of soft tissue surrounding the area. (*Courtesy of* Yasutsugu Miwa, DVM, PhD, Tokyo, Japan.)

mammal patients, especially in complicated or comminuted fractures. In addition, a CT scan provides images that allow 3D reconstruction, which may be useful to facilitate successful fracture repair.[16]

TREATMENT
Preoperative Consideration

Before fracture repair it is vital to ensure that the patient is stable. The administration of analgesics, anti-inflammatories, and antibiotics may be necessary depending on the specific case. Intravenous or subcutaneous fluid therapy and appropriate analgesia,

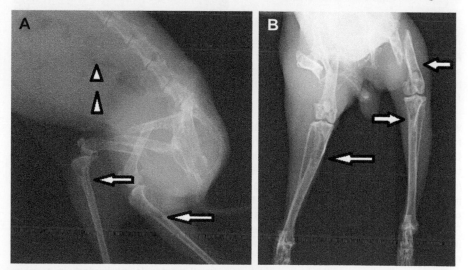

Fig. 6. Orthogonal radiographs of a female rabbit with suspected pathologic fractures caused by metastatic disease. Note the abnormal bone density on the femur (*arrows*) and mineralization of the uterus (*arrowhead*). (*A*) Lateral view and (*B*) craniocaudal view. (*Courtesy of* Yasutsugu Miwa, DVM, PhD, Tokyo, Japan.)

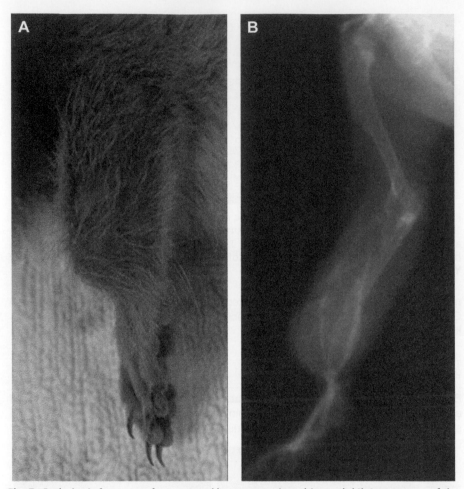

Fig. 7. Pathologic fractures of a suspected bone tumor in a chipmunk (*A*) Appearance of the affected limb. (*B*) Radiograph of the affected limb. The swelling lesion (*A*) was a suspected bone tumor with a pathologic fracture (*B*). (*Courtesy of* Yasutsugu Miwa, DVM, PhD, Tokyo, Japan.)

wound care, bandaging, and nutritional support should be provided for patient comfort, to decrease further injuries, to decrease the incidence of infection, and to improve the patient's condition and consequently the overall prognosis. The authors have traditionally used buprenorphine (20–50 μg/kg, subcutaneous [SC], every 6–12 h [q6–12 h]),[26–28] which appears to have no adverse effect on gastrointestinal motility in healthy rabbits, and meloxicam (0.1–1.0 mg/kg, SC or orally, q12–24 h provided correct renal perfusion is maintained) as multimodal analgesia[26–29]; methadone (0.1–3 mg/kg) has gradually replaced buprenorphine in more painful conditions because it provides the benefits of a pure μ-agonist while having fewer side effects than morphine.[30,31]

Other medications routinely used in exotic small mammals, particularly in herbivorous species, are prokinetics such as ranitidine and/or metoclopramide, to minimize secondary gastrointestinal stasis. The management of stress is also important. Handling should be reduced to a minimum, and prey species should be always hospitalized away from stressful smells, noises, and visual contact with predatory species. If infection is suspected, broad-spectrum antibiotic therapy should be initiated until bacteriologic results are available.

Fracture Management

Orthopedic conditions may be managed with various approaches and techniques, including conservative management (eg, cage rest, bandages, and splints) and/or surgical approaches (eg, intramedullary pins, external skeletal fixators, and bone plates). Recently, differing orthopedic equipment has become commercially available in a wide range of sizes, some being suitable for use in smaller patients.

The selection of the method of fracture repair should be based on the animal species, character, age, fracture type, location and duration of the fracture, owner compliance, cost, the practitioner's surgical expertise, and the equipment available. Given the relatively limited bibliography available, the clinician must have an open vision and adaptability in order to decide between the suitable treatment options for each individual case. Extrapolation from other species is sometimes the only option available, although it is necessary to consider the anatomic and physiologic particularities of each species.

Cage Rest/Confinement

Cage rest is crucial in the preoperative and postoperative period, and cage rest itself is one of the choices of fracture treatment in specific cases. Restriction of the patient activity is important, but it can be challenging to accomplish in certain species and, in some instances, a minor and tolerable degree of welfare compromise must be accepted to achieve the best final outcome. In some circumstances it can be difficult to find the right balance between providing a minimum space to ordinary life but restricting overexercise by limiting the space to run (and jump) around. Any exercise wheels, climbing platforms, or tubing should be removed during the convalescence period. Providing the owner with the right information on how to restrict the animal's activity and the importance of the follow-up are vital, and as relevant as the treatment therapy itself, as some owners will confine animals in excessively small cages such as travel cages, whereas others will not restrict the animal activity, leading to possible further complications and undesired outcomes.

Cage rest might be considered the treatment of choice in some fractures when the fracture is aligned or relatively stable, or the patient's size significantly limits surgical options and external coaptation is not feasible. Fractures of proximal long bones, such as the femur and the humerus, where the proximal joint (thoracic and pelvic girdle) cannot be immobilized by external coaptation, and which are surrounded by large muscles, are occasionally cured by second intention if proper cage rest occurs, especially in young patients (in particular those aged a few weeks or months old) (**Fig. 8**). In these cases, most patients will recover and live normally showing minor deformities, which can be recognized only on radiographs (**Fig. 9**). However, the clinician must accept the risks of fractures resulting in severe deformation and/or even nonunion, and involve the client in the informed decision-making process.

External Coaptation/Bandages

External coaptation includes the use of splints, casts, and other bandages. This method is a rapid and relatively inexpensive technique that can be performed with minimal equipment.

The indications for these methods include the fixation of closed fractures distal to the elbow or stifle joints, as immobilization of the joint located immediately distal

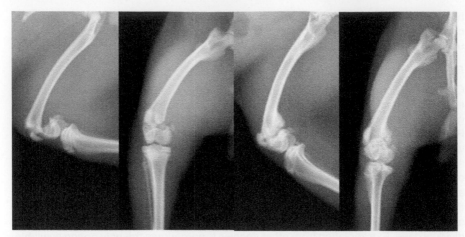

Fig. 8. Radiographic follow-up of a distal femoral fracture in a 5-month-old male rabbit treated by manual reduction of the fracture under general anesthesia and cage rest, at initial presentation and at 30 days follow-up (lateral and craniocaudal views). (*Courtesy of* Yasutsugu Miwa, DVM, PhD, Tokyo, Japan.)

and proximal to the affected bone, with at least 50% contact between proximal and distal fragment ends, may be achieved. They are also especially indicated in young animals and/or greenstick fractures (**Figs. 10–13**). This method is also indicated as a temporary treatment of fractures before surgery to provide hemostasis, avoid further soft-tissue damage and edema, prevent bone fragments from penetrating the skin and becoming contaminated, and increase animal comfort. External coaptation may be also used in combination with internal fixations such as intramedullary (IM) pins to prevent rotational movement after surgery.

The authors prefer to use relatively soft and light materials such as cast padding, roll gauze, and bandage tape for external coaptation in small exotic mammals.

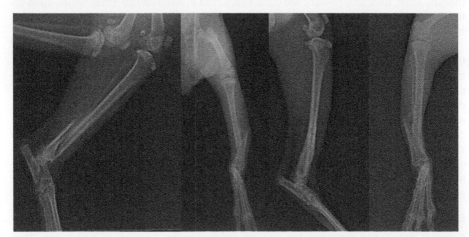

Fig. 9. Radiographic follow-up of a tibial fracture in a 4-month-old female rabbit at initial presentation and 21 days later. Because of the patient's nervous temperament, it was elected to treat by cage rest alone. The fracture healed by second intention within 2 months, at initial presentation and at 30 days' follow-up (lateral and craniocaudal views). (*Courtesy of* Yasutsugu Miwa, DVM, PhD, Tokyo, Japan.)

Traditionally Robert Jones bandages have been applied to small exotic mammals. However, they are not ideal for small patients because they do not provide enough stability. Alternatively, the authors have used Altmann tape splints, a technique described for long bone fractures (particularly in tibiotarsus) in birds. This technique is ideal for the smaller patients (<200 g) such as hamsters (**Fig. 14**), but has been also used in the treatment of fractures and luxations in large patients.[32] Using this technique, although the knee or the elbow are usually immobilized, the limb can be left in a physiologic position (**Fig. 15**), allowing the animal to stand and use the limb, in contrast to a Robert Jones or modified Robert Jones type bandage, whereby the affected limb should be extended and thus might decrease the patient's quality of life and cause stress, especially in those cases affecting the hind limbs of rabbits, hamsters, and hedgehogs (**Fig. 16**). A digital aluminum-foam splint can also be used in combination with the bandage to provide additional stability to the fracture.

It is recommended to apply the bandage and/or splint under sedation or general anesthesia to allow adequate alignment and prevent pain and further injuries. The fracture site should be clipped and examined for wounds and, if present, additional care such as debridement, flushing, and hydrocolloid bandages should be considered.

After placing the bandage or splint, the toes should be observed for swelling for a minimum of 24 hours, and the bandage must be kept clean and dry during the duration of the whole treatment period. The bandage should be replaced if there is swelling of the toes and/or signs of irritation or if any discharge is present. Patient activity should be restricted with cage confinement and the Elizabeth collar may be used, although its use should be avoided, if possible, particularly in species that practice cecotrophy, as it may prevent the normal ingestion of cecotrophs, or in prey species, as narrowing their vision field could result in stress.

The follow-up care includes regular re-examinations of the bandage, evaluation of the patient's appetite and general condition, and postoperative radiographs indicated periodically throughout the healing process. The devices are usually removed within 4 to 6 weeks based on the radiographic findings. Long-term limb immobilization makes rehabilitation difficult. After removing the device, cage rest should be continued for a few weeks until complete healing of the fracture is confirmed on radiographs.

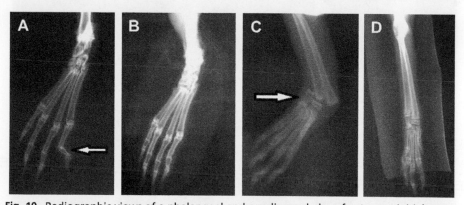

Fig. 10. Radiographic views of a phalangeal and a radius and ulnar fracture at initial examination (*arrows* in *A* and *C*) and following manual reduction and placement of external coaptation (*B,D*). External coaptation of distal limbs in rabbits is a rapid, inexpensive technique especially for fractures of the distal limbs (*arrows* in *A* and *C*). (*Courtesy of Yasutsugu Miwa, DVM, PhD, Tokyo, Japan.*)

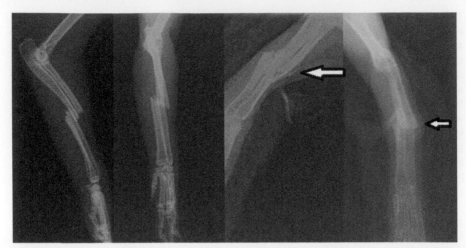

Fig. 11. Radiographic follow-up of a radioulnar fracture in a 1-year-old male rabbit treated with external coaptation at initial presentation and day 60. (*Courtesy of* Yasutsugu Miwa.)

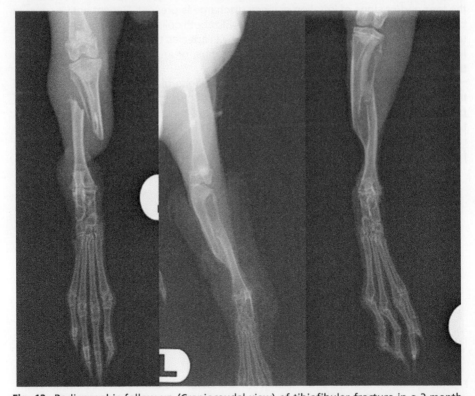

Fig. 12. Radiographic follow-up (Craniocaudal view) of tibiofibular fracture in a 3-month-old female rabbit treated with external coaptation at initial presentation and days 30 and 60. Synostosis was confirmed in 30 days (2) and the fracture was cured within 60 days. (*Courtesy of* Yasutsugu Miwa, DVM, PhD, Tokyo, Japan.)

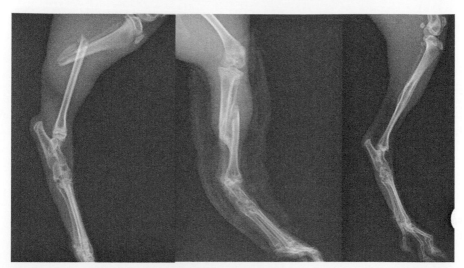

Fig. 13. Radiographic follow-up (lateral view) of tibiofibular fracture in a 3-month-old female rabbit treated with external coaptation at initial presentation and days 30 and 60. Synostosis was confirmed in 30 days (2) and the fracture was cured within 60 days. (*Courtesy of* Yasutsugu Miwa, DVM, PhD, Tokyo, Japan.)

Inappropriate application of the external coaptation cannot only impede healing of the fracture but can also become a cause of other fractures owing to the added weight of the coaptation, which can restrict the movement of the patient and also may act as a fulcrum at the fracture site.

INTERNAL FIXATION
Intramedullary Pins

IM pins are relatively inexpensive and require minimal tissue exposure for insertion, and are easy to apply and in a relatively short time compared with other internal fixations (**Fig. 17**).

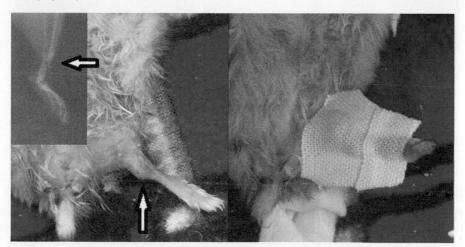

Fig. 14. Djungarian hamster with a tibial fracture (*arrows*) treated with Altmann method. (*Courtesy of* Yasutsugu Miwa, DVM, PhD, Tokyo, Japan.)

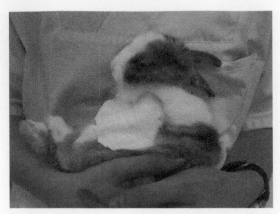

Fig. 15. Altmann tape splint applied to a rabbit with a traumatic elbow luxation. (*Courtesy of* Minh Huynh.)

IM pins can be used for stabilization of diaphyseal fractures, and have also been used in combination with external coaptation to stabilize certain luxations (**Fig. 18**). Although IM pins provide axial alignment and bending stability, they are not stable against rotation and shear forces. Moreover, long bones of limbs are curved in some exotic mammal species (**Fig. 19**). Because of these facts, it is occasionally difficult to insert the pins of recommended diameter (which is 60%–70% of the medullary canal diameter in dogs) in exotic mammals. IM pin insertion carries certain risks, such as causing further fractures if fissures have not been noticed, cracking of the affected bone, and/or interfering with the medullary blood supply. Additionally there is a risk of arthritis if the pin is placed through a joint. In some cases, large IM pins will impair the application of pins for an external fixator. Pin loosening or bone fractures related to

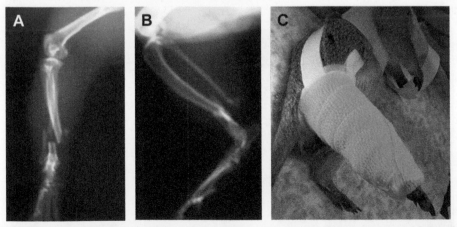

Fig. 16. External coaptation of tibiofibular fracture in a prairie dog (craniocaudal [*A*] and lateral [*B*] radiographs and aspect following bandaging [*C*]). Robert Jones bandages interfere with patient's locomotion (*C*) because the affected limb is immobilized in extension. This disadvantage is more problematic in species with short limbs such as prairie dogs, hamsters, and hedgehogs. (*Courtesy of* Yasutsugu Miwa, DVM, PhD, Tokyo, Japan.)

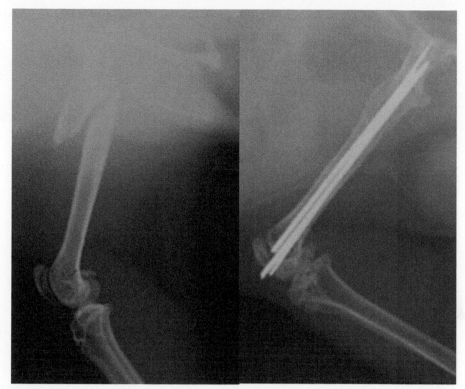

Fig. 17. Radiographic follow-up of a femoral fracture in a chinchilla treated with 3 IM pins at initial presentation and 2 months' follow-up. Note that the femoral bone of the chinchillas is straight in comparison with other species. (*Courtesy of* Yasutsugu Miwa, DVM, PhD, Tokyo, Japan.)

inserted pins are other possible postoperative risks in a rabbit with thin cortex and powerful muscles (**Figs. 20** and **21**), even in successful surgeries.

These shortcomings may be overcome with the concurrent use of other fixations such as external coaptation, ESF, and cerclage wire. Their combination with an ESF, commonly known as "tie-in" or hybrid external fixator, is one of the most used and versatile techniques.

IM pin in combination with a cerclage wire has been used by one of the authors to treat fractures of the calcaneus bone in rabbits. This technique is more likely to be successful in closed fractures; unfortunately, many are open fractures that carry a worse prognosis.[21]

External Skeletal Fixation

ESF has numerous advantages and is a popular treatment option for small exotic mammals because of its relatively low cost and easier application compared with other surgical options such as plating. ESF eliminates bending, rotational, and shearing forces, and maintains fracture apposition with minimal damage to soft tissue and vasculature.[25] In addition, ESF allows access to any potential wounds for further treatment in open-wound fractures, and can be applied to comminuted fractures. ESF can also be applied to smaller patients such as hamsters, using hypodermic needles (see **Fig. 18**). This method does not interfere with joint function, allows the patient to

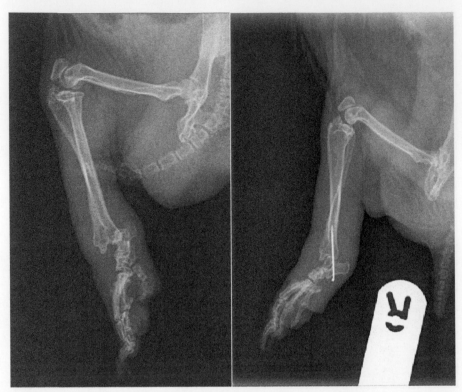

Fig. 18. Tarsocrural luxation in a common hedgehog (*Erinaceus europaeus*) treated using a hypodermic 21-gauge needle used as an extra-articular pin. (*Courtesy of* Daniel Calvo Carrasco, LV, CertAVP (ZooMed), MRCVS, United Kingdom.)

stand and use the affected limb shortly after surgery, and is easily removed once the fracture has healed. Based on these advantages, ESF has been used widely and might even be the most common method of fracture repair in small exotic mammals. There are different types of ESF—using connecting bars and rods, the FESSA system, and in combination with acrylic resins—to join the pins with external and IM pins.

This technique is the preferred choice of one of the authors (D.C.C.) for those fractures whereby the tie-in fixator (TIF) cannot be used because of the inability to place the IM pin, such as radial and ulnar fractures.

Damage to the fixator (which may get caught), premature pin loosening, and pin-tract infections are potential complications of ESF.[25] Premature pin loosening is common in rabbits because of their thin cortices, and breaks and bending of the pins are occasionally seen in such patients owing to the limitation of using small-diameter pins (**Fig. 22**). Ideally, threaded pins should be preferred to smooth pins, and the applied pins should penetrate both cortices (the lateral and medial bone cortices), if possible applied at a certain angle to minimize premature pin loosening. Threaded pins increase pin contact with bone, thus increasing fixator stiffness and decreasing premature pin loosening.

Basic principles for applying ESF are similar in all species. The pin diameter should not exceed 25% to 30% of the bone diameter and a minimum of 2 pins is recommended for each fragment, aiming at the maximum number of pins across the bone fragments spreading the forces along the bone (**Figs. 23 and 24**) and increasing stiffness

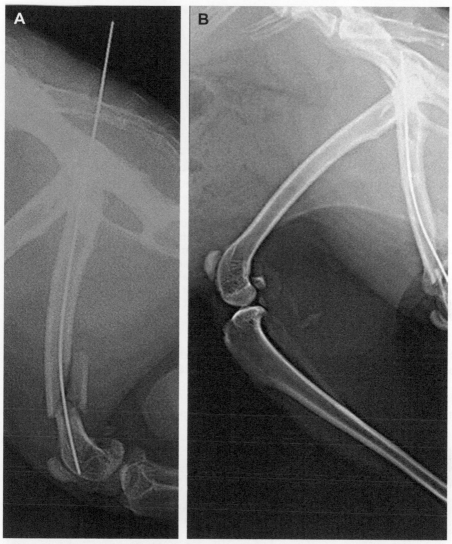

Fig. 19. (*A*) Radiograph of fractured femur in a rabbit, as well as the contralateral limb. (*B*) Femoral bones of rabbits are curved, and it is difficult to insert the recommended diameter pins of dogs in rabbits. (*Courtesy of* Yasutsugu Miwa, DVM, PhD, Tokyo, Japan.)

of the construction. However, it is often difficult to insert more than 2 pins per fragment because of the limited size of these species. It is recommended to use a low-speed power drill to prevent thermal injury rather than a high-speed power drill, as well as to avoid creating larger holes by hand insertion. However, hand insertion with hand chucks should be considered when the power drill produces excessive movements to the affected bone or in smaller patients such as small rodents.

The authors prefer to use resin or acrylic polymer for replacement rods and connecting bars, which are too heavy for small patients (**Fig. 25**). Another significant advantage is the versatility and adaptability of the method, which can be easy molded to

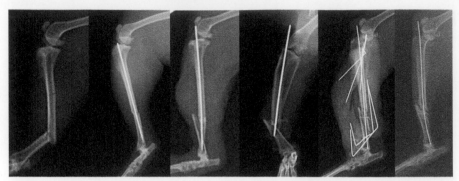

Fig. 20. A case of tibial fracture treated with combination IM pin and ESF after IM pin fixation failed. Two-year-old female (lateral views). 1, preoperative radiograph; 2, postoperative radiograph on day of operation; 3, postoperative radiograph 4th day; 4, postoperative radiograph 7th day; 5, postoperative radiograph 7th day; 6, post–pin removal radiograph (3 months later). Two fracture sites of tibia were confirmed (1), and 1.2-mm diameter IM pin was used for surgical reduction (2). However, splitting of the distal tibia and pin loosening was confirmed (3) and worsened (4). The IM pin was then changed to one of 0.7-mm diameter and an ESF device was added to provide additional holding power (5). The patient was weight bearing normally after the removal of ESF device, although remodeling of the distal lesion was incomplete so the IM pin was left in place (6). (*Courtesy of* Yasutsugu Miwa, DVM, PhD, Tokyo, Japan.)

the shape required. These materials can be used as a temporary connecting bar before the final connection during surgeries (**Fig. 26**).

The distance between the limb and the connecting materials should be minimized to increase biomechanical stiffness and decrease the fixator weight, while the space left must be sufficient to accommodate postoperative soft-tissue swelling and to provide

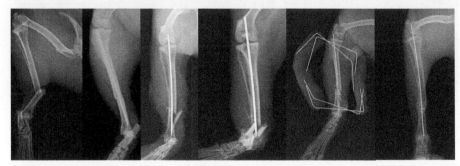

Fig. 21. A case of tibial fracture treated with combination IM pin and ESF after IM pin fixation failed. Two-year-old female (craniocaudal views). 1, preoperative radiograph; 2, postoperative radiograph on day of operation; 3, postoperative radiograph 4th day; 4, postoperative radiograph 7th day; 5, postoperative radiograph 7th day; 6, post–pin removal radiograph (3 months later). Two fracture sites of tibia were confirmed (1), and 1.2-mm diameter IM pin was used for surgical reduction (2). However, splitting of the distal tibia and pin loosening was confirmed (3) and worsened (4). The IM pin was then changed to a 0.7-mm diameter pin and an ESF device was added to provide additional holding power (5). The patient was weight bearing normally after the removal of the ESF device, although remodeling of the distal lesion was incomplete so the IM pin was left (6). (*Courtesy of* Yasutsugu Miwa, DVM, PhD, Tokyo, Japan.)

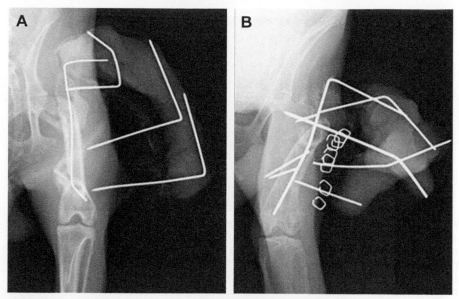

Fig. 22. Premature pin loosening is relatively common, especially with a half-pin style (*A*), in rabbits because of their thin cortices, and bending and breaking pins (*B*) are occasionally seen in those patients because of the limitation of using small-diameter pins. (*Courtesy of Yasutsugu Miwa, DVM, PhD, Tokyo, Japan.*)

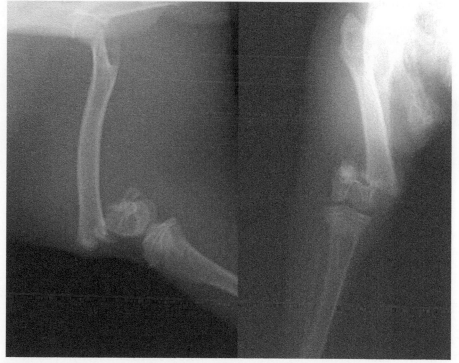

Fig. 23. Radiographs of a distal fracture of the femur in a 4-month-old rabbit. (*Courtesy of Yasutsugu Miwa, DVM, PhD, Tokyo, Japan.*)

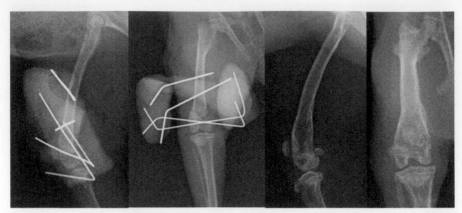

Fig. 24. Postoperative radiograph and post–pin removal radiograph of the rabbit of **Fig. 23**. After the open reduction, the fracture site was fixed with ESF with 2 of each in proximal and distal fragments. The most proximal pin was a half pin with a threaded pin because of consideration of the anatomic feature of rabbits. Other pins were full pin with nonthreaded pins. The fracture was cured and the ESF was removed on 38th day postoperatively. (*Courtesy of* Yasutsugu Miwa, DVM, PhD, Tokyo, Japan.)

the space to allow the use of bone cutters when the fixator is removed without causing iatrogenic soft tissue or further fractures.

Following surgery, the fixator should be wrapped without adherent pads or elastic tape. This bandaging helps prevent the fixator from becoming caught, which can lead to disruption of the fixator and fracture.

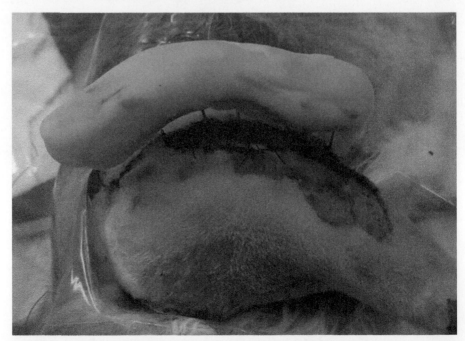

Fig. 25. Both authors prefer to use resin or similar-based products such as acrylic polymer as a replacement of the metallic connecting bars and clamps, which are too heavy for small patients. It also has great versatility and can be adapted to each individual case. (*Courtesy of* Yasutsugu Miwa, DVM, PhD, Tokyo, Japan.)

After discharge, periodic checking of the bandage and the fixator are continued until pin removal. Pins can be removed if sufficient bony callus bridging between fracture sites is confirmed on 2 different views on radiographs. If necessary, staged removal of pins can be used to gradually increase the load on the bone in a process called dynamization or dynamic destabilization.

"Tie-In" or "Hybrid" External Fixator

The TIF or "hybrid" external fixator consists of the external union of the IM pin with the ESF pins, either by a long IM pin bend 90° twice, to make it run parallel to the affected bone externally, or with a connecting bar. One of the authors (Y.M.) has experienced several postoperative problems such as pin loosening, pin bending, pin breakage, and nonunion in the past when using IM pins and simple ESF. After switching to the TIF, the rate of these postoperative problems decreased remarkably, and this method became the author's first choice for fracture repair in small mammals, with the exception of bone plates when feasible in larger patients.

The TIF is the preferred method of one of the authors (D.C.C.) to repair femoral, humeral, and tibial fractures, if allowed by the size of the patient.

Certain bones of small exotic mammals are not only small but also have the tendency to be curved, such as the femur (see **Fig. 19**). Therefore, the authors recommend the use of relatively small-diameter IM pins; the authors tend to place the IM pins retrogradely whenever possible, exteriorizing the IM pin via the proximal fragment. External fixation pins are then inserted to fix the fracture sites for additional stiffness. After applying the IM pin and the ESF device, the proximal end of the IM pin and the fixation pins of ESF are connected ("tie-in") with resin materials (**Figs. 27–29**). This method provides more stiffness and prevents pin loosening during the healing period.

Because the goal of the combined technique of ESF with intramedullary pins is to provide antirotational stability, a single pin per bone fragment is meant to be sufficient. In birds, the 2 + 2 pin construction has been proved to be stiffer than 1 + 1 pin construction.[33] Therefore, the authors prefer to insert more at least 2 pins per fragment whenever possible in exotic small mammals, because the cortex of these species is thin and pin loosening is more likely to happen, and the available medullar pin diameter

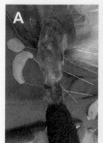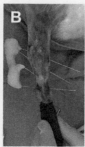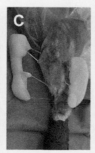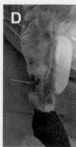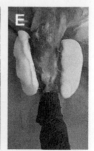

Fig. 26. Temporary connecting bar during surgery. (*A*) Temporary connection of 2 pins in distal and proximal parts, respectively. (*B*) Temporary connection of distal and proximal connections after reduction of fracture. (*C*) The final connection applied to the medial aspect. (*D*) The temporary connection was removed. (*E*) The final connection applied to the lateral aspect. Materials such as resin can be used as a temporary connecting bar (*A–C*) before the final connection (*D, E*) during surgery. (*Courtesy of* Yasutsugu Miwa, DVM, PhD, Tokyo, Japan.)

is limited (**Fig. 30**). A retrospective study performed in femoral fractures in rabbits repaired using the TIF technique demonstrated a good outcome in most cases, and although not uncommon most complications could be managed.[34]

Recently, a combination of internal and external fixation has been used to stabilize the fractured calcaneus in a rabbit. An IM pin combined with a type IIa transarticular external fixator achieved a full recovery.[9]

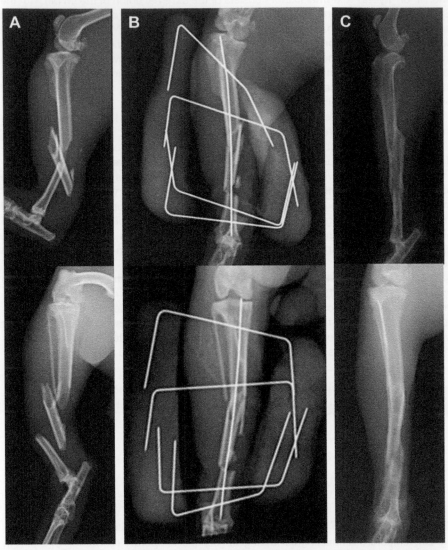

Fig. 27. Fig. 25 IM pin and ESF fixation of tibial fracture in a 5-year-old male rabbit. (*A*) Preoperative radiograph. (*B*) Postoperative radiograph. (*C*) Post–pin removal radiograph. 1, lateral view; 2, craniocaudal view. Two-site fracture with a piece of bone fragment (*A*) was fixed with IM pin and ESF combination. IM pin arranges the alignment of the affected bone and ESF works as a fixator. The fracture was cured and pins were removed 3 months later (*C*). (*Courtesy of* Yasutsugu Miwa, DVM, PhD, Tokyo, Japan.)

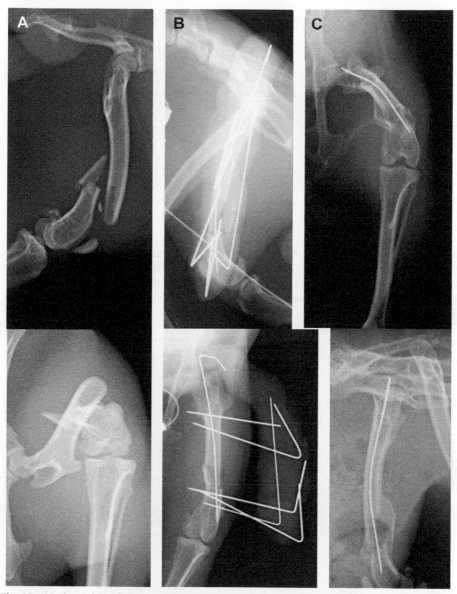

Fig. 28. IM pin and ESF fixation of femoral bone fracture in a 4-year-old male rabbit. (*A*) Preoperative radiograph. (*B*) Postoperative radiograph. (*C*) Post–pin removal radiograph. 1, lateral view; 2, craniocaudal view. Femoral fracture (*A*) was fixed with IM pin and ESF combination. IM pin arranges the alignment of the affected bone and ESF works as a fixator, and IM pin and ESF were tied in. The fracture was cured and ESF device was removed 2 months later (*C*). (*Courtesy of* Yasutsugu Miwa, DVM, PhD, Tokyo, Japan.)

Bone Plate Fixation

There are significant advantages of bone plate fixation, including the rigid internal fixation that provides anatomic alignment without interfering with joint function and

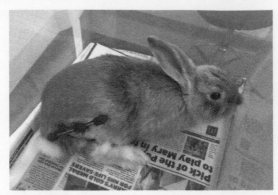

Fig. 29. Appearance of a TIF in a rabbit with a femoral fracture. (*Courtesy of* Daniel Calvo Carrasco, LV, CertAVP (ZooMed), MRCVS, United Kingdom.)

allowing early return to function with little postoperative care.[35] Based on these facts, bone plate fixation has been used in dogs and cats as the first-choice treatment, with constant evolution of the literature available as well as improved designs. However, this technique presents limitations when it comes to applying it to exotic small

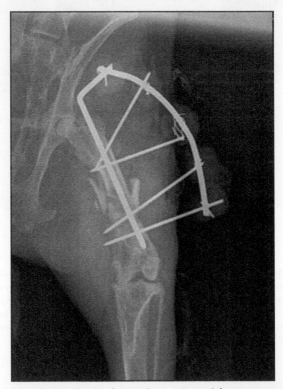

Fig. 30. Craniocaudal radiograph of a femoral comminuted fracture repaired with a 2 + 2 TIF in a rabbit. (*Courtesy of* Daniel Calvo Carrasco, LV, CertAVP (ZooMed), MRCVS, United Kingdom.)

mammals, owing to the small size of the bones and the thin cortices in small exotic mammals, as well as being technically difficult to perform and requiring surgical expertise and specialized equipment. Additionally there are other disadvantages such as the disruption of periosteal blood supply, a significant increase in the risk of wound infection, and prolonged surgical time.[25] The most significant difficulty or complication of bone plating is the cortical size, which leads to bone shattering while implanting the screws, as well as difficulty in holding the retaining power of screws after surgery. Bone plating has been historically reported to often fail, which based on one of the authors' experience (Y.M.) is often due to bone collapse rather than implant break in rabbits. Based on these aspects, the bone plate has not been a first choice of fracture treatment in small exotic mammals.

It has been reported that plating in these species often overprotects a fracture, preventing load sharing and causing subsequent delayed healing or nonunion.[17,25] There are also reports revealing a significant reduction in bone strength 12 weeks after plating, and plate removal at 6 weeks after surgery was recommended in laboratory tibial osteotomies cases.[25,35,36]

Despite these disadvantages, bone plating remains a useful technique to be considered.

Locking Compression Plate

There are many different designs of plates, including DCP (dynamic compression plate), LCDCP (limited-contact dynamic compression plate), and LCP (locking compression plate). LCP has the unique feature of the presence of a threaded plate hole that couples with a threaded screw head. The threaded head of the screw locks firmly in the reciprocal threaded plate hole and provides angular stability and better stiffness of fixation than conventional plates. LCP also respects the periosteum and maintains blood supply because it is not pressed against the bone, whereas conventional plates gain stability by friction as the screw presses the plate against the cortex.[37] LCPs have been used successfully in the treatment of osteoporotic fractures whose cortices are thin in humans, and the usefulness of LCPs is also reported in rabbits.[38,39] LCPs function more like an external fixator rather than a conventional plate; the plate functions as a connecting bar and the screw functions as a threaded fixator pin, and the whole construction is covered by soft tissues and skin, with the advantage of reduced postoperative care and potential complications in comparison with external fixations. In addition, LCP does not need the precise bending of plates to the shape the affected bone, because upon tightening the plate is not pressed against the bone.

Owing to the thin cortices and increased risk of bone shattering while drilling and screwing into rabbit bones, it is considered that smaller pitch screw with minimum number of screws and longer plate is ideal, as well as placing the screws as close as possible to the epiphysis area, which has thicker cortices to reduce the risk of complications.

Combination of Bone Plates and Wiring

Research on bone regeneration using rabbits as an animal model has been recently carried out by the laboratory team of the University of Tokyo.[40] In this research, a cortical mid-diaphyseal segmental bone defect (length, 10 mm) was created and the affected bone was fixed with bone plate. During the preliminary research, failure of the bone fixation was confirmed in 19 of 50 (38%) animals (**Fig. 31**). The failure of the bone fixation was confirmed to be linked to the fissured fracture originating from the screw holes in all 19 cases, and fissures between screw holes were found even in the case with good callus formation, which was detected on radiographs (**Fig. 32**). After these results, the combined method based on the use of bone plates and wirings was applied.[41] The failure rate decreased to 6% (1 of 19 rabbits) after using this combined method (**Fig. 33**).

The combined method for rabbits was different from those used in dogs and cats; the wire was applied after the bone plating, as the plate was wrapped with circumferential wires to reinforce the fixation. The rate of fixation failure dramatically decreased after using this method in rabbits, although it is not generally recommended in dogs and cats.[41]

The principle of fracture fixation combining bone plates and screws was that the screw-tightening moment leads to surface pressure between the plate and bone, and the friction created in the plate-bone contact zone stabilized the bone fragment. Because of these aspects, the thickness of cortices is important in increasing the tightening and holding power. Given that the cortices of rabbit bone are thin these

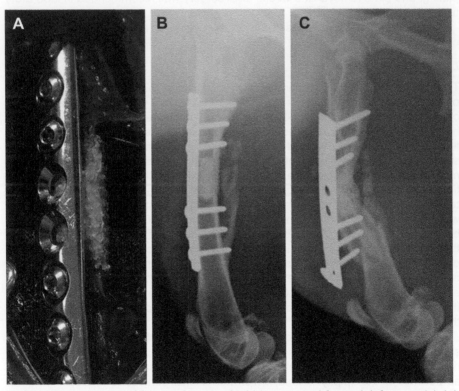

Fig. 31. The percentage of failure of repair of rabbit segmental femoral defects model. (*A*) Surgical views. (*B*) Postoperative radiograph 2 weeks later. (*C*) Postoperative radiograph 4 weeks later. A cortical mid-diaphyseal segmental defect (length 10 mm) was created in 50 male Japanese white rabbits weighing 3.0 to 4.5 kg (aged 18 weeks) for the purpose of evaluation of biomaterials. The created lesion was fixed with an 8-hole stainless bone plate (2.7 mm/2.0 mm Cut-To-Length Plate Synthes Vet, Tokyo, Japan). The fixation failure was confirmed in 35% of cases within 4 weeks after the surgery. All cases failed because of new fractures starting from the screw holes although there were no cases of implant damage. Based on these facts, rabbit cortical bone seems to lack the strength to hold bone screws and prevent drawing power. (*Courtesy of* Muneki Honnami, DVM, PhD, Tokyo, Japan/unpublished data as preliminary research, 2010.)

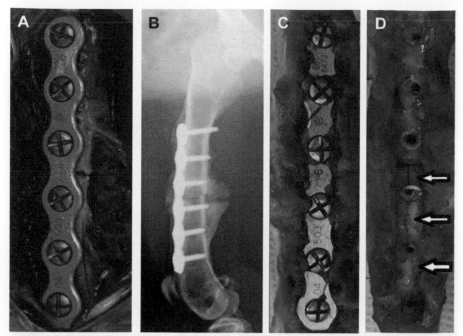

Fig. 32. The bone crack starting from the screw hole. (*A*) Surgical views. (*B*) Postoperative radiograph after 4 weeks. (*C, D*) Autopsy findings. One case of the same research of **Fig. 31** (*A*) Bone healing with periosteal callus was noted on radiograph. (*B*) Although the implant device was not broken (*C*), cracks (*arrows*) were confirmed between screw holes (*D*). (*Courtesy of* Muneki Honnami, DVM, PhD, Tokyo, Japan/unpublished data as preliminary research of reference, 2010.)

powers are limited, but the loading stress to the screw hole might be dispersed using wires, and thus the fissure rate might be decreased.

Based on these findings and considerations, we applied this method to clinical cases achieving relatively good results (**Figs. 34–37**). One of the authors (Y.M.) prefers to use this method in rabbits of advanced age and/or in rabbits whose character is restless, because the postoperative care of ESF will be difficult in these cases. Although the author has used this technique only in rabbits, it may be useful in other species.

Transfixation Pin Splinting

This technique, which consists in ESF or transcutaneous pins joined to an external cast or splint encasing the affected limb, has been widely used in larger species. It has the advantages of being relatively noninvasive and can be used on comminuted fractures of the distal limb. Recently this technique has been successfully used to treat a tibial and radius and ulna fractures in 2 rabbits.[8]

Amputation

Owing to the limited interaction that some owners have with their small exotic mammal pets, because of either nocturnal habits (such in hamsters) or the natural tendency to hide signs of illness of certain prey species, some lesions are not noticed until they are chronic. With open fractures, by the time they are presented they carry a very poor

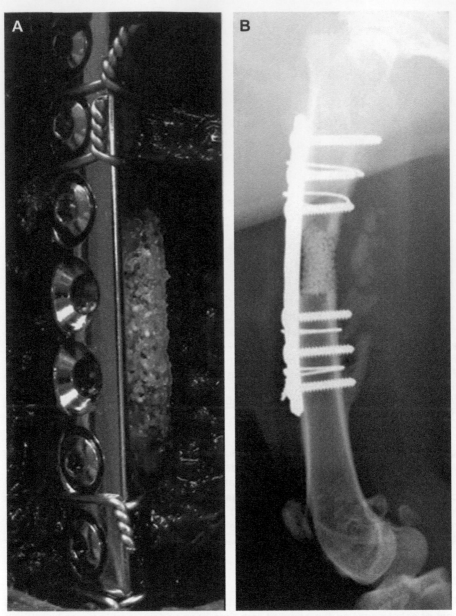

Fig. 33. The segmental femoral defects model of rabbit. (*A*) Surgical views. (*B*) Postoperative radiograph. The rate of fixation failure decreased to 6% from 35% after 4 cerclage wires (0.6 mm) were added to the same model. Note the cerclage wire pressing the plate to the bone. It was thought that the fracture starting from the screw holes was prevented because wires decentralized the weight stress to the plate, and the pressure to the screw hole was decreased. (*Courtesy of* Muneki Honnami, DVM, PhD, Tokyo, Japan/unpublished data as preliminary research of reference, 2010.)

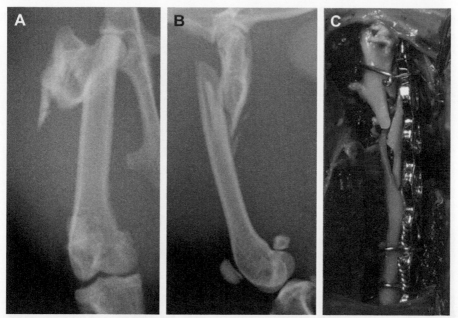

Fig. 34. Case 1 of bone plating. (*A, B*) Preoperative radiograph. (*C*) Operative view. Three-year-old male Netherlands dwarf rabbit weighing 1.35 kg was referred because of proximal femoral compound fracture (*A, B*). The fracture was fixed with a locking plate, 6 screws, and 3 wires (*C*). (*Courtesy of* Yasutsugu Miwa, DVM, PhD, Tokyo, Japan.)

prognosis because of severe damage or necrosis, as well as infection (**Fig. 38**). Amputation is indicated in those patients with unmanageable trauma, severe infection, severe neurologic damage, and pathologic fractures such as bone tumors.

In some cases, amputation is chosen because of limited funds or when the client does not wish to accept the potential failure risk of attempting surgical repair. Those

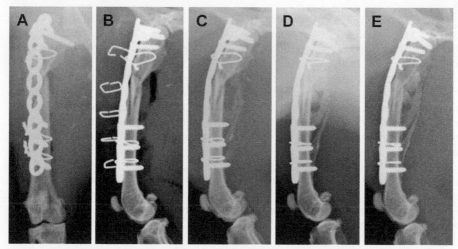

Fig. 35. Postoperative follow-up of case 1 of bone plating. Postoperative radiographs immediately after (*A, B*) and at 3 weeks (*C*), 7 weeks (*D*), and 11 weeks (*E*). (*Courtesy of* Yasutsugu Miwa, DVM, PhD, Tokyo, Japan.)

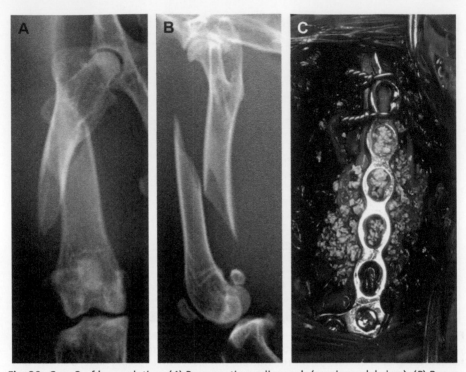

Fig. 36. Case 2 of bone plating. (*A*) Preoperative radiograph (craniocaudal view). (*B*) Preoperative radiograph (lateral view). (*C*) Operative view. Ten-year-old, spayed female Netherlands dwarf rabbit weighing 1.6 kg was referred because of spiral fracture of femur (*A, B*). The fracture was fixed with a locking plate, 3 screws, and 2 wires (*C*). Granular artificial bone (Osferion, Olympus) and bFGF (basic fibroblast growth factor; Kaken Pharmaceutical) was applied for stimulation of osteogenesis because of her age. (*Courtesy of Yasutsugu Miwa, DVM, PhD, Tokyo, Japan.*)

patients that because of their nature will not be able to be correctly managed and, therefore, provided with adequate postoperative care are also reasonable candidates for amputation.

Based on the authors' experience, most small exotic mammals can adapt well to the amputation of one limb except some species with short legs and heavy weight such as guinea pigs and hedgehogs. In those short-legged species, decubitus (pressure ulcer) and/or moist dermatitis of the amputated lesions are occasionally seen after surgery (**Fig. 39**). Ferrets usually tolerate amputation despite having short legs.

Amputation techniques are similar to those in dogs and cats. The authors prefer to amputate the front limb at the site of midhumeral level or remove it with the scapula, and the hind limb at the site of midfemoral to one-third level. Amputation should be performed thorough normal tissue and proximal to the diseased tissue, and the creation of a long dangling stump should be avoided.[25]

It is recommended to use epidural analgesia and local nerve blocks, especially in rodent species, to avoid chewing of the surgical wound postoperatively.

The idea of an animal existing as an amputee has very negative emotional connotations for some owners, who worry about the quality of life after surgery. Thus, it is

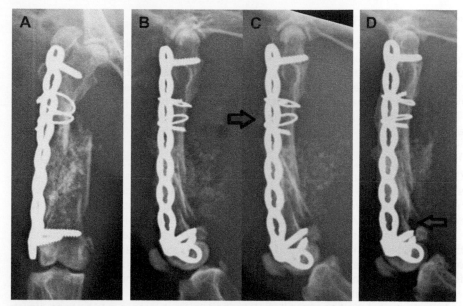

Fig. 37. Postoperative follow-up of case 2 of bone plating. Postoperative radiographs imme-diately after (*A, B*) and at 2 weeks (*C*) and 8 weeks (*D*). Mild callus formation was noted after 2 weeks (*C: arrow*) without any implant deformation. Callus formation increased and bridging callus formation (*D: arrow*) was confirmed. Osteogenesis likely occurred with ra-diodensity remarkably increased (*D: arrowhead*), although granular artificial bone density decreased time-dependently (*C, D*). (*Courtesy of* Yasutsugu Miwa, DVM, PhD, Tokyo, Japan.)

important to inform the owner that most cases, especially those with painful and inconveniently affected legs, may obtain a better quality of life and recover their appe-tite and normal activity after the surgery. It is helpful to show some photos or videos of previous cases of the same species before the owner chooses amputation.

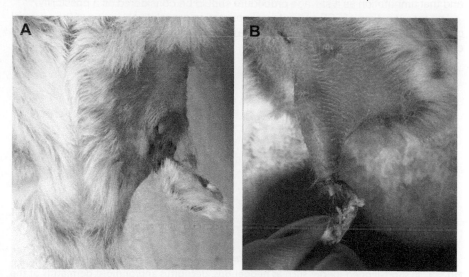

Fig. 38. Amputation of affected limb. Daily interactions are often limited in small exotic mammals, so the fracture can be days to weeks old (*A, B*). These affected limbs should be amputated. (*Courtesy of* Yasutsugu Miwa, DVM, PhD, Tokyo, Japan.)

PELVIC AND SPINAL FRACTURES

Lesions on the lumbosacral region (L6–L7) are common in rabbits and usually result from trauma of the spine following inadequate handling; if the patient struggles while being restrained and kicks, this may result in spinal fracture or dislocation. Prognosis depends on the severity of the lesion, but to the authors' knowledge no specific treatment exists other than supportive care. Chronic cases carry a poor prognosis.

Pelvic fractures in rabbits have been treated successfully by cage rest by one of the authors (D.C.C.).

Luxations

Coxofemoral luxations in rabbits have been treated by a femoral head and neck excision. This technique is well described and has been used successfully by one of the authors regularly, with a speedy recovery and minimal postoperative care.[42] More recently, a rabbit has been successfully treated using toggle-pin fixation.[10]

Elbow luxation has been described as the most common luxation observed in rabbits.[43] This condition can be treated conservatively in early cases, and with circumferential suture prostheses in chronic cases.[12,32] This technique has also been used in ferrets with elbow luxation (Jaume Martorell, personal communication) and in rabbits with tarsocrural luxation.[44]

A similar technique has also been described to treat tarsocrural luxations, which consisted in creating transosseous tunnels where the medial long collateral ligament originates (medial malleolus) and inserts (talus) in order to pass a suture through them in a figure-of-8 pattern to replace the function of the damaged ligament.[7]

Postoperative Care

Small exotic mammals carry a higher risk of postoperative complications than dogs and cats; most of them are highly active, and given their already explained anatomic particularities and the predisposition of certain species to self-trauma, owners should be informed that, even despite excellent surgical care being provided, a nonunion may occur and that amputation as a salvage procedure should be considered as a possibility.[25]

The recovery time of ESF and external coaptation are relatively long and the owners' cooperation and dedication is probably the most relevant factor in minimizing potential complications.

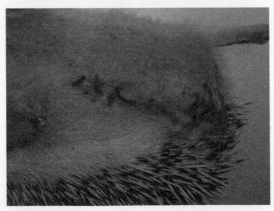

Fig. 39. In short-legged species such as hedgehogs, decubitus and/or moist dermatitis of the amputated lesions are occasionally seen after the amputation. (*Courtesy of* Yasutsugu Miwa, DVM, PhD, Tokyo, Japan.)

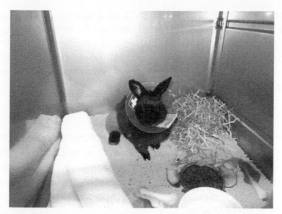

Fig. 40. Postoperative care. The most important time is awaking from the anesthesia. We usually instruct an experienced staff member to stay and monitor the patient during this period until the patient can stand by itself safely. Photo shows the soft and nonslip flooring with rolled towel to support the incompletely awake patient. (*Courtesy of* Yasutsugu Miwa, DVM, PhD, Tokyo, Japan.)

Postoperative management includes exercise restriction, analgesics, bandage and fixator care, and nutritional supplementation, among others. Analgesics should be given before surgery and a few days after surgery, depending on the patient's activity (**Fig. 40**). Exercise restriction is performed by cage rest (confinement) and client compliance is a key factor for success. Strict cage rest usually is continued for 4 to 6 weeks after surgery. The owner and the clinician should check the toes for swelling or discharge during the follow-up period, and external bandaging should be removed and the limb and surgical site examined if necessary. During the treatment period, the animal's appetite and fecal production and activity should be monitored closely, and appropriate supportive care such as analgesia and nutritional support should be given if needed (**Fig. 41**).

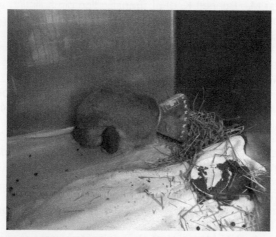

Fig. 41. Postoperative care. The animal was hospitalized for a few days postoperatively to check appetite, surgical wound, bandages, and general physical condition. (*Courtesy of* Yasutsugu Miwa, DVM, PhD, Tokyo, Japan.)

The bandage should be rechecked every 1 to 2 weeks and radiographs may be repeated every 4 to 5 weeks to evaluate healing. In some cases, this procedure may require heavy sedation or anesthesia to avoid iatrogenic problems.

Implants and/or bandages are removed after confirmation of adequate healing based on radiographic findings. Exercise restriction is still recommended for 4 weeks after removal of the fixator to prevent the fracture reoccurring.

SUMMARY

Orthopedics in small exotic mammals is constantly under research. Many exotic small mammals kept as pets are also used as experimental models, and the clinician must be aware of the new research constantly being undertaken. Extrapolation from larger species is a useful source of information but must be conducted carefully. The anatomic and physiologic particularities of each species should always be considered when elaborating a treatment plan.

REFERENCES

1. DeCamp CE, Johnston SA, Déjardin LM, Schaefer SL. Fractures: classification, diagnosis, and treatment. In: DeCamp CE, Johnston SA, Déjardin LM, et al, editors. Brinker, Piermattei and Flo's. Handbook of small animal orthopedics and fracture repair. 5th edition. St. Louis (MO): Elsevier; 2016. p. 24–152.
2. Periat J. Femoral fracture repair in two Guinea pigs. Exotic DVM 2008;10(1):3–6.
3. Pead MJ, Carmichael S. Treatment of a severely comminuted fracture in a rabbit using a Kirschner-Ehmer apparatus. J Small Anim Pract 1989;30:579–82.
4. Conn M. Tibial fracture in a guinea pig. Exotic DVM 2000;2(5):5–6.
5. Aguilar J, Mogridge G, Hall J. Femoral fracture repair and sciatic and femoral nerve blocks in a Guinea pig. J Small Anim Pract 2013;55(12):635–9.
6. Macedo AS, Goulart MA, Alievi MM, et al. Tibial osteosynthesis in a guinea pig (Cavia porcellus). Arq Bras Med Vet Zootec 2015;67(1):89–93.
7. Sabater M, Calvo Carrasco D. Surgical correction of traumatic tarsocrural joint luxation in a rabbit (Oryctolagus cuniculus). Journal of Exotic Pet Medicine 2019;29:154–8.
8. Ciwko E, Sadar MJ, Bennett K, et al. Transfixation pin splinting as an alternative external coaptation method in domestic rabbit (Oryctolagus cuniculus). J Exot Pet Med 2018;27(4):31–7.
9. Volait-Rosset L, Pignon C, Manou M, et al. Surgical management of a calcaneus fracture in a pet rabbit. J Exot Pet Med 2019;29:110–4.
10. Marinkovich M, Sánchez Migallón-Guzman D, Hawkins MG, et al. Open reduction and stabilization of a luxated coxofemoral joint in a domestic rabbit (Oryctolagus cuniculus) using a toggle-pin fixation. J Exot Pet Med 2019;30:43–9.
11. Pignon C, Vallefuoco R, Krumeich N, et al. Surgical repair of a pelvic fracture in a ferret (Mustela putorius furo). J Exot Pet Med 2014;23(1):96–100.
12. Calvo Carrasco D, Minier K, Shimizu N, et al. Surgical management of a traumatic elbow luxation with circumferential suture prostheses in a rabbit (Oryctolagus cuniculus). J Exot Pet Med 2018;27(3):38–42.
13. Wilson A, Sanchez-Migallon Guzman D, Keller D, et al. Medical management of multiple traumatic vertebral subluxations and fractures in a rabbit (Oryctolagus cuniculus). J Exot Pet Med 2012;21(2):172–80.
14. Liatis T, Gardini A, Café Marçal V, et al. Surgical treatment of a vertebral fracture caused by osseous plasmacytoma in a domestic ferret (Mustela putorius furo). J Exot Pet Med 2019;29:202–6.

15. Barron HW, McBride M, Martinez-Jimenez D, et al. Comparison of two methods of long bone fracture repair in rabbits. J Exot Pet Med 2010;19(2):183–8.
16. Sasai H, Fujita D, Seto E, et al. Outcome of limb fracture repair in rabbits: 139 cases (2007-2017). J Am Vet Med Assoc 2018;252(4):457–463.
17. Zehnder A, Kapatkin AS. Orthopedics in small mammals. In: Queensberry KE, Carpenter JW, editors. Ferrets, rabbits, and rodents clinical medicine and surgery. 3rd edition. St. Louis (MO): Elsevier Saunders; 2016. p. 472–84.
18. Available at: https://www.pfma.org.uk/pet-population-2018.
19. Reuter JD, Ovadia S, Howell P, et al. Femoral fracture repair and postoperative management in New Zealand white rabbits. Contemp Top Lab Anim Sci 2002; 41(4):49–52.
20. Sasai H, Fujita D, Tagami Y, et al. Characteristics of bone fractures and usefulness of micro-computed tomography for fracture detection in rabbits: 210 cases (2007-2013). J Am Vet Med Assoc 2015;246(12):1339–44.
21. Langley-Hobbs S, Harcourt-Brown N. Fracture management. In: Harcourt-Brown F, Chitty J, editors. BSAVA manual of rabbit surgery, dentistry and imaging. Gloucester (UK): BSAVA; 2013. p. 283–304.
22. Metsemakers WJ, Schmid T, Zeiter S, et al. Titanium and steel fracture fixation plates with different surface topographies: Influence on infection rate in a rabbit fracture model. Injury 2016;47(3):633–9.
23. Arens D, Wilke M, Calabro L, et al. A rabbit humerus model of plating and nailing osteosynthesis with and without Staphylococcus aureus osteomyelitis. Eur Cell Mater 2015;30:148–61.
24. Rich GA. Rabbit orthopedic surgery. Vet Clin North Am Exot Anim Pract 2002; 5(1):157–68.
25. Helmer PJ, Lightfoot TL. Small exotic mammal orthopedics. Vet Clin North Am Exot Anim Pract 2002;5(1):169–82, vii-viii.
26. Miller AL, Ricardson CA. Rodent analgesia. Vet Clin North Am Exot Anim Pract 2011;5(1):81–92.
27. Flecknell P. Analgesics in small mammals. Vet Clin North Am Exot Anim Pract 2018;21(1):83–103.
28. Flecknell P. Analgesia of small mammals. Vet Clin North Am Exot Anim Pract 2001;4(1):47–56.
29. Deflers H, Gandar F, Bolen G, et al. Influence of a single dose of buprenorphine on rabbit (Oryctolagus cuniculus) gastrointestinal motility. Vet Anaesth Analg 2018;45(4):510–9.
30. Erichsen HK, Hao JX, Xu XJ, et al. Comparative actions of the opioid analgesics morphine, methadone and codeine in rat models of peripheral and central neuropathic pain. Pain 2005;116:347–58.
31. Johnson-Delaney CA, Hartcourt-Brown F. Analgesia and postoperative care. In: Harcourt-Brown F, Chitty J, editors. BSAVA manual of rabbit surgery, dentistry and imaging. Gloucester (UK): BSAVA; 2013. p. 26–38.
32. Calvo Carrasco D, Huynh M. Non invasive technique for reduction of an elbow luxation in a rabbit (Oryctolagus cuniculus). Proceedings of the 1st International Conference on Avian, Herpetological & Exotic Mammal Medicine. 2013. p. 309. Available at: https://www.vetion.de/eaav/member/content/ICARE_2013_Proceedings_complete_n.pdf.
33. Van Wettere AJ, Redig PT, Wallace LJ, et al. Mechanical evaluation of external skeletal fixator–intramedullary pin tie-in configurations applied to cadaveral humeri from red-tailed hawks (Buteo jamaicensis). J Avian Med Surg 2009;23: 277–85.

34. Calvo Carrasco D, Skarbek A, Shimizu N. Retrospective study of femoral fracture repair with tie-in fixator (TIF) in rabbits (*Oryctolagus cuniculus*). Proceedings of the ExoticsCon Conference. 2018. p. 773. Available at: https://www.aav.org/page/proceedingslibrary.
35. Terjesen T. Bone healing after metal plate fixation and external fixation of the osteotomized rabbit tibia. Acta Orthop Scand 1984;55:69–77.
36. Terjesen T. Plate fixation of tibial fractures in the rabbit Correlation of bone strength with duration of fixation. Acta Orthop Scand 1984;55:452–6.
37. Sommer C, Schutz M, Wanger M. Internal fixator. In: Rudei TP, Buckley RE, Moran CG, editors. AO principles of fracture management, vol. 1, 2nd edition. Davos (Swtizerland): AO Publishing; 2007. p. 321–35.
38. Ring D, Kioen P, Kadzielski J, et al. Locking compression plate for osteoporotic nonunions of the diaphyseal humerus. Clin Orthop Relat Res 2004;425:50–4.
39. Ueno H, Uto S, Seo K, et al. Usagi no kossetu: locking plate wo mochiita seihuku. J Exo Anim Pract 2016;8(1):56–64.
40. Honnami M, Choi S, Liu I, et al. Repair of rabbit segmental femoral defects by using a combination of tetrapod-shaped calcium phosphate granules and basic fibroblast growth factor-binding ion complex gel. Biomaterials 2013;34:9056–62.
41. Wang L, Fan H, Zhang ZY, et al. Osteogenesis and angiogenesis of tissue-engineered bone constructed by prevascularized β-tricalcium phosphate scaffold and mesenchymal stem cells. Biomaterials 2010;31:9452–61.
42. Coleman KA, Palmer RH, Johnston MS. Femoral head and neck osteotomy for surgical treatment of acute craniodorsal coxofemoral luxation in rabbits. J Exot Pet Med 2015;24:178–82.
43. Ertelt J, Maierl J, Kaiser A, et al. Anatomical and pathophysiological features and treatment of elbow luxation in rabbits. Tierarztl Prax Ausg K Kleintiere Heimtiere 2010;38(4):201–10.
44. Calvo Carrasco D, Sabater Gonzalez M, Shimizu N, et al. Surgical management of traumatic tibio-tarsal joint luxation with circumferential suture prostheses in two rabbits (*Oryctolagus cuniculus*). Proceedings of Icare Conference. 2016. p. 755.

Animal Models of Osteoarthritis in Small Mammals

C. Iván Serra, Ldo Vet, PhD*, Carme Soler, Lda Vet, PhD

KEYWORDS

• Osteoarthritis • Animal model • Mouse • Guinea pig • Rat • Rabbit

KEY POINTS

• Osteoarthritis is characterized as a chronic disease that affects the joint cartilage, as well as subchondral bone, synovial membranes, and periarticular tissues.
• Animal models play a key role for understanding the pathophysiology of the disease and for the evaluation of new therapeutic tools.
• Osteoarthritis models can be classified into spontaneous or induced models.

INTRODUCTION

Osteoarthritis (OA) is the most common joint disease affecting the human population, as well as most mammals. Around 630 million people worldwide are thought to have this condition, with an estimated annual health care cost in the United States of around 185 billion US dollars.[1–3]

OA is characterized as a chronic disease that affects the joint cartilage, but also the subchondral bone, synovial membranes, and periarticular tissues.[4] Likewise, although it has been traditionally defined as a non-inflammatory disease, current evidence suggests that inflammation plays a fundamental role in its pathogenesis.[5]

Nevertheless, because the pathologic process is still not fully understood, the study of OA is still a challenge. Consequently, the use of animal models is critical for the study of both its pathogenesis and the efficacy of the various therapeutic tools.[6,7] The ideal model would include the following characteristics: (1) it should be reproducible in a suitable time frame; (2) include all the early stages of the disease; (3) involve all the joint tissues (as in humans); (4) use an animal species that is easy to handle and house, reasonably inexpensive, and that allows different genetic, biochemical, and imaging biomarkers to be evaluated; and finally (5) the results should be transferable to

Department of Animal Medicine and Surgery, UCV Veterinary Hospital, Faculty of Veterinary and Experimental Sciences, Universidad Católica de Valencia San Vicente Mártir, Valencia, Spain
* Corresponding author. Avda. Francia N°1 1ªT-4°B, Valencia 46023, Spain.
E-mail address: ci.serra@ucv.es

Vet Clin Exot Anim 22 (2019) 211–221
https://doi.org/10.1016/j.cvex.2019.01.004
1094-9194/19/© 2019 Elsevier Inc. All rights reserved.

vetexotic.theclinics.com

the particularity of the pathology and therapeutics of human medicine.[1,8] The reality is that, unfortunately, this ideal model does not exist.

Although there is no "gold standard" experimental model, the correct selection of the model to use is essential. To that end, the authors recommend that the following points are taken into consideration: (1) the OA stage on which the researcher wishes to work, (2) the extension of the lesion that requires study (focal or generalized), (3) the treatment effects to be evaluated, (4) the target tissues to be studied (eg, cartilage, membrane, synovial fluid, bone), and (5) the variables to be analyzed.[9] Similarly, it is essential to apply the principle of the 3 Rs (replacement, reduction, and refinement) before starting the study.[6]

The many OA models described can be classified into 2 large categories: spontaneous models (including naturally developing and genetic models) and induction models (surgically or by injection).[3] In general terms, the spontaneous models enable the study of the pathogenetic mechanisms of OA development, have a high economic cost, and require a long period of time to achieve their objectives. In contrast, induction models achieve early and reproducible models of OA that allow the assessment of the effects of various treatments, but preclude the researcher from studying the likely pathogenetic development of the disease usually seen in humans.[3–6] Small mammals (mice, rats, Guinea pigs, and rabbits) are the most widely used models for the study of the pathogenesis and pathophysiology of the disease, mainly because these models have more rapid disease progression, and are relatively inexpensive and easy to handle. However, the effect of treatments in these models is not considered transferrable to humans.[10] Accordingly, larger animal models (dogs, sheep, goats, horses, and pigs) are used in preclinical studies for evaluating the clinical processes and their treatment in this disease.[3,4,7,11]

Regarding the evaluation of these OA models, as well as their response to different therapies, histopathology has been traditionally considered the method of choice. Nevertheless, new evaluation methods including image analysis methods (eg, MR imaging and computed tomography scan), evaluation of local (eg, synovial fluid) and systemic (eg, serum or urine) biomarkers, and biomechanical assays of joint tissues, have been standardized in recent years.[3,4,12]

The aim of this paper is to provide a general description of the main experimental models of OA in small mammals, stating their advantages and limitations, and to show the evaluable variables in each of them. Thus, the authors hope to help the researchers to choose the most appropriate model for their study and the clinicians to improve their pathology understanding.

TYPES OF MODELS

The types of animal models of OA currently used are classified mainly into spontaneous or induced models. The spontaneous models include those OA in which the disease develops naturally (primary OA) and those generated by models with genetic abnormalities. In contrast, induced models of OA are those that arise from a surgical procedure or intra-articular injection.[3,6,7]

Below, we will describe the various models used in small mammals, discussing their advantages and limitations, as well as the indications and considerations to consider for each of them.

Spontaneous Animal Models of Osteoarthritis

These types of models are characterized mainly by their slow evolution, which leads to very lengthy study periods with their resultant economic costs; however, from a pathophysiological point of view, there is an excellent correlation with the natural progression of OA in humans.[6]

These models can be further subdivided into 2 types: those that occur naturally or those that occur as a result of genetic manipulation of the individual.

Naturally developing models of Osteoarthritis

These types of models are usually developed in small mammals, mainly mice and Guinea pigs (although rabbits are also an interesting species for such studies), and are generally used to evaluate the pathogenesis of this disease.[13] They have also been of interest for their usefulness in assessing the effect of age, diet, sex, and other characteristics on the evolution of the osteoarthritic process.[7,14]

Among these, the Dunkin Hartley Guinea pig is the most commonly used due to its incidence of OA, early age of onset, and its histopathological similarities with human primary idiopathic OA.[15,16] It is important to consider that, although lesions can be observed in the central region of the medial tibial plateau at 3 months of age, it is recommended to work with 12- to 18-month-old individuals in which lesions in the medial compartment of the knee (medial femoral condyle and medial tibial plateau) are observed in almost 100% of individuals.[3,15] In this respect, the Guinea pig has been the most widely used model to evaluate inflammatory biomarkers related with this disease.[17]

The next natural model in terms of importance is the rat; specifically, it has been used with satisfactory results to correlate OA and chondrocyte metabolism.[18] In these types of models, and in genetically modified models, high-fat diets are also used, together with exercise limitation, to induce obesity, which exacerbates the osteoarthritic lesions.[19]

Within the small mammals, the rabbit seems to be an interesting natural model, reaching OA rates of around 70% in the knee and hip in adulthood in the individuals studied. It has been suggested that this model may be of interest in tissue bioengineering.[20,21] In the authors' experience, this species has also shown a high rate of focal osteochondral lesions in the lateral femoral condyle in young developing individuals.

Genetic models of Osteoarthritis

These types of models have helped to better understand the genetic bases of OA and their effect on the pathogenesis of the disease.[9,22,23] Genetic modification for the study of this type of pathology has been performed mainly in mice, although there is also a rat model of overexpression of interleukin-1β for evaluating pain.[9] It should be taken into account that these transgenic models can be used to potentiate the development of an osteoarthritic process and to protect the joint from the development of this abnormality.[24] Thus, we find models such as the CBA mouse, which is considered resistant to the development of spontaneous OA,[25] and others such as STR/ort and C57BL/6 mice, which are considered predisposed to its development.[26]

These models that predispose the animal to the development of OA are usually the result of modifications in genes involved in: degradation of the cartilage matrix (Tnc-1, Adamts5(cat), Jaffa, Sulf1−/−, Sulf2−/−, Col9a1−/−); chondrocyte differentiation or apoptosis (S100a9−/−, Epas1+/−); subchondral bone metabolism (Frzb−/−); and at the inflammatory mediator level (Cd59a−/−, Fgf2−/−, Tnfrsf11 b+/−).[9,24]

Nevertheless, although these last models can develop the disease naturally, it is common to stimulate or accelerate the onset of the abnormality using induction methods, thereby shortening the onset times and exacerbating the disease stages.[27]

Finally, it should be remembered that, despite the advantages of these models, the significant inter-animal variability in the development of the disease, as well as the high costs of housing for long study periods, condition the use of these models. Likewise, because the disease developed in humans is associated with polygenic pathologies, and most of these models act on specific genes, results should be extrapolated with caution.[28]

Induction Models of Osteoarthritis

Models of induced OA represent better the secondary OA, generally post-traumatic, observed in humans. The aim of the induction methods is to generate joint instability, altered joint mechanics or an inflammatory process that alters the cell metabolism at a local level.[3,4,6] It should be remembered that most induction methods, primarily surgical, produce a combination of the previous factors. The high inter-individual repeatability, together with rapid onset and progression of the disease, explain the wide use of these models nowadays.[4]

Below is a description of the most common models used in small mammals, as well as their characteristics and more specific indications.

Surgical induction models

When working with a surgical model, the research team must: (1) have specific knowledge of the anatomy of the species on which they are going to work, (2) know the biomechanics of the joint, (3) be proficient in the aseptic and surgical technique that allows the desired model to be accurately produced, and (4) be familiar with the anesthetic and analgesic management of the species. If these aspects are mastered, the morbidity and mortality of the experimental animals are considerably reduced, resulting in better welfare for them, a lower economic cost of the study, and greater homogeneity in the lesion model by preventing iatrogenic damage during the procedure.

The main surgical models are mainly based on the generation of joint instability, the change of load distribution of the joint, or the creation of focal defects (chondral and/or osteochondral defects).

Models of joint instability

Anterior cruciate ligament transection Anterior cruciate ligament transection is a model that has traditionally been used in large animals, and which was later incorporated into small mammals, mainly rabbits, rats, and mice, and considered the most widely used today.[7,29] This type of model induces changes in the physiology of the chondrocytes, destruction of cartilage, and formation of osteophytes.[3]

The model is produced by arthrotomy (medial or lateral) or arthroscopy. After direct visualization of the anterior cruciate ligament, it is completely transected (transection by blind lance is not recommended). Several authors mention the need to dislocate the patella to expose the ligament, but, in the authors' experience, this procedure is not necessary, thereby minimizing concomitant lesions[4] (**Fig. 1**). It is essential to confirm complete transection of the ligament, using the drawer test as an intra-surgical check.

The type of degeneration and time of development of the alterations (4 weeks for first cell changes and 8–12 weeks for cartilage degradation and osteophyte formation) (see **Fig. 1**) makes it the model of choice for pharmacologic studies.[30]

One of the surgical induction models of OA that has been described by various authors is ovariectomy. The development of the disease is attributed to the fact that estrogen reduction has a negative impact on the quality of bone and cartilage. Although the pathogenesis of this model is not fully known, it is not a model that is recommended in therapeutic trials.[6]

Finally, several authors suggest combining lesions in other structures at the same time as cruciate ligament transection, to accelerate the degenerative processes and

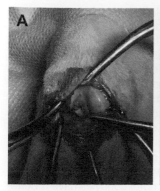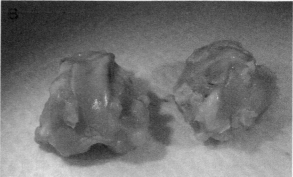

Fig. 1. Intra-operatory image of the anterior cruciate ligament of a rabbit before its transection (A). Macroscopic lesions 12 weeks following induction of a rabbit anterior cruciate ligament rupture (B). (*Courtesy of* Iván Serra, Ldo, Vet, PhD, Valencia, Spain.)

achieve more advanced lesions. These procedures include transection of the patellar ligament, posterior cruciate ligament and medial/lateral collateral ligament, and total and partial meniscectomies.[29,31]

Meniscal destabilization Meniscal destabilization is achieved by transection of the medial meniscotibial ligament, producing mild joint instability.[32] This model is commonly used for pathophysiological studies of OA, as well as to evaluate drug responses for pain control.[33] With this model of injury, the first osteoarthritic changes at macroscopic examination are obtained as early as 2 weeks, by the presence of osteophytes.[19,27]

Collateral ligament transection Collateral ligament transection, primarily the medial ligament, is a model that is generally produced in association with other models of injury (eg, meniscal or anterior cruciate ligament) to increase the presence of joint abnormalities. These types of lesions have been used in chondroprotection studies.[4,34]

Models of abnormal load distribution (meniscal injury) There are many methods for inducing meniscal injuries, including: partial or total meniscectomy (medial and/or lateral), medial meniscal tear, and medial meniscal transection.[6,19] It is very important to bear this in mind when designing the study and being aware of the lesions the researcher expects to obtain, because the type of model used determines the grade and evolution of OA. Although these models are considered to produce compartmental alteration of the load distribution on the articular cartilage and subchondral bone, there are also authors who attribute a certain component of joint instability to these injuries.[7]

Partial medial meniscus lesions and destabilization of the medial meniscus are the most commonly used models of meniscal injury, achieving the first abnormalities at 4 weeks, with evident progression of the OA at 8 and 12 weeks.[35] The lesion is generally produced on the medial meniscus, as this is the area that suffers most mechanical stress. This does not apply in the rabbit, because, mechanically, the area of greatest load distribution is the lateral compartment, so producing the meniscal lesions laterally is recommended.[04]

Models for generating focal defects (chondral/osteochondral defects) Focal chondral lesions are used to evaluate joint cartilage repair locally, minimizing inflammation of other tissues and thus limiting the onset of generalized joint lesions.[36] Spontaneous healing of these injuries involves the appearance of fibrocartilaginous tissue, whose biomechanical characteristics cannot be compared with those of articular hyaline cartilage. For this reason, this type of animal model has been the gold standard in tissue bioengineering, allowing the healing response to be evaluated in various therapies within regenerative medicine (eg, stem cells, growth factors, platelet-rich plasma), together with the use of different biomaterials (different types of scaffolds). [37–41] It has also been used, albeit to a lesser extent, to evaluate various drugs, such as hyaluronic acid. [42]

When generating this type of injury, the researcher must bear in mind not only the individual on which he or she is going to work, but it is also crucial to decide the location within the joint, as well as the size of the defect in terms of depth and diameter. [43,44] The effect of the location in the healing of these defects is attributed, among other factors, to regional variation in the cell morphology and composition of the extracellular matrix, as well as to differences in the ability of each joint region to withstand mechanical stress. Thus, we can observe how injuries in the region of the femoral condyles have a better prognosis than those suffered in the femoral trochlea. [45]

Superficial chondral defects, those that do not cross the tidemark, are not often used as animal models, because their natural tendency is to become full thickness defects. [46] On the other hand, the diameter of the lesion is certainly considered critical, because lesions that are too small can regenerate spontaneously. For this reason, lesions in small mammals should be no less than 3 mm, with lesions of 4 to 5 mm recommended in these species. [3,47]

To produce these types of defects, the authors recommend the use of specific instruments for harvesting osteochondral material that allow the injury to be homogenized, in diameter and depth, in all study individuals.

Non-surgical induction models

Intra-articular injection Used in pain studies, this induces cell apoptosis and joint degeneration. It is mainly an inflammatory model.

Chemical induction models include those that use the injection of a toxic or inflammatory compound directly into the joint as a triggering mechanism. These models have been traditionally used in studies with drugs to treat pain and inflammation because of their simplicity and repeatability, and because they can work within short periods. [7] Nevertheless, one drawback of these models is that they do not reproduce the pathophysiological mechanism characteristic of secondary OA in humans; thus, they have basically been used in studies on the response to pain and inflammation. [6]

At present, the most commonly used model is induction with monosodium iodoacetate (MIA), which has been gaining ground on the most traditionally used agent, papain. [48] Other agents used in the induction of OA include collagenase, carrageenan, and Freund's adjuvant. [6,9]

Monosodium iodoacetate Monosodium iodoacetate is an agent that inhibits the aerobic pathway of cell glycolysis, consequently inducing cell death by inhibiting glyceraldehyde-3-phosphate dehydrogenase activity in the chondrocytes. [49] The onset of joint lesions with this model is very early, and histologic lesions can be seen as soon as 1 to 3 days post-MIA injection. [49]

Although the onset of spontaneous pain, hyperalgesia, and allodynia are among its principal effects, this type of model has been used mainly for conducting pain studies, and for evaluating the pain response to various treatments. [50] It should also be taken into account that the appearance and severity of clinical signs and lesions are dose dependent. The authors of this paper use doses of 0.4 mg of MIA per joint in their research, obtaining obvious cartilaginous and synovial lesions at study times also in the medium term (**Fig. 2**). Several authors report 1 mg as the maximum effective dose. [49]

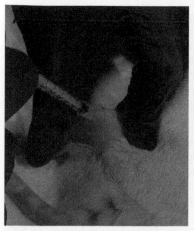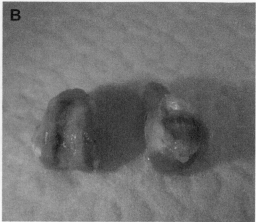

Fig. 2. Intra-articular injection procedure of MIA in a rat (*A*). Macroscopic appearance of the joint surface 8 weeks following injection (*B*). (*Courtesy of* Iván Serra, Ldo, Vet, PhD, Valencia, Spain.)

Papain Papain is a proteolytic enzyme that degrades the proteoglycans in the cartilaginous matrix, thus modifying its capacity for water retention and, consequently, its biomechanical characteristics.[6] The grade of the lesions developed also seems to be related with the dose administered.[51] Although papain has been historically used as a model of OA, showing moderate grades of OA in short times (3 weeks), today it has mainly been replaced by MIA.[52]

Collagenase Intra-articular administration of collagenase combines an inflammatory model of OA with an instability model. This joint instability is produced due to lesions of structures containing collagen type I, which in these structures are mainly the tendons and ligaments. This model achieves rapid joint instability, which translates into obvious cartilaginous lesions at 3 weeks and subchondral bone lesions at 6 weeks.[6,52]

Administration of quinolones The systemic administration of quinolones has been shown to cause degeneration of the joint cartilage and tendons during the individual's development, and involves irreversible loss of proteoglycans, chondrocytes, and extracellular matrix.[34,53] Superficial cartilaginous lesions appear very early (from day 1 in developing Guinea pigs), but lesion of deeper layers is not easily achieved.[34]

Non-invasive post-traumatic models The use of invasive models of OA, either surgical or by injection, involves the use of aseptic techniques and depends on the ability of the researcher when it comes to generating the model. This characteristic determines the repeatability of the model, and sometimes even the viability of the experiment.[6] It is for this reason that non-invasive models arose with the intention of filling these gaps.

Thus, non-invasive models can trigger post-traumatic OA by the application of external mechanical loads, without causing a break in the skin or affecting the joint capsule. These models are completely aseptic, and eliminate the consequences of invasive procedures on the rest of the joint tissues.[1] In particular, however, these methods reproduce a large number of specific clinical situations in the development of OA, so that they can be studied from onset through to later stages of the process.[1] The methods for developing non-invasive post-traumatic OA used in animal models are the following.

Intra-articular fracture of the tibial plateau This model was first described in 2007, and represents an injury secondary to a high-energy trauma; it is ideal for studying the early changes that occur in OA.[54] The injury is achieved using an instrument (ELF 3200, Bose, Eden Praire, MN) that keeps the individual (described in mice) anesthetized in position with the knee flexed at 90°, on which a high-energy impact is applied with a wedge-shaped indentor. The compression force applied is 55 N at a rate of 20 N/s, although the severity of the injuries will depend on the strength and frequency of the loads applied.[1,7,54]

Cyclic tibial compression of articular cartilage This model consists of applying forces that simulate the axial weight loads supported by the limb, subjecting the knee to stress because of its tendency to cranial displacement of the tibia with respect to the femur, which restricts the anterior cruciate ligament.[1] The magnitudes commonly used in mice are between 4.5 and 9 N, with a total of 1200 cycles/d for 5 days.[55]

The repeated action of these weight loads generates changes at the level of the subchondral bone because of its tendency to adapt to the new mechanical scenario. This model has also been used to generate articular cartilage injuries, simulating chronic models of injury due to overuse/overloading of joints.[55,56]

Anterior cruciate ligament rupture via tibia compression overload This method uses the same type of compression loads as the previous models, but with a greater peak force (12 N) applied in a short period of time (500 mm/s), causing rupture of the anterior cruciate ligament. This type of anterior cruciate ligament injury follows a very similar mechanism to that reported during sports in human medicine.[57,58]

For this reason, this model is ideal for the study of early osteoarthritic changes, and their response to treatment in cases of low-energy trauma.[59,60]

SUMMARY

The use of small mammals as experimental models of osteoarthritis has been shown to play a key role for understanding the pathophysiology of the disease and for the evaluation of new therapeutic tools. It is essential to understand the advantages and limitations of each existing model, because, as we have seen, there are many animal models of OA, and not all represent the different types of OA that exist. Only in this way is it possible to design an experiment that can meet the expectations and objectives pursued. Finally, the choice of species is crucial, as the age of the individuals at the start of the study, their sex, and the nutritional and environmental conditions in which they are kept, all affect the onset and progression of OA, as well as the tissue's capacity for repair.

REFERENCES

1. Christiansen BA, Guilak F, Lockwood KA, et al. Non-invasive mouse models of post-traumatic osteoarthritis. Osteoarthritis Cartilage 2015;23(10):1627–38.
2. Kotlarz H, Gunnarsson CL, Fang H, et al. Insurer and out-of-pocket costs of osteoarthritis in the US: evidence from national survey data. Arthritis Rheum 2009; 60(12):3546–53.
3. McCoy AM. Animal models of osteoarthritis: comparisons and key considerations. Vet Pathol 2015;52(5):803–18.
4. Teeple E, Jay GD, Elsaid KA, et al. Animal models of osteoarthritis: challenges of model selection and analysis. AAPS J 2013;15(2):438–46.

5. Garner BC, Stocker AM, Kuroki K, et al. Using animal models in osteoarthritis biomarker research. J Knee Surg 2011;24:251–64.
6. Lampropoulou-Acadamidou K, Lelovas P, Karadimas EV, et al. Useful animal models for the research of osteoarthritis. Eur J Orthop Surg Traumatol 2014; 24(3):263–71.
7. Kuyinu EL, Narayanan G, Nair LS, et al. Animal models of osteoarthritis: classification, update, and measurement of outcomes. J Orthop Surg Res 2016;2:11–9.
8. Little CB, Smith MM. Animal models of osteoarthritis. Curr Rheumatol Rev 2008;4: 175–82.
9. Little CB, Zaki S. What constitutes an "animal model of osteoarthritis" - the need for consensus? Osteoarthritis Cartilage 2012;20:261–7.
10. Pelletier J, Boileau C, Altman RD, et al. Experimental models of osteoarthritis: usefulness in the development of disease-modifying osteoarthritis drugs/agents. Therapy 2010;7(6):621–34.
11. Aigner T, Lohmander S. OAC histopathology supplement. Osteoarthritis Cartilage 2010;18(Suppl 3):S1–122.
12. Poole R, Blake S, Buschmann M, et al. Recommendations for the use of preclinical models in the study and treatment of osteoarthritis. Osteoarthritis Cartilage 2010;18:S10–6.
13. Kyostio-Moore S, Nambiar B, Hutto E, et al. STR/ort mice, a model for spontaneous osteoarthritis exhibit elevated level of both local and systemic inflammatory markers. Comp Med 2011;61(4):346–55.
14. Bijlsma JW, Berenbaum F, Afeber FP. Osteoarthritis: an update with relevance for clinical practice. Lancet 2011;377(9783):2115–26.
15. Jimenez PA, Glasson SS, Trubetskoy OV, et al. Spontaneous osteoarthritis in Dunkin Hartley Guinea pigs: histologic, radiologic, and biochemical changes. Lab Anim Sci 1997;47(6):598–601.
16. Kraus VB, Huebner JL, De Groot J, et al. The OARSI histopathology initiative: recommendations for histological assessments of osteoarthritis in the Guinea pig. Osteoarthritis Cartilage 2010;18(suppl 3):S35–52.
17. Hueber JL, Kraus VB. Assessment of the utility of biomarkers of osteoarthritis in the guinea pig. Osteoarthritis Cartilage 2006;14(9):923–30.
18. Pasold J, Osterberg A, Peters K, et al. Reduced expression of Sfrp1 during chondrogenesis and in articular chondrocytes correlates with osteoarthritis in STR/ort mice. Exp Cell Res 2013;319(5):649–59.
19. Fang H, Beier F. Mouse models of osteoarthritis: modelling risk factors and assessing outcomes. Nat Rev Rheumatol 2014;10:413–21.
20. Arzi B, Wisner ER, Huey DJ, et al. A proposed model of naturally occurring osteoarthritis in the domestic rabbit. Lab Anim (NY) 2011;41(1):20–5.
21. Arzi B, Wisner ER, Huey DJ, et al. Naturally-occurring osteoarthritis in the domestic rabbit: possible implications for bioengineering research. Lab Anim 2012; 41(1):20–5.
22. Miller RE, Lu Y, Tortorella MD, et al. Genetically engineered mouse models reveal the importance of proteases as osteoarthritis drug targets. Curr Rheumatol Rep 2013;15(8):350.
23. Little CB, Hunter DJ. Post-traumatic osteoarthritis: from mouse models to clinical trials. Nat Rev Rheumatol 2013;9(8):485–97.
24. Moskowitz RW, Altman RD, Hochberg MC, et al. Experimental models of osteoarthritis. In: Moskowitz RW, Goldberg VM, Hochberg MC, editors. Osteoarthritis: diagnosis and medical/surgical management. 4th edition. Philadelphia: Lippincott Williams & Wilkins; 2007. p. 107–25.

25. Poulet B, Westerhof TA, Hamilton RW, et al. Spontaneous osteoarthritis in Str/ort mice is unlikely due to greater vulnerability to mechanical trauma. Osteoarthritis Cartilage 2013;21(5):756–63.
26. Glasson SS. In vivo osteoarthritis target validation utilizing genetically-modified mice. Curr Drug Targets 2007;8(2):367–76.
27. Kamekura S, Hoshi K, Shimoaka T, et al. Osteoarthritis development in novel experimental mouse models induced by knee joint instability. Osteoarthritis Cartilage 2005;13(7):632–41.
28. Pitsillides AA, Beier F. Cartilage biology in osteoarthritis - lessons from developmental biology. Nat Rev Rheumatol 2011;7:654–63.
29. Kamekura S, Hoschi K, Shimoaka T, et al. Osteoarthritis development in novel experimental mouse models induced by knee joint instability. Osteoarthritis Cartilage 2005;13:632–45.
30. Piskin A, Gulbahar MY, Tomak Y, et al. Osteoarthritis after meniscectomy in rats. A histological and immunohistochemical study. Saudi Med J 2007;28(12): 1796–17802.
31. Hayami T, Pickarsi M, Zhuo Y, et al. Characterization of articular cartilage and subchondral bone changes in the rat anterior cruciate ligament transection and meniscenctomized models of osteoarthritis. Bone 2006;38(2):234–43.
32. Welch ID, Cowan MF, Beier F, et al. The retinoic acid binding protein CRABP2 is increased in murine models of degenerative joint disease. Arthritis Res Ther 2009;11(1):R14.
33. Miller RE, Tran PB, Das R, et al. CCR2 chemokine receptor signaling mediates pain in experimental osteoarthritis. Proc Natl Acad Sci U S A 2012;109(50): 20602–7.
34. Bendele AM. Animal models of osteoarthritis. J Musculoskelet Neuronal Interact 2001;1(4):363–76.
35. Knights CB, Grentry C, Bevan S. Partial medial meniscectomy produces osteoarthritis pain-related behaviour in female C57BL/6 mice. Pain 2012;153:281–92.
36. Masterbergen SC, Marijnissen AC, Vianen ME, et al. The canine groove model of osteoarthritis is more than simply the expression of surgically applied damage. Osteoarthritis Cartilage 2006;14(1):39–46.
37. Serra CI, Soler C, Carrillo JM, et al. Effect of autologous platelet-rich plasma on the repair of full-thickness articular defects in rabbits. Knee Surg Sports Traumatol Arthrosc 2013;21:1730–6.
38. Bornes TD, Adesida AB, Jomha NM. Mesenchymal stem cells in the treatment of traumatic articular defects: a comprehensive review. Arthritis Res Ther 2014; 16(5):432.
39. Berninger MT, Wexel G, Rummeny EJ, et al. Treatment of osteochondral defects in the rabbit's knee joint by implantation of allogenic mesenchymal stem cells in fibrin clots. J Vis Exp 2013;75:e4423.
40. Duan P, Pan Z, Cao L, et al. The effects of pore size in bilayered poly(lactide-co-glycolide) scaffolds on restoring osteochondral defects in rabbits. J Biomed Mater Res A 2014;102(1):180–92.
41. Iulian A, Dan L, Camelia T, et al. Synthetic materials for osteochondral tissue engineering. Adv Exp Med Biol 2018;1058:31–52.
42. Figueroa D, Espinosa M, Calvo R, et al. Treatment of acute full-thickness chondral defects with high molecular weight hyaluronic acid: an experimental model. Rev Esp Cir Ortop Traumatol 2014;48(5):261–6.
43. Ahern BJ, Parvizi J, Boston R, et al. Preclinical animal models in single site cartilage defect testing: a systematic review. Osteoarthritis Cartilage 2009;17(6):705–13.

44. Cook JL, Hung CT, Kuroki K, et al. Animal models of cartilage repair. Bone Joint Res 2014;3(4):89–94.
45. Kreuz PC, Seinwaschs MR, Erggelet C, et al. Results after microfracture of full thickness chondral defects in different compartments in the knee. Osteoarthritis Cartilage 2006;14:1119–25.
46. McNulty MA, Loeser RF, Davey C, et al. Histopathology of naturally occurring and surgically induced osteoarthritis in mice. Osteoarthritis Cartilage 2012;20(8): 949–56.
47. Flanigan DC, Harris JD, Brockmeier PM, et al. The effects of lesion size and location on subchondral bone contact in experimental knee articular cartilage defects in a bovine model. Arthroscopy 2010;26(12):1655–61.
48. Bentley G. Articular cartilage studies and osteoarthritis. Ann R Coll Surg Engl 1975;57(2):86–100.
49. Bove SE, Calcaterra SL, Brooker RM, et al. Weight bearing as a measure of disease progression and efficacy of anti-inflammatory compounds in a model of monosodium iodoacetate-induced osteoarthritis. Osteoarthritis Cartilage 2003; 11(11):821–30.
50. Schuelert N, McDougall JJ. Grading of monosodium iodoacetate-induced osteoarthritis reveals a concentration-dependent sensitization of nociceptors in the knee joint of the rat. Neurosci Lett 2009;465(2):184–8.
51. Miyauchi S, Machida A, Onaya J, et al. Alterations of proteoglycan synthesis in rabbit articular cartilage induced by intra-articular injection of papain. Osteoarthritis Cartilage 1993;1(4):253–62.
52. Van der Kraan PM, Vitters EL, van de Putte LB, et al. Development of osteoarthritic lesions in mice by "metabolic" and "mechanical" alterations in the knee joints. Am J Pathol 1989;135(6):1001–4.
53. Sendzik J, Lode H, Stahlman R. Quinolone-induced arthropathy: an update focusing on new mechanistic and clinical data. Int J Antimicrob Agents 2009; 33(3):194–200.
54. Furman BD, Strand J, Hembree WC, et al. Joint degeneration following closed intraarticular fracture in the mouse knee: a model of posttraumatic arthritis. J Orthop Res 2007;25(5):578–92.
55. Poulet B, Hamilton RW, Shefelbine S, et al. Characterizing a novel and adjustable non-invasive murine knee joint loading model. Arthritis Rheum 2011;63(1): 137–47.
56. Melville KM, Robling AG, Van der Meulen MC. In vivo axial loading of the mouse tibia. Methods Mol Biol 2015;1226:99–115.
57. Christiansen BA, Andersoon MJ, Lee CA, et al. Musculoskeletal changes following non-invasive knee injury using a novel mouse model of post-traumatic osteoarthritis. Osteoarthritis Cartilage 2012;20(7):773–82.
58. Lockwood KA, Chu BT, Anderson MJ, et al. Comparison of loading rate-dependent injury modes in a murine model of post-traumatic osteoarthritis. J Orthop Res 2014;32(1):79–88.
59. Onur TS, Wu R, Chu S, et al. Joint instability and cartilage compression in a mouse model of posttraumatic osteoarthritis. J Orthop Res 2014;32(2):318–23.
60. Khorasani MS, Diko S, Hsia AW, et al. Effect of alendronate on post-traumatic osteoarthritis induced by anterior cruciate ligament rupture in mice. Arthritis Res Ther 2015;17:30.

Fracture Management in Avian Species

Daniel Calvo Carrasco, LV, CertAVP (ZooMed), MRCVS[a,b,*]

KEYWORDS

- Orthopedics • Avian • External skeletal fixator • Fracture • External coaptation

KEY POINTS

- The general principles of fracture management in birds are the same as in mammals or reptiles.
- The principal objective in avian orthopedics is to restore and maintain longitudinal, lateral, and rotational alignment of the affected bones during the required time to allow healing while causing the minimum iatrogenic damage to both skeletal and soft tissues.
- The avian clinician must be prepared to think laterally and assess each case individually, taking into account the unique characteristics of the fracture, the temperament of the species and the individual, its lifestyle, and the desired outcome.

INTRODUCTION

Orthopedic conditions, particularly fractures, are a common presentation in avian practice.[1,2] Other orthopedic conditions seen in avian patients include luxations, degenerative joint diseases, and developmental abnormalities. These conditions may occur owing to trauma, an underlying pathologic disorder, and/or inadequate management during the rearing process. Articular orthopedic disorders are covered in Mikel Sabater González's article, "Avian Articular Orthopedics," in this issue.

The general principles of fracture management in birds are the same as in mammals or reptiles. However, anatomic and physiologic particularities resulting in different biomechanics and pathologies should be considered when dealing with orthopedic conditions in birds.

Historically, there has been a relatively limited amount of scientific material available describing avian orthopedics. However, recent advances in orthopedic techniques fully evaluated in nonavian species, have been recently extrapolated with or without modification to avian orthopedic procedures.

Disclosure Statement: The author has nothing to disclose.
[a] Great Western Exotics, Vets Now Swindon, UK; [b] Wildfowl & Wetlands Trust (WWT), Newgrounds Lane, Gloucestershire, England, Gloucester GI2 7BT, United Kingdom
* Wildfowl & Wetlands Trust (WWT), Newgrounds Lane, Gloucestershire, England, Gloucester GL2 7BT, United Kingdom.
E-mail address: danicalvocarrasco@gmail.com

The avian clinician must be prepared to think laterally and assess each case individually, taking into account the unique characteristics of the fracture, as well as the temperament of the species and the individual, its lifestyle, and the desired outcome. All this should be considered during the decision making process, which should involve the owner or career of the patient. The clinician should always aim for a result as close as possible to the original functional anatomy. The degree of perfection required for postoperative return to normal function will be dictated by the species and the lifestyle of the patient.[3]

The principal objective in avian orthopedics is to restore and maintain longitudinal, lateral, and rotational alignment of the affected bones during the required time to allow healing while causing the minimum iatrogenic damage to both skeletal and soft tissues. The surgical approach should cause minimal trauma to the soft tissues, including the delicate nerves and vascular supply. More rapid recoveries and fewer complications are associated with better protection of soft tissues, shorter surgical times, and good overall patient management.[4]

Additionally, the bipedal nature of avian species should be considered during the immediate postoperative and recovery periods when a pelvic limb is involved, because impaired function of the pelvic limb will create additional strain and weight-bearing on the contralateral leg.[4]

INITIAL STABILIZATION AND TRIAGE

Traumatized birds are usually presented in shock. Patient stabilization requires restoring the normal circulation and oxygen exchange, and establishing pain control, as well as to prevent any further damage (including dehydration) of the traumatized tissues. The initial physical examination has to be adapted to the stability status of the patient, and certain aspects of the examination may have to be delayed until the patient is more stable. Ideally, the animal should be examined fully, including a careful and thorough palpation of the whole skeletal system and a complete ophthalmic examination, before potentially obtaining orthogonal radiographs. Sedation or general anesthesia may be required, and this measure should only be performed when the patient is stable enough to tolerate these procedures safely.

Birds tend to go through the same early compensatory phase of shock as dogs and might be presented with tachycardia in early stages of shock, in contrast with small mammals like cats or rabbits.[5] Critically ill birds have a low physiologic reserve of metabolites that, combined with their basal high metabolic rate and the increased metabolic demand associated with illness provokes, means that fluid therapy and nutritional support should be provided as soon as possible.[6] However, it should be remembered that, to the prevent refeeding syndrome, assisted feeding should not be initiated until the hydroelectrolitic imbalances of the patient have been corrected. Antimicrobial treatment should be given where there is a loss of asepsis or if an implant is required.

Birds presented with hemorrhage, head trauma, or fractures should be examined immediately.[7] However, physical restraint should be limited as much as possible because the stress associated with it may result in further decompensation of the avian patient.[8]

One of the challenges that avian clinicians face is finding the balance between stabilizing the patient, obtaining a diagnosis, and avoiding exacerbating shock and stress through patient handling and treatment administration. After the initial assessment of the patient initial stabilization must be prioritized over a thorough examination and further diagnostics.[9] An additional challenge in wildlife cases is to determine the long-term prognosis for the individual as early possible, to avoid an unnecessary compromise of the patient welfare and the waste of limited resources in those cases carrying a poor prognosis. Many factors have to be considered in the decision making process to establish the more suitable treatment option associated with the best possible prognosis: species, life style, fracture type, concomitant injuries, underlying preexisting conditions, surgeon expertise and experience, available equipment and rehabilitation facilities, and economic resources.[10]

Wound management and soft tissue preservation throughout triage and treatment will help to prevent the loss of bone viability and improve the long-term prognosis.[9] This author recommends further reading for emergency medicine and critical care of avian species.[7,8,11]

OCULAR CONSIDERATIONS IN THE TRIAGE OF AVIAN TRAUMA PATIENTS

It is important to remember that ocular damage is common in avian trauma cases, owing to countercoup forces on the head and resultant traction to the retinal insertion of the pecten. Hemorrhage in the anterior chamber will clear rapidly but, if present in the posterior segment, it is likely to be associated with retinal detachment or hemorrhage around the pecten. Hemorrhage in the posterior segment takes weeks or even longer to clear and is often associated with long-term loss of retinal function, which potentially precludes the wildlife patient's release back to the wild. However, a recent retrospective study evaluating ocular trauma in raptors concluded that even relatively severe cases (especially in diurnal birds) can potentially recover.[12] Such cases may benefit from the injection of tissue activator plasminogen into the anterior chamber (under general anesthesia) 48 hours after insult, which may be repeated if necessary once or twice at 48-hour intervals.[13]

FRACTURE ASSESSMENT

As mentioned, orthogonal views of the suspected affected area(s) should be performed. If injuries of the thoracic girdle are suspected, the clinician should consider performing a caudoventral–craniodorsal oblique radiographic view obtained at 45° to the frontal plane (H view) in addition to the ventrodorsal view, to decrease the risk of misdiagnosing fractures. Similarly, fractures of the femoral head may not be noticed with orthogonal views and advanced imaging or different projections may be required.[14,15]

Fractures are currently classified according to different systems, including causal factors, location, morphology, communication with an external wound (open or closed), and their severity.[16] It is important to notice the implications that a specific characteristic has on the other aspects that define the fracture; for example, a severely displaced fracture is more likely to be open than closed. The classification system is particularly helpful not only to describe the fracture, but also to understand its nature as well as the factors that may have contributed to its development, such as bone quality and physiologic status.

The characteristics and nature of the fracture (eg, location or type) have a direct impact on the choice of treatment.[9] The robustness of the fixator required is directly influenced by the load sharing across the bone, as well as by the strength, durability, and capacity of the fixing construction to support bending, rotational, and compressive forces. The different treatment options, of increasing robustness, are: cage rest, external coaptation, intramedullary (IM) pin alone, external skeletal fixator (ESF) type I, ESF type II, and tie-in or hybrid ESF (involving an ESF and an IM pin attached together).

Fractures are classified as open when there is exposure of 1 or more bone fragments, and are considered contaminated (**Fig. 1**). Closed fractures, those in which the skin is intact, are less likely to become infected. Fractures can be simple

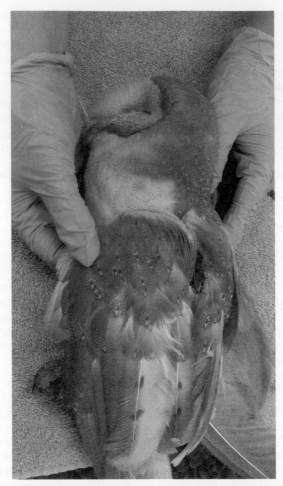

Fig. 1. Wild Barn Owl (*Tyto alba*) with an open contaminated fracture of the humerus.

(2 fragments) or comminuted (>2 fragments), also called multifragmental. Long bone fractures are described by the location of the fracture (proximal, midshaft, and distal). Diaphyseal (shaft) long bone fractures are described with reference to the direction of the fracture line in relation to the shaft of the bone (transverse, oblique, spiral, or comminuted), as well as by the location of the fracture (proximal, midshaft, or distal). Contrarily, epiphyseal fractures (those involving the epiphysis) may be classified as Salter Harris (I–IX) depending on whether the growth plate is still open or not. Fractures affecting short, sesamoid, or irregular bones follow a different classification. The displacement of a fracture is always defined in terms of the distal fragment in relation to the proximal fragment. Fractures may involve the loss of axial alignment (lateral or medial), angulation (varus or valgus), or rotation (internal or external), or a change in length (proximal migration, distraction, or impaction).

TREATMENT OPTIONS

During triage and stabilization, temporary stabilization with conservative techniques is indicated. Initial external coaptation should be placed immediately after triage, to prevent further trauma and pain until a different definitive treatment is planned. Definitive treatment occurs after the initial stabilization phase and may involve 1 or more surgical techniques, combined or not with external coaptation and/or cage rest. It is important to have a full understanding of the bird's husbandry requirements to appropriately managed the case through the convalescent period. It must be remembered that the treatment aim is to facilitate a full and early recovery of the physiologic function of the affected limb (including joints and tendons) without adversely affecting the healing process. In this author's opinion, a wing strapped up in a manner that prevents normal joint function should not be left immobilized for longer than 48 hours after surgery to minimize the risk of developing a diminished joint range of motion.

CONSERVATIVE MANAGEMENT: CAGE REST AND EXTERNAL COAPTATION

This author considers that external coaptation techniques are, although limited and generally speaking accepted to carry a worse prognosis, often poorly understood by the general practitioner, underestimated, and not used to their full potential. Surgical treatment options are better known within the avian veterinary community, and wet laboratories and other training sessions are routinely offered in conferences. However, probably not enough attention is paid to training less experienced avian veterinarians about the different conservative options available.

As mentioned, cage rest is often part of the initial stabilization. It can also be the treatment of choice for certain types of fractures and patients who are not suitable candidates for external coaptation or surgical repair, such as very small birds or those with pelvic fractures.

It is of vital importance to house the inpatient in a suitable enclosure during the recovery period; often, a reduced space is provided to minimize physical activity. However, it is important to consider the animal welfare and the local legislation. Under UK law (Animal Welfare Act 2006), it is unacceptable to house a bird in an enclosure small enough to prevent full wing extension in all 3 dimensions, although such confinement is permitted when a bird is undergoing treatment by a veterinary surgeon. If the prevention of wing extension is required for healing, a better alternative would be to combine cage rest and external coaptation, decreasing the movement of the affected limb only. A simple method commonly used by this author is to tape the tip of the wings together over the back in a physiologic position, which significantly restricts the movement of the wings, without completely immobilizing the thoracic limb (**Fig. 2**). This technique is used to avoid further trauma, either alone or after surgical repair, and can be left in place for weeks.

External coaptation may also be used for long-term treatment. It is easy to apply and is less expensive than surgical options. Such techniques are not appropriate for all

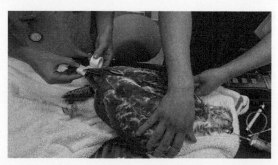

Fig. 2. Wing taping on a wild buzzard (*Buteo buteo*) with an aligned close ulnar fracture.

situations. The joints located proximally and distally to the fracture site must be immobilized[17] to achieve an effective immobilization. Also, this technique may not be suitable for those fractures in which an increase of bending and torsional forces to the fracture site might occur.[9] Despite most external coaptation options are not particularly challenging to perform, these techniques are frequently applied under sedation or general anesthesia to decrease the patient's stress and iatrogenic damage.

It is important to remember that the use of coaptation alone for fracture management is often accompanied by poorer outcomes and severe complications when compared with other treatment options.[9] However, in some instances, it may be the treatment of choice (or elected); factors to consider may have already been mentioned, and include funds available, infection, severely comminuted fractures, and the existence of severe trauma to the soft tissue surrounding the bone.

Dressings and bandages should never be placed across the leading edge of the propatagium owing to the risk of causing pressure necrosis.[3] Equally, compressive bandages across the celomic cavity should be very carefully placed and monitored, owing to the high risk of air sac compression and the risk of suffocation. Once in place, the bandage or splint should be monitored carefully, because it may provoke abrasions of the surrounding skin or swelling of the distal aspect of the bandaged limb, even if the bandage remains in place correctly.

Some conservative techniques are considered as the preferred technique for specific fractures, such as metacarpal fractures[18] and for fractures of the tibiotarsus and tarsometatarsus of small birds.[19,20]

Different methods of external coaptation are currently used in avian patients, some of them extrapolated from mammalian species, and 2 (nearly) exclusive avian techniques: the figure-of-eight bandage and the Altmann's tape splint.

Thoracic Limb

Figure-of-eight bandage

This bandage configuration (**Fig. 3**) immobilizes the distal wing. Bandaging is initiated on the ventral aspect between the radius, ulna, and humerus; brought round to cover the elbow/distal humerus; and passed dorsally over the wing until the digits, then ventrally to reach the starting point covering the end of the bandage. After a second loop, the bandage is directed forward along the ventral surface toward the distal aspect of the radius and ulna, loops around the dorsal aspect of the carpometacarpus, and finally back to the starting point to close the figure-of-eight.

After a few more complete loops, the second layer of cohesive flexible bandage can be applied to secure the bandage. It can be used as a temporary option, in

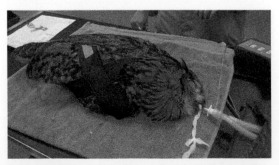

Fig. 3. Figure-of-eight bandage in a Eurasian eagle-owl (*Bubo bubo*).

combination with certain surgical approaches, or as a single definitive treatment. The technique is used to immobilize and stabilize fractures located distally from the elbow, as well as to prevent soft tissue damage. It does not immobilize the shoulder or the humerus; however, it does immobilize the elbow. This bandage should be applied carefully, because it might damage the propatagium and its ligament. Excessive pressure on the propatagium must be avoided, and bandage changes and physiotherapy every few days are needed to avoid joint stiffening. An interval of 48 to 72 hours is recommended by some authors.[9] Ideally, this bandage should be applied in 2 layers (a conforming stretch bandage and a cohesive flexible bandage), with the exception of very small birds, in which a cohesive flexible bandage is applied alone.

Body wrap

This bandaging method is used to immobilize the whole wing in normal resting position temporarily. Different methods have been described. With a small modification, this bandage enables the wings to be kept immobilized attached to the body without causing any restriction or compression of the air sacs. Other than for the initial stabilization of wing fractures, it can also be used to immobilize the wing for thoracic girdle fractures.

Aluminum foam-backed splint

These splints have a 2-mm-thick aluminum base, covered with a padding of foam along one side. They are lightweight and flexible, and can be shaped to fit each case. Aligned simple fractures of the radius or ulna can be treated with external coaptation using an aluminum foam-backed splint with drilled holes (to enable placement of suture material through the splint). This splint is anchored with sutures around the primary feathers, which are firmly attached to the periosteum, thereby anchoring the splint firmly to the bone. This technique carries a higher risk of promoting synostosis than surgical repair, and should not be used if there is significant misalignment of the fractured bone or if both bones are fractured. Other clinicians have also reported great success in the treatment of certain carpometacarpal fractures, especially in small birds, with this technique.

Curve edge splint

Semirigid casting tape or other moldable materials, such as thermoplastic, can be used to cover distally from the carpometacarpus, on the dorsal aspect or dorsal and ventral aspects.[21] A figure-of-eight bandage or a body wrap can be used in combination to maintain the splint in place after it has been taped to the distal wing.

Pelvic Limb

Altmann's tape splint

This technique is indicated for long bone fractures of the hind limb where the joint above and below can be included; although not ideal, this technique can also be attempted in very distal femoral fractures in small birds. A recent retrospective study in birds up to 200 g body weight reported that the majority of cases (>90%) had an acceptable outcome.[20] This author has used this technique in heavier birds successfully (**Fig. 4**) when surgical fixation was not feasible. The feathers of the area should be plucked before the application of the tape. The clinician must consider that plucking is a painful stimulus,[22] and should be performed after correct analgesia has been provided and, ideally, under general anesthesia. The Altmann's tape splint technique consists of 2 or more (often several) layers of adhesive tape, placed in a sandwich fashion with the fracture bone in the middle of the sandwich, and reinforced with tissue glue to increase rigidity.[2] The strips of tape are placed after fracture reduction and with the

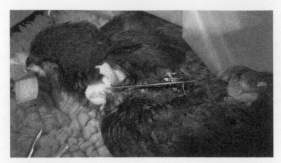

Fig. 4. ESF tie-in for a humeral fracture of a Sparrow hawk (*Accipiter nisus*).

hind limb held in the normal perching position, with the knee and tarsus–metatarsus joints slightly flexed (**Fig. 5**). The 2 strips are placed across the whole length of the affected bone, overlapping and extending to the proximal and distal joints, both laterally and medially. The sheets are then adhered to each other and tightened around the leg using hemostat forceps, followed by the application of tissue glue and trimming of excess tape. The use of cyanoacrylate-based glue allows a smaller tape size.

Aluminum foam-backed splint
This splint foam can be used to temporarily treat tibiotarsus fractures, lacing the splint cranially and caudally, shaped to fit and immobilize the proximal (knee) and distal (tibiotarsus–tarsometatarsus joint) joints. This technique is used in larger bird species in which the Altmann's tape splint will not provide enough stability. Ideally, the splint should be placed both cranially and caudally (2 pieces). Alternatively, 2 tongue depressors with soft bandaging can also be used (**Fig. 6**).

Syringe barrel splint
This technique can be used for long bone fractures such as tibiotarsal or tarsometatarsal fractures. The syringe to be used varies depending on the size of the affected bone. Both ends of the syringe barrel are cut off and the syringe barrel is cut longitudinally. A layer of conforming stretch bandage is placed over the affected limb. The syringe barrel is placed over the fractured bone and secured proximally and distally with tape in a sandwich fashion.

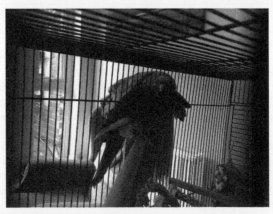

Fig. 5. The Altmann's tape splint technique.

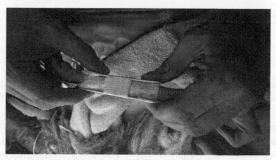

Fig. 6. Splint in a green stick fracture of a juvenile red-legged seriema (*Cariama cristata*).

Ball bandages

Ball bandages consist of a ball of cotton wool or similar material placed in the palmar aspect of the feet that are maintained in position with a flexible bandage. It keeps the digits in a semiextended position, and it allows for certain movements that may help to prevent the entrapment of the nerve within the callus.

Recently, a polyvinyl chloride piping device was used to stabilize the pathologic bilateral femoral fractures in a Maroonbellied Conure (*Pyrrhura frontalis*), which braced the bird's feet at the level of the perch and supported its upper body weight via a breast plate, thus maintaining the bird in a physiologically appropriate perching position. The conure was ambulatory and returned to normal function after 3 weeks of external coaptation with this device.[23]

Psittacines and some birds of prey may be particularly likely to interfere with bandages and external coaptation, and this situation must be prevented or addressed if it occurs. Psittacines often require a collar to stop them from chewing at or removing bandages or even self-mutilating; note that the collar itself may represent a significant stressful factor for the avian patient. As with bandages and splints, different materials are available. The collar most commonly used by this author is based on a foam pipe lining, which can be easily customized to fit the individual bird (see **Fig. 5**). In some individuals, when the foam collar is not enough to prevent self-mutilation or picking of the bandage, a plastic disc collar can be incorporated (see **Fig. 6**).

Conversely, certain birds will better tolerate a felt collar. This author recommends using light sedation and hospitalization of the bird for the initial 24 hours after the collar has been placed, because some patients will be significantly distressed, vocal, and may not eat during this period.[24] In some accipiter species, particularly Harris hawks (*Parabuteo unicinctus*), a blob of dental acrylic in the beak is useful to prevent the bird from picking at the bandage.[25]

It is also important to prevent damage of the flight feathers, both of the wings (remiges) and of the tail (retrices), particularly in wild birds intended to be released. Tail covers made of old radiographic film are used while birds are hospitalized, and birds should be provided adequate perches at the right heights.

SURGICAL OPTIONS

The surgical treatment options are more widely used within avian practice; traditionally, the main treatment option has been the tie-in or hybrid fixator (TIF), which consists of the combination of an IM pin joined to an external fixator. This technique is versatile, light, and suitable for most long bone fractures in birds. More recently, bone plating has increased its popularity and recent publications have demonstrated that it can be used with good outcomes, even in relatively small avian patients.

INTRAMEDULLARY PINS

The use of an IM pin is a relatively easy to apply treatment method that provides good longitudinal stability, counteracting bending forces. However, it has not effect against rotational forces, which limits its sole use. IM pins are more commonly used as part of the already mentioned TIF, or in combination with external coaptation. IM pins can be placed from the fracture site (retrograde placement) or pointing toward the fracture site from either the proximal or distal aspect of the bone (normograde placement). This author prefers a retrograde placement, whenever possible, because open reduction of the fracture provides a better understanding of the extension of the lesions, although it requires gentle handling of the tissues to avoid further trauma (**Fig. 7**). Other investigators advise normograde placement[9] to decrease soft tissue disruption of the fracture site. It is important to avoid iatrogenic damage to certain joints, such as the elbow, the tarsal joint, and the stifle, whereas other joints, such as the carpal–phalangeal joint, could be penetrated by the IM pin without serious limitation to flight. IM pins can be partially exteriorized and fixed, allowing for removal after the fracture has healed fully. This method has been used in a number of long bones, including the radius, the ulna, the tibiotarsus, and the major metacarpal bone (**Fig. 8**).

EXTERNAL FIXATORS

External fixators (types I and II) are the most widely used in avian orthopedics, in which all the elements are found within the same 2-dimensional planes. This method prevents tensile and compression as well as rotational movements, but has moderate resistance to bending forces. Pins that go through both cortices and exteriorize in 1 side (type I) or both (type II) are connected to 1 (type I) or 2 (type II) external bars.

Different types of pins can be used, including Steinmann pins (smooth pins usually with a trocar point in both ends), Kirschner wires (possess pointed pins), and threaded pins. The difference between a pin and a wire is the diameter (0.9–1.5 mm, wire; 1.5–6.5 mm, pins). Threaded pins could have a positive or a negative profile; threads are cut into the shank of the pin for varying lengths, usually near the tip. In mammals, negative profile pins are generally avoided because they have less holding power than positive profile pins, and do not have any benefit to smooth pins; threads simply glide through the hole without engaging the bone[26] and can more easily break at the thread–pin interface.[27] However, negative threaded pins have been shown to possess

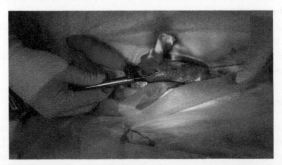

Fig. 7. Retrograde IM placement in a tibiotarsal fracture of a Gyr falcon (*Falco rusticolus*).

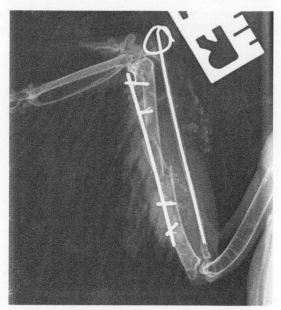

Fig. 8. IM pin in a fractured radius of a Sparrow hawk (*Accipiter nisus*).

a greater holding power than smooths pins in a study performed with common buzzards (*Buteo buteo*).[28] The holding power of threaded pins seem to vary between bones and the location within the pitch of the threat. A study on humerus and tibiotarsus of common buzzards (*Buteo buteo*) demonstrated differences on the extraction force depending on the location within the same bone, as well as a higher holding power with a lower treat pitch,[29] whereas threaded pins showed more pull-out strength in the ulna than in the femur in a different study, and no differences observed related to pin location along the ulna and the femur when considering the same pin type.[28]

Positive profile pins have a greater diameter than negative profile pins in the threaded area. Partially threaded positive-profile ESF half-pin (IMEX Veterinary, Inc, Longview, TX) have been reported to provide good cortical anchoring,[9] but owing to the larger diameter than negative profile pins, are not always a suitable option for smaller patients.

Type I external fixators are usually used as part of a TIF, and will be discuss elsewhere in this article. Type II external fixators are used most commonly used for the tarsus–metatarsus fracture, using partially centrally threaded pins, which should be carefully placed to avoid entrapment of the extensor tendons (cranially) and the flexor tendons (caudally).

The circular or ring external fixator is also an external fixator but surrounds the affected bone across the whole circumference, and has been used in a yellow-naped amazon (*Amazona ochrocephala auropalliata*)[30] and a sacred ibis (*Thresjiornis aethiopicus*)[31] successfully

TIE-IN OR HYBRID FIXATOR

This technique, which consists on the combination of a type I ESF with an IM pin, is considered the most versatile and effective method to treat avian fractures. The

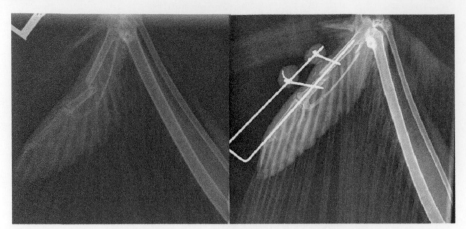

Fig. 9. Preoperative and postoperative radiographs of a major carpal bone fracture in a common European kestrel (*Falco tinnunculus*).

combination of the IM and ESF provides stability in the 3 dimensions, while it remains light, relatively inexpensive, and allows the bird to stand in a physiologic position. The connecting bar has to be located in the dorsal aspect of the bones within the thoracic limb, and in the lateral aspect of the femur and the tibiotarsus for obvious anatomic reasons (**Fig. 9**). One of the main limitations of this technique is the requirement of the IM to exit the bone to connect with the rest of the ESF, which makes it unsuitable for those straight bones in which both joints should not be affected, such as the tarsus–metatarsus. However, in sigmoidal shaped bones, such as the humerus or the femur, the IM pin can exit the bone before reaching the distal elbow joint or the pelvis.

Different systems are available commercially, including the FESSA system, or specifically design systems with pins, connecting bars and clamps or rods. The author prefers choice is joining the ESF pins and the connecting bar polymethylmethacrylate or epoxy putty, after initial stabilization with a cable wire (see **Fig. 4**). This method allows flexibility and does not require all the pins to be in exactly the same plane and in a 90° angle. It is also a simple and economical alternative because it eliminates the need for connecting bars and clamps.

This technique has been used to treat humeral, ulnar, femoral, and tibiotarsal fractures, but has only been studies in tibiotarsal fractures. In a retrospective study on wild birds of prey, most tibiotarsal fractures were successfully managed by surgical reduction and stabilization with a 1 + 1 (1 pin on each fragment) TIF.[32] Similar outcomes were seen in a retrospective study on pet birds[33] using a 2 + 2 structure (**Fig. 10**), which has been proven to provide significantly increased the stiffness in torque (110%) and compression (60%), and the safe load in torque (107%) and compression (50%) compared with a 1 + 1 strructure[34] (see **Fig. 9**). In the configuration with 2 fixation pins, placing the proximal pin distally in the proximal bone segment significantly increased the stiffness in torque (28%), and the safe load in torque (23%) and in axial compression (32%).[34]

BONE PLATES

Bone plates provide stability against shear forces and rotation when compared with IM pins. The use of surgical plates in avian practice is limited by multiple factors, such as the bone affected, the type of fracture, the size of the bone (eg, generally

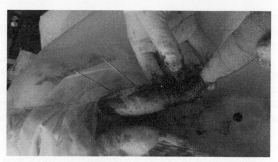

Fig. 10. A 2 + 2 TIF in a tibiotarsal fracture of a Gyr falcon (*Falco rusticolus*).

presenting thinner cortices than mammals), the size of the plate, and the cost of the equipment. Bone plating is generally considered as a useful method for midshaft humeral, midshaft femoral, tibiotarsal, and coracoid fractures in large birds.[35] However, few research studies have been published regarding the use of bone plates in birds. An experimental study in pigeons comparing 3 miniplate systems for ulnar and radial fracture stabilization (1.3-mm adaptation plates, 1.3-mm limited contact system [adaptation plate with washers], and 1.0-mm maxillofacial miniplates) reported a 33% rate of screw loosening and failure for the adaptation plates, bending of all the maxillofacial miniplates, and 100% of success when using 1.3-mm adaptation plates.[36] Another experimental study in pigeons evaluated 2 miniplate systems and figure-of-eight bandages for the stabilization of experimentally induced ulnar and radial fractures concluding that 1.3-mm adaptation plates and 1-mm compression plates meet the requirements for avian bone fracture repair of the ulna in birds weighing less than 500 g and that their use in combination with a figure-of-eight bandage might benefit fracture healing.[37] Ex vivo biomechanical evaluation of pigeon cadaver intact humeri and ostectonized humeri stabilized with caudally applied 1.6-mm titanium screw locking plates or 1.5-mm stainless steel dynamic compression plates concluded that increased torsional strength may be needed before plate repair can be considered as the sole fracture repair method.[38] A deeper review of technological advances in bone plating for avian species will be published in the next issue of this journal.

AMPUTATION

Amputations are indicated when the damage to the limb is beyond repair. This method is only considered for pet birds, because no wild animal should be released if it has a clear disadvantage compared with any other member of its own species. Historically, it has been believed that amputations of the hind amputations are well-tolerated in small light birds, but a recent case report in a Blue-and-gold Macaw (*Ara ararauna*) coped well for more than a year and died of unrelated reasons.[39] This author prefers to do a (mid to a third) femur amputation whenever is possible to avoid future trauma to the stamp if the patient uses it to stand on it; however, stifle disarticulation has been recently described as an alternative to transfemoral limb amputation.[40]

In regard to thoracic limb amputations, a novel technique for scapulohumeral amputations has also been recently described in a case series of 3 birds.[41]

SKULL FRACTURES

A single case of growing skull fracture has been reported in birds. The thin, soft nature of the skull combined with the high growth rate of young avian species increases the likelihood of fracture expansion rather than healing. A computed tomography scan of the skull of an immature red-tailed hawk (*Buteo jamaicensis*) revealed a large, calvarial defect with skin and subcutaneous tissue covering a protruding section of dura mater surrounded by dense fibrous tissue. Surgical repair consisted of accessing and incising the dura mater to expose the cerebral cortex, removing the fibrous adherences surrounding, covering the dural defect with sterile, processed swine intestinal submucosa and a sheet of sterile polypropylene mesh that was sutured to the surrounding temporalis muscle and subcutaneous tissue and routine suture of the skin. The bird recovered from surgery without complications and could be released back into the wild.[42]

The editors of this issue had the opportunity to be involved in the management of a calvarial fracture in a Harris hawk (*P unicinctus*) presented with ataxia, unilateral blindness, and soft tissue swelling in the calvarial region. Surgery was performed by Dr Neil Forbes to decompress the brain and reposition the displaced calvarial fragments into a more normal position. The bird recovered well from surgery but remained unilaterally blind.

A trauma-induced aneurysmal bone cyst was surgically excised from the calvarium of a cockatiel (*N hollandicus*).[43]

REFERENCES

1. Howard DJ, Redig PT. Analysis of avian fracture repair: implications for captive and wild birds. Proceedings of the Annual Conference of the Association of Avian Veterinarians. 1993. p. 77–83. Available at: https://www.aav.org/global_engine/download.aspx?fileid=F7F7D013-9807-4C1E-9D20-15DBB242F44E&ext=pdf.
2. Helmer P. Orthopaedic disorders. In: Harrison GJ, Lightfoot TL, editors. Clinical avian medicine, vol. II. Palm Beach (FL: Spix Publishing; 2006. p. 761–74. Available at: https://www.ivis.org/advances/harrison/toc.asp.
3. Forbes NA. Raptors. In: Mullineaux E, Keeble E, editors. BSAVA manual of wildlife casualties. 2nd edition. Gloucester (United Kingdom): BSAVA; 2016. p. 398–420.
4. Redig PT, Ponder J. Orthopaedic surgery. In: Samour J, editor. Avian medicine. 3rd edition. St Louis, (MO): Elsevier; 2016. p. 321–58.
5. Riley J, Barron H. Wildlife emergency and critical care. Vet Clin North Am Exot Anim Pract 2016;19:613–26.
6. Brown AJ, Drobatz KJ. Triage of the emergency patient. In: King LG, Boag A, editors. BSAVA manual of canine and feline emergency and critical care. 2nd edition. Gloucester (United Kingdom): BSAVA; 2007. p. 1–7.
7. Sabater González M, Calvo Carrasco D. Emergencies and critical care of commonly kept fowl. Vet Clin North Am Exot Anim Pract 2016;19:543–65.
8. Stout JD. Common emergencies in pet birds. Vet Clin North Am Exot Anim Pract 2016;19:513–41.
9. Ponder JB, Redig P. Orthopaedics. In: Speer B, editor. Current therapy in avian medicine and surgery. St Louis (MO): Elsevier; 2016. p. 657–67.
10. Best D, Mullineaux E. Basic principles of treating wildlife casualties. In: Mullineaux E, Best D, Cooper JE, et al, editors. BSAVA manual of wildlife casualties. 1st edition. Gloucester (United Kingdom): British Small Animal Association (BSAVA); 2003. p. 6–28.
11. Hildreth CD. Preparing the small animal hospital for avian and exotic animal emergencies. Vet Clin North Am Exot Anim Pract 2016;19:325–45.
12. Scott DE. A retrospective look at outcomes of raptors with ocular trauma. Proceedings of ExoticsCon Conference, 2015. p.103. Available at: https://www.aav.org/global_engine/download.aspx?fileid=F7F7D013-9807-4C1E-9D20-15DBB242F44E&ext=pdf.

13. Korbel RT. Disorders of the posterior eye segment in raptors, examination procedures and findings. In: Lumeij JT, Remple JD, Redig PT, et al, editors. Raptor biomedicine III. Lake Worth (FL): Zoological Education Network; 2000. p. 179–93.
14. Visser M, Hespel AM, De Swarte M, et al. Use of a caudoventral-craniodorsal oblique radiographic view made at 45° to the frontal plane to evaluate the pectoral girdle in raptors. J Am Vet Med Assoc 2015;247(9):1037–41.
15. Burgdorf-Moisuk A, Whittington JK, Bennett A, et al. Successful Management of simple fractures of the femoral neck with femoral head and neck excision arthroplasty in two free-living avian species. J Avian Med Surg 2011;25(3):210–5.
16. DeCamp CE, Johnston SA, Déjardin LM, et al. Fractures: classification, diagnosis, and treatment. In: DeCamp CE, Johnston SA, Déjardin LM, et al, editors. Brinker, Piermattei and Flo's handbook of small animal orthopedics and fracture repair. 5th edition. St Louis (MO): Elsevier; 2016. p. 24–152.
17. Harasen G. External coaptation of distal radius and ulna fractures. Can Vet J 2003;44:1010–1.
18. Murray M, Tseng F. Management of metacarpal fractures in free-living raptors. Proceedings of the 33rd Annual Conference of the Association of Avian Veterinarians, 2012. p. 283–4. Available at: https://www.aav.org/global_engine/download.aspx?fileid=419AF0DD-CACC-4B8D-99BD-7DE6C55BA8F4&ext=pdf.
19. Bueno-Padilla I, Arent LR, Ponder JB. Tips for raptor bandaging. Exotic DVM 2011;12(3):29–47.
20. Wright L, Mans C, Olsen G, et al. Retrospective evaluation of tibiotarsal fractures treated with tape splints in birds: 86 Cases (2006-2015). J Avian Med Surg 2018; 32(3):205–20.
21. Scott DE. Orthopaedics. In: Scott DE, editor. Raptor medicine, surgery and rehabilitation. 2nd edition. Wallingford (United Kingdom): Cabi; 2016. p. 165–209.
22. Gentle MJ, Hunter LN. Physiological and behavioural responses associated with feather removal in Gallus gallus var domesticus. Res Vet Sci 1991;50(1):95–101.
23. Shakeri JS, Lightfoot TL, Raffa GF. Novel nonsurgical approach to stabilization of bilateral pathologic femoral fractures in an egg-laying Maroon-bellied conure (Pyrrhura frontalis). J Avian Med Surg 2016;30(2):179–86.
24. Van Zeeland Y, Friedman SG, Bergman L. Behavior. In: Speer B, editor. Current therapy in avian medicine and surgery. 1st edition. St Louis (MO): Elsevier; 2016. p. 177–251.
25. Smith SP, Forbes NA. A novel technique for prevention of self-mutilation in three Harris' hawks (Parabuteo unicinctus). J Avian Med Surg 2009;23(1):49–52.
26. Piermattei DL, Flo GL, DeCamp CE. Handbook of small animal orthopedics and fracture repair. 4th edition. St Louis (MO): Saunders/Elsevier; 2006. p. 100–18.
27. Harasen G. Orthopedic hardware and equipment for the beginner: part 1. Pins and wires. Can Vet J 2003;52:1025–6.
28. López García M, López Beceiro AM, Valcárcel Juárez V, et al. Holding power of three different pin designs in the femur and ulna of the common buzzard (Buteo buteo). J Zoo Wildl Med 2011;42(4):552–7.
29. Castiñeiras Pérez E, Segade Seoane M, Villanueva Santamarina B, et al. Comparison of holding power of three different pin designs for external skeletal fixation in avian bone: a study in common buzzard (Buteo buteo). Vet Surg 2008;37(7): 702–5.
30. Johnston MS, Thode HP 3rd, Ehrhart NP. Bone transport osteogenesis for reconstruction of a bone defect in the tibiotarsus of a yellow-naped Amazon parrot (Amazona ochrocephala auropalliata). J Avian Med Surg 2008;22(1):47–56.

31. Kinney ME, Gorse MJ, Anderson MA. Circular external fixator placement for repair of an open distal tarsometatarsal fracture in an African sacred ibis (*Thresjiornis aethiopicus*). J Zoo Wildl Med 2015;46(4):957–60.
32. Bueno I, Redig PT, Rendahl AK. External skeletal fixator intramedullary pin tie-in for the repair of tibiotarsal fractures in raptors: 37 cases (1995-2011). J Am Vet Med Assoc 2015;247(10):1154–60.
33. Calvo Carrasco D, Shimizu N, Zoller G, et al. Retrospective study on 35 tibiotarsal fracture repairs with external skeletal fixato-intramedullary pin Tie-In in pet birds. Proceedings of the Icare Conference, 2017. p. 764. Available at: https://www.aav.org/global_engine/download.aspx?fileid=F7F7D013-9807-4C1E-9D20-15DBB242F44E&ext=pdf.
34. Van Wettere AJ, Redig PT, Wallace LJ, et al. Mechanical evaluation of external skeletal fixator-intramedullary pin tie-in configurations applied to cadaveral humeri from red-tailed hawks (*Buteo jamaicensis*). J Avian Med Surg 2009;23(4):277–85.
35. Sanchez Migallón Guzman D, Bubenik LJ, Lauer S, et al. Repair of a coracoid luxation and a tibiotarsal fracture in a bald eagle (Haliaeetus leucocephalus). J Avian Med Surg 2017;21(3):1082–6742.
36. Gull JM, Saveraid TC, Szabo D, et al. Evaluation of three miniplate systems for fracture stabilization in pigeons (Columba livia). J Avian Med Surg 2012;26(4):203–12.
37. Bennert BM, Kircher PR, Gutbrod A, et al. Evaluation of two miniplate systems and figure-of-eight bandages for stabilization of experimentally induced ulnar and radial fractures in pigeons (Columba livia). J Avian Med Surg 2016;30(2):111–22.
38. Darrow BG, Biskup JJ, Weigel JP, et al. Ex vivo biomechanical evaluation of pigeon (Columba livia) cadaver intact humeri and oestectomized humeri stabilised with caudally applied titanium locking plate or stainless steel nonlocking plate constructs. Am J Vet Res 2017;78(5):570–8.
39. Summa N, Boston S, Eshar D, et al. Pelvic limb amputation for the treatment of a soft-tissue sarcoma of the tibiotarso-tarsometatarsal joint in a blue-and-gold macaw (*Ara ararauna*). J Avian Med Surg 2016;30(2):159–64.
40. Ozawa S, Mans C. Stifle disarticulation as a pelvic Limb amputation technique in a Cockatiel (*Nymphicus hollandicus*) and a Northern Cardinal (*Cardinalis cardinalis*). J Avian Med Surg 2017;1:33–8.
41. Latney L, Runge J, Wyre N, et al. Novel technique for scapulohumeral amputations in avian species: a case series. Isr J Vet Med 2018;73(1):35–45.
42. Heatley JJ, Tully TN Jr, Mitchell MA, et al. Trauma-induced aneurysmal bone cysts in 2 psittacine species (Cacatua alba and Nymphicus hollandicus). J Zoo Wild Med 2004;35(2):185–96.
43. Rush EM, Shores A, Meintel S, et al. Growing skull fracture in a red-tailed hawk (Buteo jamaicensis). J Zoo Wild Med 2014;45(3):658–63.

Avian Articular Orthopedics

Mikel Sabater González, LV, CertZooMed, DECZM (Avian), MRCVS

KEYWORDS

• Avian • Articular • Orthopedic • Surgery • Luxation

KEY POINTS

• Luxations and subluxations occur infrequently in birds compared with other orthopedic conditions.
• Avian joints present unique anatomic conformations.
• Luxations and subluxations can be managed conservatively or surgically.
• The extrapolation of surgical techniques described in nonavian species to avian ones is not always successful due to anatomic differences.

INTRODUCTION

The term joint luxation refers to the complete displacement of a bone from the joint, whereas in a subluxation the bone is only partially displaced and some contact between the 2 articular surfaces still occurs. In most avian species, luxations occur infrequently compared with other orthopedic conditions.[1] A comprehensive review of the frequency, etiology, clinical presentation, diagnosis, and treatment of luxations in birds is published in 2014.[2]

The aim of this article was to describe from an orthopedic point of view the different types of luxations reported in birds, the surgical treatment, and, whenever possible, the potential limitations and complications related to these procedures.

CORACOID LUXATIONS

The coracoid, the scapula, and the clavicle comprise the avian thoracic girdle. The coracoid articulates proximally with the sternum and distally with the humerus, clavicle, and scapula. Coracoid luxations are uncommon in birds.[3] Unilateral caudoventral luxation of the left coracoid, affecting its distal articulation with the clavicle and its proximal articulation with the sternum, has been reported in a bald eagle (*Haliaeetus leucocephalus*) that presented also with a tibiotarsal fracture.[3] A ventral approach to coracoid was achieved by performing an incision over the clavicle and extending it along the cranial half of the sternum, which was followed by the severing and caudal

Disclosure Statement: The author has nothing to disclose.
Exoticsvet, Marques de San Juan 23-5, Valencia 46015, Spain
E-mail address: exoticsvet@gmail.com

retraction of the superficial and deep pectoral muscles from the cranial attachment to the clavicle.[3] The luxation affecting the coracoid-sternum articulation was repaired by using a T-plate and a dynamic compression plate placed side by side. The luxation affecting the coracoid and the clavicle was repaired with 2 cerclage wires passed through the coracoid around the clavicle. The bird was released 105 days after the first surgery.[3]

SHOULDER JOINT ORTHOPEDICS

The shoulder joint is formed by the *facies articularis humeri* and the ellipsoid head of the humerus. The *facies articularis humeri* is composed of 2 separated articular surfaces: the *processus glenoidalis* of the coracoid, the major component of the facies, and the *facies articularis scapularis*. The joint capsule comprises the *fibrocartilago humeroscapularis* incorporated into its dorsal section, the *ligamentum acrocoracohumerale* that connects the acrocoracoid process with the transverse groove on the proximal cranial aspect of the humerus, the *ligamenta scapulohumeralia* extending between the scapula and the humerus and 2 intracapsular ligaments, covered in synovial folds. The surrounding musculature provides additional support to the joint capsule to prevent an excessive rotation of the humerus.[1,4] The supracoracoideus muscle and tendon are best developed in birds with a slow flapping flight, in those that hover and those with a rapid jump take off (eg, pheasants).[5]

As an ellipsoid joint, the shoulder has a wide range of movement. In the resting position with the humerus adducted, it lies along the trunk, whereas during gliding flight, it is abducted by up to 90°.[4] In hummingbirds, the wing can rotate almost 180° at the shoulder joint, providing lift but no thrust during hovering flight.[4]

In a study involving 49 wild birds with fractures of the shoulder girdle, 15 of them presented shoulder luxation.[6] Despite the shoulder joint is well-supported by muscle and ligaments, the tendon of the supracoracoideus muscle is sometimes stripped from the muscle belly. The tendon rupture provokes an upward subluxation of the head of the humerus.[5] Shoulder luxation is often accompanied by osseous fractures (eg, humerus or coracoid) and sometimes by brachial plexus avulsion. Although the signs of avulsion of the roots of the brachial plexus are predominantly those of radial nerve paralysis at the level of the shoulder, multiple nerve deficits (including Horner syndrome) may be observed.[7] Electromyography and nerve-conduction studies are useful when evaluating suspected cases of brachial avulsion.[7]

Close reduction and external coaptation (bandaging the wing to the body) for 10 to 14 days may be effective for mild cases. Open reduction may be attempted when close reduction is not possible. A dorsal surgical approach is preferred and requires a longitudinal incision of the *dermotensor patagii*. The prognosis is considered poor for severe luxations (eg, those in which the tendon is unable to recover its function after luxation reduction) in individuals requiring complete flight restoration. Reluxation after treatment is common.[8]

ELBOW LUXATION

The avian elbow is a shallow synovial joint consisting of 3 joints enclosed by a single capsule: the humeroradial joint composed of the dorsal condyle of the humerus and the humeral cotyla of the radius, the humeroulnar joint composed of the ventral and dorsal condyle of the humerus and the ventral and dorsal cotyla of the ulna, and the proximal radioulnar joint composed of the radial incisure of the ulna and ulnar articular surface of the radius. Within the capsule, the radioulnar meniscus is located between the dorsal humeral condyle and the dorsal cotyla of the ulna. Stability of the joint is achieved by a weak capsule, the dorsal and ventral collateral ligaments, the cranial cubital ligament, and the tendon of the muscle *flexor carpi ulnaris.*[1]

Movement of the elbow joint consists mainly of flexion and extension. The extension of the elbow results in the longitudinal displacement of the radius with respect to the ulna, which provokes the concordant extension of the carpus and, if fully extended, the rotation of the bones of the antebrachium about the longitudinal axis.[1]

The prevalence of elbow luxation in raptors presented to 2 different rescue centers was 12% (8/65) and 2% (11/568).[9,10] A different study reported 18 elbow luxations in 239 wing fracture cases.[6] According to 2 different case series in raptors, the most common type of luxation was caudodorsal (62.5% [5/8] and 8% [11/12]) followed by the caudal (37.5% [3/8] and 8.3% [1/12]).[9,10] Ventral luxation is possible when the radius is fractured.[9] In these case series, 3 of 12 and 3 of 7 individuals presenting with elbow luxations were released back to the wild.[9,10]

Under general anesthesia, the proximal radius and ulna are held with one hand, whereas the distal humerus is held with the other. Then, the elbow is flexed to counteract the forces of the scapulotriceps muscle, which tends to pull the ulna caudally. After this, the radius and ulna are rotated internally with pressure on the proximal radius to bring the radial head into alignment with the dorsal condyle. If the radius and ulna and their transverse ligament are intact, the ulna should return into place as the elbow is extended.[9]

One red-tailed hawk (*Buteo jamaicensis*) and one bald eagle (*H leucocephalus*) responded well to close reduction of the luxation and 7 days of wing bandage.[9] Open surgical reduction through a ventral approach may be difficult because of the presence of blood vessels and nerves in the area. In case of caudodorsal or dorsal luxation, a dorsal approach to the elbow joint has been described.[10] The dorsal approach avoids the various nerves, arteries, and veins that cross and branch at the elbow joint ventrally. The feathers are plucked from the distal humerus to the middle of the antebrachium dorsally. A curvilinear incision should be made over the distal end of the humerus, extending distally between the radius and ulna and taking care not to damage the branches of the radial nerve or the insertion of the *tensor propatagialis* (*pars brevis*) tendon. The supinator muscle is transected near its end on the humerus, allowing access to the elbow joint.[11] Once the luxation is corrected, additional stability to the joint could be provided by suturing the origin of the *extensor digitorum communis* tendon to the insertion of the biceps tendon.[10] Then the transected supinator muscle can be sutured again. If the elbow remains stable, a figure-of-8 bandage should be applied for 7 to 12 days.[9] If contrarily, the elbow is unstable, external fixation is recommended.

Multiple options for external fixation have been reported. A great horned owl was treated with a type I external fixator composed of 3 Kirschner (K) pins inserted in the dorsal aspect of the distal humerus, 3 more in the dorsal aspect of the proximal radius, and 1 more in the dorsal aspect of the proximal ulna, all of them bent at right angles and connected with methyl methacrylate for 7 days.[9] In a peregrine falcon and an eastern screech owl, 2 pins were inserted in the dorsal humerus and 2 in the dorsal ulna, then 1 plastic tube was placed to connect the 2 humeral pins and another to connect the 2 ulnar pins, and a bent pin was used to connect both tubes in a partially extended angle before the tubes were filled with methyl methacrylate, stabilizing the external fixator.[10] A female prairie falcon was treated with a type II external fixator consisting of 1 K-pin placed in the humerus and another one in the ulna, connected dorsally and ventrally with methyl methacrylate crossbars for 12 days.[9] In those cases in which the bone may be not suitable for pin placement because of small size or high risk of potential fracture, a figure-of-8 may be of utility as reported in a merlin (*Falco columbarius*).[10] Following removal of bandages or external fixators, a 3-stage progressive physical therapy may be instituted: (1) passive range of motion, (2) active and active assisted range of motion, and (3) free flight for endurance.[9]

CARPOMETACARPAL AND METACARPOPHALANGEAL JOINT LUXATIONS

The bones comprising the joints of the carpus are the radius, the ulna, the radial carpal, the ulnar carpal, and the carpometacarpus. The intercarpal meniscus is located between the radial and ulnar carpal bones. Numerous ligaments interconnect the bones of the carpal joint. The carpus functions as a hinge joint that is extended and flexed in synchrony with the elbow in response to the sliding movements of the radius and ulna during the extension and flexion of the elbow.[1] Sporadic cases of carpal joint luxation have been reported.[2] Carpal luxations can be treated with a figure-of-8 bandage for 7 to 12 days or with open reduction and type I external skeletal fixation (ESF).[2] Open reduction of carpal dislocations are done through a ventral approach.[11] Natural healing has been reported in a canvasduck.[2]

The alular, major, minor digits articulate with the carpometacarpus by means of synovial metacarpophalangeal joints. The major digit presents also an interphalangeal joint. The articulations of the major and minor digits function as hinge joints, whereas the alular digit can move in multiple directions.[1] The management of metacarpophalangeal joint luxations in a bald eagle (*H leucocephalus*) and a red-tailed hawk (*B jamaicensis*) with closed reduction and stabilization with a type 1 external skeletal fixator alone or in conjunction with a splint did not restore joint stability and resulted in an unsatisfactory outcome.[12] However, a juvenile prairie falcon (*Falco mexicanus*) and an adult female great horned owl (*Bubo virginianus*) with dorsal luxations of the metacarpophalangeal joint were treated with type I external fixator to achieve arthrodesis, and this allowed them to restore full flight capacity. The ventral surgical approach to the joint was used.[12]

COXOFEMORAL JOINT

The coxofemoral joint is diarthrodial. In the coxocapital joint, the fibrocartilaginous acetabular *labrum* articulates with the head of the femur and is anchored to the acetabular socket by the ligament of the femoral head. In the coxotrochanteric joint, the antitrochanter articulates with the articular surface of the femoral neck and the trochanter restricting abduction of the limb and reducing bending stress on the femur.[4] The stability of the coxofemoral joint is maintained by the articular capsule, multiple ligaments, and the surrounding muscles. Multiple ligaments attach the ilium, ischium, and pubis to the femur.[4] The ventral collateral and the round ligament play major roles for the proper position of the femoral head in the acetabulum, especially in noncursorial species (eg, psittacines, hawks, falcons, owls, and pigeons) with a gliding hinge joint that primarily moves in a cranial-caudal plane.[13] Contrarily, a ball-socket–type joint is present in cursorial species (eg, ratites).[14] The sciatic nerve, artery, and vein course along the caudal aspect of the femur, whereas the femoral nerve, artery, and vein are found cranial and medial to the femur. The femoral and ischiatic veins often anastomose medially along the proximal one-fourth of the femur. The obturator nerve is deep medially to the proximal femur.[13]

Coxofemoral joint luxation is more common in birds weighing up to 1 kg.[2] Luxations are usually craniodorsal to the acetabulum with the knee displaced laterally almost at a 90° angle, although cranioventral luxations may occur.[11,15] If closed reduction is possible and the joint remains stable, a spica-type splint may be effective.[13] If open reduction is necessary, an incision is made from the wing of the ilium caudally around the trochanter major and continued distally along the caudal aspect of the femur, as needed. The *iliotibialis cranialis* and *iliotibialis lateralis* muscles are separated longitudinally from the *iliofibularis* muscle and retracted. Then, the *iliotrochantericus caudalis* is incised near its insertion, exposing the acetabulum, and the joint capsule is incised along the acetabular rim.[13] If reduction is achieved in a species with a gliding hinge-type coxofemoral joint, a nonabsorbable suture may be passed through the trochanter major and then passed through the dorsal rim of the ischium, caudal to the acetabulum, and another suture may be passed from the trochanter major to the dorsal rim of the ilium, cranial to the acetabulum, and then both sutures are tightened and tied with a surgeon's knot.[13,14] The use of these sutures may not be appropriate in species with a ball and socket-type coxofemoral joint.[14] Alternatively, nonabsorbable suture can be passed from the lateral aspect to medial aspect of the femoral head and neck, and then though the dorsal rim of the acetabulum, as has been reported in a black-crowned night heron (*Nycticorax nycticorax*).[15] A different surgical technique in which a K-pin is introduced through the acetabular protuberance and then through the greater trochanter to create tunnels for a prosthetic ligament made of nonabsorbable woven multifilament suture tied in a figure-of-8 pattern has been reported in 2 cormorants (*Phalacrocorax carbo*).[16] Then, the joint capsule is closed in a simple interrupted pattern, the caudal iliotrochanteric muscle is sutured to its attachment at the trochanter major, and the cranial and lateral bellies of the *iliotibialis* muscle are reapposed in a simple continuous pattern. Skin is closed in a simple interrupted pattern and a spica-type splint is applied.[13] The use of a transarticular pin or a prosthetic ligament of the femoral head anchored with a toggle pin behind the acetabulum are techniques reported in other species but dangerous in birds because of the location of the kidney within the pelvis directly adjacent to the acetabulum.[13]

If reduction of the coxofemoral joint fails, femoral head and neck ostectomy may be considered. The lateral approach is used for the open reduction and stabilization of the coxofemoral joint or for excision arthroplasty of the femoral head. The femoral head and neck are transected with an osteotome or oscillating saw, and the remaining bone edges smoothed with a rongeur or a file. Stabilizing sutures, described before, are used to prevent external rotation of the femur. Muscle layers are closed as previously described. Following femoral ostectomy, early use of the leg is encouraged to create a fibrous pseudoarthrosis.[11]

FEMOROTIBIAL JOINT

The knee joint consists of 4 individual synovial intercommunicating joints enclosed by a joint cavity. The medial femoral condyle articulates with the medial meniscus and tibiotarsus. The lateral femoral condyle articulates with the lateral meniscus, tibiotarsus, and fibula. The femoropatellar joint is the articulation of the patellar sulcus with the patella. The patella is incorporated onto the cnemial crest in gaviiforms, ciconiforms, and podicipediforms.[17] An ossified patella is not observed in the emu.[18] The proximal tibiotarsus articulates with the fibular head. The lateral and the medial menisci augment the congruence of the femorotibial joint. The main supporting structures of the stifle joint are the joint capsule, medial and lateral collateral ligaments, cranial and caudal cruciate ligaments, menisci, joint capsule, and the tendon of the musculi femorotibiales and the musculature surrounding it. The medial collateral ligament originates in the medial femoral condyle and inserts on the medial aspect of the proximal tibiotarsus; the lateral collateral ligament originates in the lateral femoral condyle and inserts on the proximal lateral fibula. The cranial cruciate ligament connects intercondylarly the caudal lateral femoral condyle with the center of the tibial plateau, whereas the caudal cruciate ligament connects the caudal femoral intercondylar groove with the posterior medial tibial condyle.[19] The cruciate ligaments restrict extension and flexion of the knee.[19]

Luxations of the femorotibial joint are common in birds and tend to occur craniolaterally, craniomedially, caudolaterally, and caudomedially with concomitant damage to the collateral and cruciate ligament, whereas meniscal damage is rarely diagnosed (**Fig. 1**).[2] The muscular contraction frequently present after luxation may difficult its correction. Muscle and nerve damage may cause paresis or paralysis of the extremity, resulting in ambulatory, perching, or gripping difficulties.[2]

Stabilization of femorotibial luxations by external coaptation or combinations or not of intra-articular and extra-articular surgical techniques have been described.

In many species (eg, psittacines), the inguinal web extends nearly to the level of the stifle, limiting the proximal extension of the external coaptation.[19] However, external coaptation may be useful in neonates or small-sized birds in which the size of the structures involved precludes surgical stabilization (**Fig. 2**). Immobilizing the legs with a semirigid foam splint has been reported in a 35-day-old cockatiel (*Nymphicus hollandicus*).[20] The author has observed functional recovery of the leg in psittacine neonates treated with external coaptation made with an Altmann tape splint.

Intra-articular repair attempts to retain postoperative mobility of the joint by directly repairing or replacing damaged ligaments to allow rapid return to function, but may be not feasible because the small size of the ligaments and associated soft tissues in small to medium avian species precludes surgical reapposition and repair (**Fig. 3**).[19] Surgical treatment for right medial femorotibiotarsal subluxation with damage to the lateral meniscus, tendon of origin of the cranial tibial muscle, and cranial cruciate ligament in a 3-month-old umbrella cockatoo (*Cacatua alba*) has been reported. A lateral parapatellar approach was selected and followed by debridement of the disrupted meniscus and reduction of the luxation. The femorotibiotarsal joint was stabilized by using a lateral extracapsular suture in a modified technique using a self-tapping cortical screw in the lateral femoral condyle and a hole through the proximal tibiotarsus. Severe osteoarthrosis of the stifle joint and persistent implant migration were confirmed radiographically 209 days after surgery. The screw was removed but ankylosis in a physiologic perching angle had already occurred.[19]

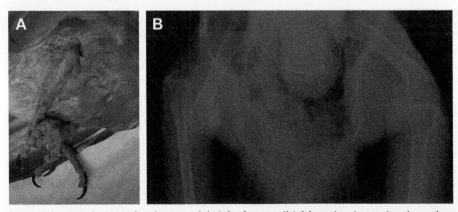

Fig. 1. (*A*) Lateral view of a dorsocaudal right femorotibial luxation in a mitred parakeet (*Psittacara mitratus*). (*B*) Craniocaudal radiographic view of the luxation. (*Courtesy of* Mikel Sabater, LV, CertZooMed, DECZM (Avian), Exoticsvet, Valencia, Spain.)

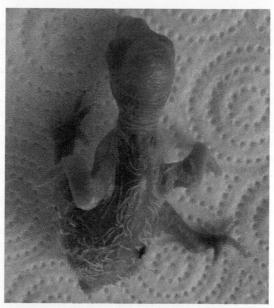

Fig. 2. Right femorotibial joint luxation in a neonate rainbow lorikeet (*Trichoglossus moluccanus*). (*Courtesy of* Mikel Sabater, LV, CertZooMed, DECZM (Avian), Exoticsvet, Valencia, Spain.)

The stabilization of a reduced stifle luxation with a transarticular ESF at a normal perching angle until periarticular fibrosis occurs, has the potential to result in more complete restoration of limb usage than external coaptation alone.[19] The proper angle must be established, because a joint fixed in an overextended angle will cause the animal to circumduct while ambulating, whereas a joint fixed in an overflexed angle will

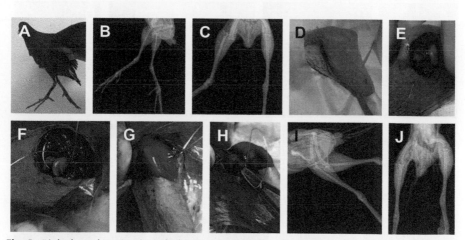

Fig. 3. Right knee luxation in a dusky moorhen (*Gallinula tenebrosa*). The collaterals and the cruciate ligaments are broken. (*A*) Luxation. (*B, C*) LL and VD radiographic projections showing the caudolateral femorotibial luxation. (*D*) Macroscopic view of the luxation. (*E*) Distal epiphysis of the right femur showing fractured cruciate ligaments. (*F*) Prosthetic (Nylon) cruciate ligament (intra-articular stabilization). (*G, H*) Circumferential prosthesis (Nylon) in the right femorotibial joint placement (extra-articular stabilization). (*I*) Postoperative LL radiographic view. (*J*) Postoperative VD radiographi view. LL, latero-lateral; VD, ventro-dorsal. (*Courtesy of* Mikel Sabater, LV, CertZooMed, DECZM (Avian), Exoticsvet, Valencia, Spain.)

cause functional shortening of the limb and alter the mechanical loads and propulsive and breaking forces on both limbs, which could also predispose to pododermatitis.[19] The perching-joint angles were radiographically investigated in cockatiels (*N hollandicus*), Hispaniolan Amazon parrots (*Amazona ventralis*), and barred owls (*Strix varia*).[21]

An extracapsular stabilization technique was used to repair cruciate ligament ruptures in a trumpeter hornbill (*Bycanistes bucinator*) and an African gray parrot (*Psittacus erithacus*). Circumferential nonabsorbable sutures passed through bone tunnels created in the distal femur and proximal tibiotarsus, mimic the function of the collateral ligaments, and allow movement of the joint but do not stabilize the cranial to caudal movement (drawer sign) (**Fig. 4**).[22] Stifle luxation repair by extracapsular articular stabilization technique with nonabsorbable suture has been reported in a white-fronted goose and a domestic pigeon.[23]

In pigeons with experimentally induced mediocaudal stifle luxation, the use of a FESSA (Fixeteur Externe du Service de Sante des Armees) hinged model maintained joint mobility (allowing physiotherapy without compromising stabilization) but resulted in reduced range of motion, regressive lameness, pododermatitis, fibrosis of the operated joint capsule, reduced synovial fluid production, excessive callus formation with osteophyte formation, and muscle atrophy of the affected limb.[24]

A craniolateral luxation in a monk parakeet (*Myiopsitta monachus*) was treated with closed luxation reduction and stabilization with one intramedullary pin inserted from the distal femur, another inserted from the proximal tibiotarsus, bent and connected in a normal perching angle (**Fig. 5**). A successful recovery of knee function was reported after pin removal, probably due to lack of articular damage.[25] Using this technique, osteomyelitis was reported as a complication of a stifle luxation repair in an adult female Solomon Island eclectus parrot (*Eclectus roratus solomonensis*), which ended requiring mid-femoral amputation of the leg as a salvage procedure.[26]

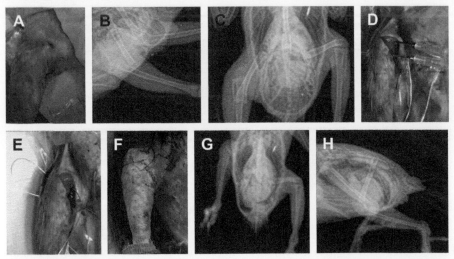

Fig. 4. (*A*) Frontal view of the right femorotibial joint luxation in an eclectus parrot (*Eclectus roratus*). (*B*) Preoperative LL radiographic projection of the luxation. (*C*) Preoperative VD radiographic projection of the luxation. (*D,E*) Circumferential prosthesis (Nylon) in the right femorotibial joint placement from a medial approach (extra-articular stabilization). (*F*) Postoperative appearance of the knee. (*G*) Postoperative LL radiographic projection of the luxation. (*H*) Postoperative VD radiographic projection of the luxation. (*Courtesy of* Mikel Sabater, LV, CertZooMed, DECZM (Avian), Exoticsvet, Valencia, Spain.)

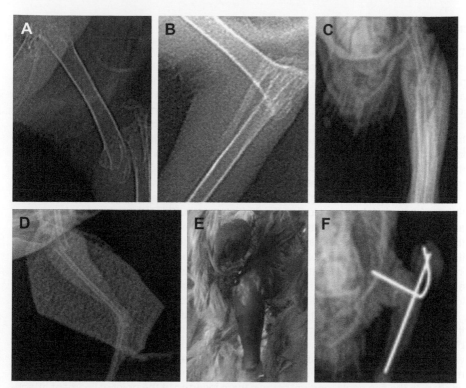

Fig. 5. Left femorotibial luxation in a cockatiel (*Nymphicus hollandicus*). (*A, B*) Radiographic projections of the right knee. (*C*) Radiograhic VD projection showing an unsuccessful correction of the luxation with an Altman's splint. (*D*) Radiograhic LL projection showing an unsuccessful correction of the luxation with an Altman's splint. (*E*) Extracapsular stabilization with 2 intramedullary pins (1 in the femur and 1 in the tibiotarsus) connected with epoxy. (*F*) Postoperative anteroposterior radiographic view (please note the diameter of the pins was excessive for this diameter of bone). (*Courtesy of* Mikel Sabater, LV, Cert-ZooMed, DECZM (Avian), Exoticsvet, Valencia, Spain.)

If severe, extensive, or irreparable damage to the joint is observed, permanent arthrodesis in a normal perching angle allows return to function of the leg as a unit and minimizes pain and discomfort. The main complication related to arthrodesis is permanent abnormal ambulation.[19] The use of a type I external fixator consisting of multiple pins inserted from the lateral aspect of the femur and tibiotarsus and connected with methylmethacrylate or thermoplastic splint material until arthrodesis was observed, has been reported in a Moluccan cockatoo (*Cacatua moluccensis*), a barn owl (*Tyto alba*) and a military macaw (*Ara militaris*).[27,28] A type II transarticular external fixator was used in a blue-fronted Amazon parrot (*Amazona aestiva*).[29]

A pilot study in domestic pigeons (*Columba livia domestica*) about the management of femorotibial luxation by coaptation splinting, intramedullary pins, external skeletal fixator, and tension bands reported that all the techniques performed represented a viable option to luxation repair and provoke minimal damage to the articular surfaces and no significant histologic differences in periarticular fibrosis tissue and bone reaction were observed among the different groups. However, decreased anesthetic and surgical duration was seen with single band tension, whereas splinting and open surgical management may increase morbidity. The formation of scar tissue to stabilize the joint requires 3 to 6 weeks.[30]

INTERTARSAL JOINT

The intertarsal joint is the synovial roll-and-glide articulation of the tibiotarsus with the tarsometatarsus. A lateral and usually also a medial C-shaped meniscus are interposed between the articulating bones and attached by ligaments to the tarsometatarsus and tibiotarsus.[4] The medial and lateral collateral ligaments restrict the movement of the joint to flexion and extension. The intercondylar tibiometatarsal ligament connects the intercondylar eminence of the tarsometatarsus with the intercondylar sulcus of the tibiotarsus, limiting the cranial-caudal sliding movement.[4] The fibrocartilaginous tibial cartilage is attached to the caudal aspect of the intertarsal joint, and presents canals for the deep flexors and grooves on its surface (eg, in hawks) or canals (eg, in parrots) for the gastrocnemius muscle and the superficial digital flexors.[4,31]

The rupture of the retaining retinaculum may provoke the displacement of the entire tibial cartilage in falcons, including the flexor tendons. The retinaculum can be sutured again.[31] The most frequent dislocation involves the tendon of the long flexor muscle of the hallux, which remains laterally displaced in the lateral aspect of the tibial cartilage. If diagnosed early, the tendon may be surgically repositioned.[31] Less frequently, the insertion of the medial gastrocnemius muscle pulls away from the tibial cartilage and allows the cartilage, the flexor tendons and the tarsometatarsus to rotate laterally (or the whole tibial cartilage displaces medially, with rotation of the tarsometatarsus).[31]

Correction with polyester fiber suture of intertarsal joint luxation due to avulsion of the tendon of the long flexor muscle of the hallux has been reported in a rooster.[32] Stability and good range of movement were achieved after treating intertarsal luxations with rupture of the lateral short and long ligaments and stretching of the medial ligament in 1 Siberian eagle owl (*Bubo bubo sibiricus*) and 1 African fish eagle (*Haliaeetus vocifer*). In the fish eagle, cortical screws were inserted at the point of ligament attachment in the tibiotarsal condyli and the tarsometatarsal cotyli (both laterally and medially), a figure-of-8 suture was placed between the screws, and a type II external fixateur was applied to stabilize the joint for 3 weeks. In the eagle owl, transcondylar pins were used instead of cortical screws.[33] Extracapsular surgical correction of the medial collateral ligament using bone tunnels and circumferential nylon suture on the medial aspect of the intertarsal joint led to a complete clinical resolution with normal return to function 2 weeks after surgery in a Pekin duck (*Anas platyrhynchos domesticus*).[34] Intertarsal joint stabilization with a braided suture and titanium button system has been reported in a bateleur eagle (*Terathopius ecaudatus*). The braided suture was passed from the lateral aspect of the intertarsal joint through 2 intraosseous tunnels created at the distal tibiotarsus and proximal tarsometatarsus. Each end of the suture was threaded through both holes of a 2-hole titanium button, passed back through each respective intraosseous tunnel, and secured with a surgeon's knot.[35] The use of an elastic transarticular external construct has been reported as a successful surgical treatment for an intertarsal joint luxation on a Harris hawk (*Parabuteo unicinctus*).[36]

Amputation can be considered a salvage procedure in small avian species (eg, canaries, budgerigars). In larger species, it frequently results in pododermatitis of the contralateral foot.[2]

METATARSAL JOINT

The metatarsal joint consists of the distal row of tarsal bones and the metatarsal bones of digits II, III, and IV. Birds with 4 digits present a syndesmosis with metatarsal I.[37] The metatarsals are incompletely fused in penguins.[37] Various ligaments extend between metatarsal I and the tarsometatarsus.[4] The metatarsophalangeal joints appear to be less susceptible to luxations and may be dislocated without ligamentous damage.[31] Therapeutic alternatives for metatarsal joint luxation include close reduction and open reduction with or without tenorrhaphy.

METATARSOPHALANGEAL AND INTERPHALANGEAL JOINT LUXATIONS

These joints are stabilized by an articular capsule, paired collateral ligaments, and a plantar ligament that reinforces the plantar aspect of the articular capsule and reduces the pressure on the flexor tendons.[4] In case of luxation, surgical correction of the tendons, ligaments, and the articular capsule may be attempted. However, when the size of the structures prevents surgical repair, arthrodesis or amputation may be considered.

LUXATIONS OF THE PTERYGOID-PARASPHENOID-PALATINE COMPLEX ('PALATINE BONE LUXATION') AND LUXATION OF THE HYOID APPARATUS

These luxations have been covered in the article written by Minh Huynh and colleagues, "Avian skull orthopedics," elsewhere in this issue.

REFERENCES

1. Maierl J, König KE, Liebich HG, et al. Thoracic limb (membrum thoracicum). In: König KE, Korbel R, Liebich HG, editors. Avian anatomy. Textbook and colour atlas. 2nd edition. Sheffield (United Kingdom): 5M Publishing Ltd; 2016. p. 45–61.

2. Azmanis PN, Wernick MB, Hatt JM. Avian luxations: occurrence, diagnosis and treatment. Vet Q 2014;34(1):11–21.

3. Sánchez-Migallón Guzman D, Bubenik LJ, Lauer SK, et al. Repair of a coracoid luxation and a tibiotarsal fracture in a bald eagle (*Haliaeetus leucocephalus*). J Avian Med Surg 2007;21(3):188–95.

4. Maierl J, König KE, Liebich HG, et al. Pelvic limb (membrum pelvinum). In: König KE, Korbel R, Liebich HG, editors. Avian anatomy. Textbook and colour atlas. 2nd edition. Sheffield (United Kingdom): 5M Publishing Ltd; 2016. p. 45–6.

5. Coles B. Surgery. In: Coles B, editor. Essentials of avian medicine and surgery. 3rd edition. Ames (IA): Blackwell Publishing; 2007. p. 142–82.

6. Schuster S, Krautwald-Junghanns M-E. Untersuchungen zu Häufigkeit, lokalisation und art von frakturen beim vogel. [[examination of the frequency, localization and type of fractures in birds]]. Giessen (Germany): Justus-Liebig Universität; 1996.

7. Smith SA. Diagnosis of brachial plexus avulsion in three free-living owls. In: Redig PT, Cooper JE, Remple D, et al, editors. Raptor biomedicine. Minneapolis (MN): University of Minnesota Press; 1993. p. 99–102.

8. Bennett RA, Altman BR. Orthopedic surgery. In: Altman BR, Clubb LS, Dorrestein GM, et al, editors. Avian medicine. 1st edition. London: Saunders; 1997. p. 733–66.

9. Martin HD, Bruecker KA, Herrick DD, et al. Elbow luxations in raptors: a review of eight cases. In: Redig PT, Cooper JE, Remple JD, et al, editors. Raptor biomedicine. Minneapolis (MN): University of Minnesota Press; 1993. p. 199–206.

10. Ackermann J, Redig PT. Surgical repair of elbow luxation in raptors. J Avian Med Surg 1997;11:247–54.

11. Orosz SE, Ensley PK, Haynes CJ. Anatomy and surgical approaches to the wing. In: Orosz SE, Ensley PK, Haynes CJ, editors. Avian surgical anatomy. Thoracic and pelvic limbs. Philadelphia: W. B. Saunders company; 1992.

12. Van Wettere AJ, Redig PT. Arthrodesis as a treatment for metacarpophalangeal joint luxation in 2 raptors. J Avian Med Surg 2004;18(1):23–9.

13. Martin HD, Kabler R, Sealing L. The avian coxofemoral joint: a review of regional anatomy and report of an open reduction technique for repair of a coxofemoral luxation. J Assoc Avian Vet 1994;8:164–72.

14. Martin D, Ritchie W. Orthopedic surgical techniques. In: Ritchie WR, Harrison JG, editors. Avian medicine principles and applications. 1st edition. Lake Worth (FL): Wingers Publishing; 1994. p. 1139–69.

15. Kim EJ, Lee JH, Kim MS, et al. Surgical repair of coxofemoral joint luxation in a wild black-crowned night heron (Nycticorax nycticorax). Jap J Vet Clin 2013; 30(1):49–52.

16. Risi E, Ordonneau D, Gauthier O. Two cases of femoral head luxations in cormorants (Phalacrocorax carbo) treated with a modified Meij-Hazewinkel-Nap technique. In: Bailey T, Chitty J, Harcourt-Brown HN, et al, editors. Proceedings of the 8th European Association of Avian Veterinarians. Congress, April 24-30, 2005. p. 190–5. Arles (France).

17. Vickaryous MK. Osteoblast and osteocyte diversity. In: Hall BK, editor. Bones and cartilage: developmental and evolutionary skeletal biology. 1st edition. London: Elsevier Academic Press; 2005. p. 328–37.

18. Regnault S, Pitsillides AA, Hutchinson JR. Structure, ontogeny and evolution of the patellar tendon in emus (Dromaius novaehollandiae) and other palaeognath birds. PeerJ 2014;2(7):e711.

19. McRee A, Tully TN, Nevarez JG, et al. A novel surgical approach to avian femorotibiotarsal luxation repair. J Avian Med Surg 2017;31(2):156–64.

20. Luparello M, Faraci L, Di Giuseppe M, et al. Correction of neonatal stifle luxation in a 35-day-old cockatiel (Nymphicus hollandicus). J Small Anim Pract 2016;57: 653–4.

21. Bonin G, Lauer SK, Sanchez-Migallón Guzmán D, et al. Radiographic evaluation of perching-joint angles in cockatiels (Nymphicus hollandicus), Hispaniolan Amazon parrots (Amazona ventralis), and barred owls (Strix varia). J Avian Med Surg 2009;23(2):91–100.

22. Chinnadurai SK, Spodnick G, Degernes L, et al. Use of an extracapsular stabilization technique to repair cruciate ligament ruptures in two avian species. J Avian Med Surg 2009;23:307–13.

23. Fukui D, Bando G, Kosuge M. Stifle luxation repair by articular stabilization technique with non-absorbable suture in a white-fronted goose and therapeutical trial in a domestic pigeon. Japanese J Zoo Wildl Med 2005;10:49–52.

24. Azmanis P. The effect of early physical therapy after experimental stifle luxation in domestic pigeons (Columba livia domestica), managed with a combination of extracapsular stabilization technique and FESSA hinged linear external skeletal fixator (FESSA-HLESF). Zurich (Switzerland): Zurich Open Repository and Archive. University of Zurich; 2011. p. 1–147.

25. Bowles HL, Zantop DW. A novel surgical technique for luxation repair of the femorotibial joint in a monk parakeet (Myiopsitta monachus). J Avian Med Surg 2002; 16:34–8.

26. Harris MC, Diaz-Figueroa O, Lauer SK, et al. Complications associated with conjoined intramedullary pin placement for a femorotibial joint luxation in a

Solomon Island Eclectus parrot (*Eclectus roratus solomonensis*). J Avian Med Surg 2007;21:299–306.

27. Rosenthal K, Hillyer E, Mathiessen D. Stifle luxation repair in a Moluccan cockatoo and a barn owl. J Assoc Avian Vet 1994;8:173–8.

28. Donato NL. Stifle arthrodesis in a military Macaw. Utilizing safe, hazardous and danger zones. Proceedings of the Association of Avian Veterinarians Annual Conference. Portland (USA), August 30 - September 1, 2000. p. 121–6.

29. Alievi MM, Hippler RA, Giacomelli L, et al. External skeletal fixation for arthrodesis of the knee joint in a parrot (*Amazona aestiva*). Cienc Rural 2001;31:1069–72.

30. Villaverde S, de la Víbora BJ, González R, et al. Management of the femorotibial luxation by coaptation splinting, intramedullary pins, external skeletal fixator and tension bands: a pilot study in domestic pigeons (*Columba livia domestica*). In: Proceedings of the 8th European Association of Avian Veterinarians. Congress, April 24-30, 2005. p. 196–202. Arles (France).

31. Harcourt-Brown HN. Orthopedic conditions that affect the avian pelvic limb. Vet Clin North Am Exot Anim Pract 2002;5:49–81.

32. Demirkan I, Kilic E. Correction of the intertarsal joint luxation in a rooster by a polyester fibre suture. Vet Cerrahi Derg 2003;9:59–61.

33. Zsivanovits P, Monks D, Forbes N. A bilateral valgus deformity of the distal wings (Angel wing) in a Northern Goshawk (*Accipiter gentilis*). J Avian Med Surg 2006; 20:21–6.

34. Baron HR, Phalen DN, Sabater González M. A novel technique for extracapsular repair of the intertarsal joint in a duck. J Avian Med Surg 2017;32(1):57–64.

35. Gjeltema J, De Voe RS, Minter LJ, et al. Intertarsal joint stabilization in a bateleur eagle (*Terathopius ecaudatus*) using a novel application of a braided suture and titanium button system. Case Rep Vet Med 2017;2017:7373242.

36. Loucachevsky T, Risi E, Potier R, et al. Use of an elastic transarticular external construct for surgical treatment of an intertarsal joint luxation on a Harris's hawk (Parabuteo unicinctus). Proceedings Joint EAZWV/AAZV/Leibniz-IZW Conference. Prague, Czech Republic, October 6–12, 2018. p. 57–8.

37. King AS, McLelland J. Skeletomuscular system. In: King AS, editor. McLelland. Birds. Their structure and function. 2nd edition. Philadelphia: Baillière Tindall; 1984. p. 43–78.

Avian Skull Orthopedics

Minh Huynh, DVM, DECZM (Avian), DACZM[a],
Mikel Sabater González, LV, CertZooMed, DECZM (Avian), MRCVS[b],*,
Hugues Beaufrére, DVM, PhD, DABVP (Avian Practice), DECZM (Avian), DACZM[c]

KEYWORDS

- Avian • Skull • Trauma • Orthopedics • Beak • Stabilization • Prosthesis

KEY POINTS

- The clinical approach to avian skull orthopedic cases starts with a physical examination and, if required, the stabilization of the bird.
- The avian jaw apparatus is complex and presents a great variability with clinical implications between species.
- The peer reviewed literature concerning the management of skull disorders in birds is relatively limited and further studies are warranted.

 Video content accompanies this article at http://www.vetexotic.theclinics.com.

INTRODUCTION

Because the avian skull is the reflection of the wide biodiversity of birds, many anatomic, morphologic, and functional variations are encountered. The main objectives of this article are to review the surgical considerations associated with the functional anatomy of the avian jaw apparatus and its variation among species, and to describe the general medical and surgical management of avian skull disorders.

ANATOMY AND KINESIS

One of the most striking features of the avian skull is the jaw apparatus, which encompasses the highly keratinized beak and a complex system of bony structures.

The beak external anatomy is made of 2 osseous projections, the *rostrum maxillare* and the *rostrum mandibulare*, covered by a horny sheath (the rhamphotheca), an analog to the lips and teeth of mammals.[1] The rhamphotheca can be divided in the rhinotheca (covers the upper beak) and the gnathotheca (covers the lower beak).[1]

The authors have nothing to disclose.
[a] Centre Hospitalier Vétérinaire Frégis, 43 Avenue Aristide Briand, Arcueil 94110, France; [b] Exoticsvet, Marques de San Juan 23-5, Valencia 46015, Spain; [c] Department of Clinical Studies, Ontario Veterinary College, University of Guelph, Guelph, ON N1G2W1, Canada
* Corresponding author.
E-mail address: exoticsvet@gmail.com

The beak originates from the epidermis and a dermis tightly attached to the periosteum of the rostrum. The stratum corneum is very thick and contains dead cells, regularly organized crystals of hydroxyapatite, phospholipids, and free calcium phosphate.[2] Hardness depends on the content of hydroxyapatite crystals and the degree of organization of the collagen fibers.[3] Keratin grows from the plates at the base of each bill and from the underlying dermis of the beak with varying contribution from the cere.[2] Keratin migrates rostrally along the surface of the beak and laterally from its vascular beds.[2]

In most terrestrial vertebrates, the movement of the jaws is restricted to a single paired joint between the mandible and the braincase. In birds, skull movements are much more complex owing to the multiple synovial joints (9–13) and syndesmotic joints (0–5) articulating the jaw.[4]

The avian skull can be described from different approaches (eg, anatomic, embryologic and kinetic). From a mechanical perspective, 4 kinematic units are distinguished[4] (**Fig. 1**):

- The upper jaw, which includes the paired premaxillary, nasal, maxillary, and sometimes the vomer and palatine bones. The so-called avian maxilla is different from its mammalian anatomic analog, which consist only in one maxillary bone.[5]
- The braincase.
- The skeleton of the palate consisting of the paired quadrate and pterygoid bones, the palatovomeral complex, and the paired jugal bars (also called the jugal arch).
- The lower jaw formed by the 2 rami of the mandible fused in a symphysis in the rostral midline.

Other elements of the skull include accessory bones (eg, in the tip of the tongue in the house sparrow [*Passer domesticus*], hyoid apparatus, columella, and scleral rings). An accessory postoccipital bone, the *os nuchale,* is present in cormorants[4,6] (**Fig. 2**).

The quadrate bones play a key role in every movement of the jaws, articulating both the lower jaw and the braincase as well as the upper and lower jaws.[4] Jaws are not independent because both are connected to the pivotal quadrate bone.[5] Any force applied will be transmitted through the apparatus, causing the movement of the bone in one direction or another.[1] The upper jaw is more or less rigid, usually moves as a whole (prokinesis), and articulates with the neurocranium by the craniofacial hinge.[1,4]

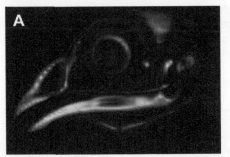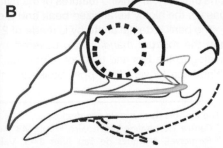

Fig. 1. Domestic fowl (*Gallus domesticus*) 3-dimensional reconstruction from a computed tomography scan. Anatomic annotation: upper jaw (*red*), palate (*blue*) composed of the jugal bars (*light blue filled*), quadrate (*light blue*), the palatovomeral complex and the pterygoid bones (*dark blue*), the mandibula (*brown*) and the brain case (*black*), scleral ossicles, and hyoid bone (*discontinuous lines*). (*Courtesy of* Minh Huynh, DVM, DECZM (Avian), DACZM, Centre Hospitalier Vétérinaire Frégis, Arcueil, France.)

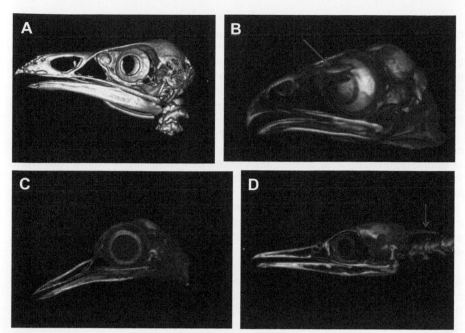

Fig. 2. Three-dimensional reconstruction from computed tomography scan in various birds. (*A*) Egyptian vulture (*Neophron percnopterus*). The maxilla and mandibula are elongated and narrow compared with avivores. (*B*) Black sparrowhawk (*Accipiter melanoleucus*). Note the prefrontal bone and superciliary bone (*red arrow*) on the craniodorsal aspect of the orbit, which compose the supraorbital ridge present in all raptors but the osprey. (*C*) Eurasian stone-curlew (*Burhinus oedicnemus*). The upper jaw is rhyncokinetic. (*D*) Little pied cormorant (*Microcarbo melanoleucos*). Note the os nuchale (*red arrow*). Most facial bones are not pneumatized in this species, and the quadrate bone has a very caudal position. (*Courtesy of* Minh Huynh, DVM, DECZM (Avian), DACZM, Centre Hospitalier Vétérinaire Frégis, Arcueil, France.)

The mandible has evolved into a single bone unit. In most birds, 7 pairs of muscle act together.[4] The *m. pterygoideus* is the main force of the jaw pulling the palatoquadrate bridge caudally and lowering the upper jaw.[4] In psittacines, a specific muscle derived from the *m. pterygoideus*, the *m. ethmomandibularis*, allows powerful biting forces and rostral movements of the lower jaw.[4] Muscle, anatomy, and innervation have been described previously.[7]

Variations of the Avian Skull and Rostrum

The development of the rostrum is independent of the development of the braincase and highly correlated with foraging methods. The incredible great morphologic variety of beaks in the class Aves results in that some species are more prone to trauma, such as long billed waders, long-legged birds, hummingbirds, or birds with very large beaks such as toucans and hornbills. In some birds, such as Charadriiformes, the upper jaw has rhynchokinetic mobility, which allows them to move a rostral part of the upper jaw[4] (see **Fig. 2**). The beak of these species presents 1 or several flexion zones within the bony structure such as the *zona elastica premaxillonasalis*.[4] Contrarily, very limited kinesis is observed in ratites, penguins, mousebirds, toucans, and hawfinches.[5]

External bony nares can be reduced or very large. In Pelecaniformes and in gannets (Suliformes), the nasal opening is lacking whereas in some other species, such as in Cathartiformes, the nares are open with a perforated intranasal septum.[4,8] In the kiwi, the nares are located at the tip of the beak and the nasal passages occupy the interior of the long tubelike rostrum.[8] A keratinized flap in the dorsal aspect of the nostril, the *operculum*, is present in some species.[8] The *operculum* of tapaculos is movable, whereas it is inverted forming a tubular structure in Procellariiformes.[8]

Some birds exhibit intermandibular mobility (eg, nightjars and pelicans).[4] Intraramal mandibular synovial joints in pelicans facilitate the swallowing of large prey. A joint has been also reported in loons, grebes, albatrosses, penguins, herons, storks, New World vultures, the great frigate bird (*Fregata minor*), and the brown booby (*Sula leucogaster*).[6]

Bones of the skull are pneumatized by air diverticula originating from the tympanic cavity (braincase) or the infraorbital sinus (other bones).[5] Pneumatization is reduced to absent in some aquatic birds, such as penguins, loons, grebes, cormorants, mergansers, and alcids.[5]

Skull osteologic differences may reflect the feeding behavior or other ecological adaptations of the species (see **Fig. 2**). Vultures have relatively long narrow curved maxillae compared with other raptors.[9] This is aimed to slice big part of meat, while the other is short and robust to produce strong bite and cut smaller pieces. Scavengers also have a deep, narrow ramus.[9] Narrow rami are probably less resistant to the twisting forces produced by struggling prey.[9] Hunting raptors have short maxillae with adductor muscle insertions further from the jaw joint. A wide maxilla and a strong symphysis would be more advantageous for a killer.[9] Piscivores have beaks with anatomic and functional characteristics closer to scavengers.[9] The position of the quadrate bones influences the opening of the beak. The more caudal the quadrates are, the more rapid the beak can close, which is especially important for insectivorous or piscivorous species.[10] Interestingly, the beak shape of nectarivorous birds such as hummingbirds and sunbirds is closely linked to the specific flowers they have coevolved with. Filtering species such as filtering ducks and flamingoes have numerous transverse lamellae on the inner tomia. Other interesting examples of beak and skull adaptations in birds are the beak conformations of crossbills, Recurvirostridae or oystercatchers, the casques of hornbills, and the hyoid apparatus of woodpeckers.

The Psittacine Skull

Psittaciformes present a wide skull variability (**Fig. 3**). Most species have a thick and short beak used to crack hard seeds and nuts. The maxillary rostrum is deep and decurved, the mandible is deep and broader than the maxilla, and strongly truncate and scoop shaped.[5] The palatines are large, bladelike, and vertically oriented.[5] Those features are particularly manifest in hyacinth macaws, who display a very large mandible and a large quadrate bone. In contrast, lories or keas have very short mandibles and an elongated slender upper beak, used for probing activity in soil and flowers.

Psittacines have a very mobile jaw apparatus with the greatest number of bony units and joints observed in avian skulls.[4] However, no flexion zones are present in their bones.[4]

In psittacines, the upper jaw bone, the pair of separate jugal bars and the pair of separate palatine bones are articulated by synovial (eg, *Ara* spp., *Cacatua* spp.) or syndesmotic joints (eg, *Poicephalus* spp.)[4] (**Fig. 4**). The craniofacial fissure

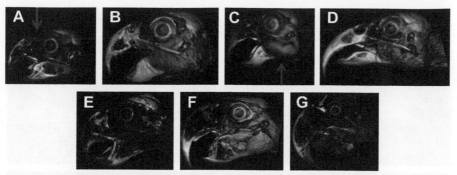

Fig. 3. Three-dimensional reconstruction from computed tomography scan in various psitta-cines. (*A*) Senegal parrot (*Poicephalus senegalus*). Note the syndesmotic craniofacial hinge in this species (*red arrow*). (*B*) African gray parrot (*Psittacus erithacus*). (*C*) Eclectus parrot (*Eclectus roratus*). The *m. pterygoideus* is prominent (*red arrow*). (*D*) Kea (*Nestor notabilis*). Note the very long and slender beak (*red arrow*). (*E*) Umbrella cockatoo (*Cacatua alba*). An *arcus suborbitalis* is present and fuse with the zygomatic process to form a temporal fenestra (*red arrow*). A true articulation is present between the jugal bars, the palatine and the upper jaw. (*F*) Green-winged macaw (*Ara chloroptera*). An arcus suborbitalis is pre-sent and fused with the zygomatic process to form a temporal fenestra (*red arrow*). The ju-gal arch is very limited (*blue arrow*). (*G*) Hyacinth macaw (*Anodorhynchus hyacinthinus*). There is no *arcus suborbitalis* (*red arrow*). Note a reinforcement of the interorbital septum (dorsocranial to the orbit) at the insertion of the ethmomandibularis (*blue arrow*). (*Courtesy of* Minh Huynh, DVM, DECZM (Avian), DACZM, Centre Hospitalier Vétérinaire Frégis, Ar-cueil, France.)

or craniofacial hinge is extremely developed, which allows a high mobility of the upper beak.[11] Additional articulations such as the pterygoid–pterygoid median articulation and the pterygoid–parasphenoid articulation, which is a diar-throsis with fibrous tissue, are involved in the sliding movement of the palatovom-eral complex.[12] The parasphenoid bone is medial and unpaired, contributes to the floor of the cranial cavity, and forms the ventral component of the interorbital septum.[5,13]

The rostral rotation of the quadrate bone pushes the pterygoid and the palatovom-eral complex and the jugal bars causing the elevation of the upper jaw.[1] Contrarily, the caudal rotation moves the upper jaw downward[1] (**Fig. 5**). The pterygoid bones artic-ulate medially forming a V-shaped depression that articulates dorsally with the parasphenoid.[12]

A suborbital arch, *arcus suborbitalis,* is present in some psittacines (eg, monk parakeet [*Myiopsitta monachus*], umbrella cockatoo [*Cacatua alba*], and green-winged macaw [*Ara chloroptera*]). Although its role is not completely under-stood, it seems to influence the bite strength[11] (see **Fig. 3**). The formation of the suborbital arch and the craniofacial hinge of parrots does not occur until the chick leaves the nest, suggesting an important role in the ability to crack hard elements.[11]

Psittaciformes present a very large mandible with a bony structure enlarged in its rostral aspect, and a thin pneumatization in its nuchal aspect in contraposition to the long, narrow, and laterally flattened mandible observed in some other birds such as galliformes or accipitriformes (**Fig. 6**).

All parrot species present a specific muscle, the *m. ethmomandibularis* and some species also present an *m. pseudomasseter*.[5,14] The *m. ethmomandibularis* originate

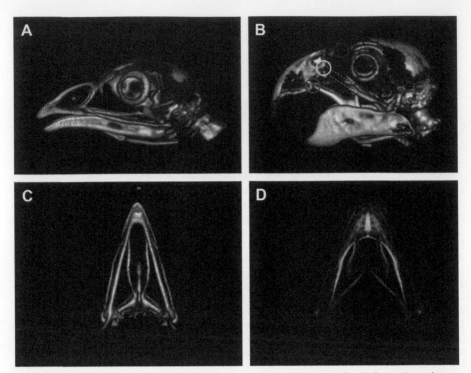

Fig. 4. Three-dimensional reconstruction from computed tomography (CT) scan in a domestic fowl (*Gallus gallus*) and an African gray parrot (*Psittacus erithacus*). (*A*) In the domestic fowl, the jugal bars and the palatine bones are fused to the upper jaw. (*B*) Three distinct joints are seen in parrots connecting the upper jaw to the brain case (*red circle*), to the jugal bar (*light blue circle*) and to the palatine bone (*deep blue circle*). The connection from the jugal bar to the upper jaw has been represented with white markings because it does not appear in the CT scan. (*C*) Ventral view of the mandibula and the palate in a domestic fowl. (*D*) Ventral view of the mandibula and the palate in an African gray parrot. (*Courtesy of* Minh Huynh, DVM, DECZM (Avian), DACZM, Centre Hospitalier Vétérinaire Frégis, Arcueil, France.)

from the *pterygoideus* and allow the rostral displacement of the lower jaw and the adduction of the lower jaw without depressing it.[4,14] The *m. pseudomasseter* derive from the *adductor mandibulae externus* and may pull the mandible forward.[8,14] A *pseudotemporalis profundus* muscle is not observed in psittacines.[14] A specific muscle attaching on the posterior portion of the orbital arch and the zygomatic process has been described in *Cyanoramphus* spp.[5]

TRAUMA MANAGEMENT

Head trauma is relatively common in wild and captive birds. Most wildlife cases are related to window collisions, gunshots, bite wounds, and road traffic accidents. Captive birds may suffer injuries from cage mates, especially biting off the rhinotheca or at the base of the gnathotheca, and other pets or predators. Other common causes of trauma include been caught by closing doors or collisions with objects.

Head trauma may lead to potential orthopedic damage, but a global assessment of the avian patient is mandatory before assessing musculoskeletal damage. Analgesia

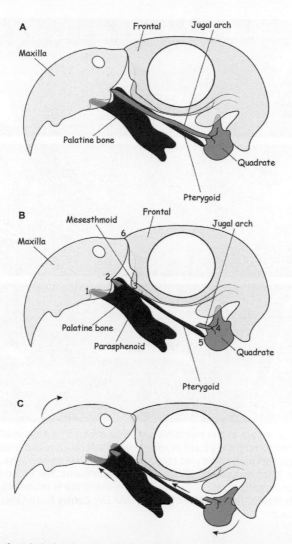

Fig. 5. (*A*) Palatofacial skeletal anatomy in psittacines. Bones linking the maxilla to the quadrate bones are highlighted in *blue*. (*B*) The jugal arch has been removed to allow visualization of articulations: 1, palatomaxillary syndesmosis, 2, craniofacial hinge, 3, pterygoid-parasphenoid-palatine complex, 4, pterygoid-quadrate articulation, 5, jugal-maxilla articulation, 6, jugal-quadrate articulation. (*C*) During cranial kinesis, the rostral rotatory movement of the quadrate pushes the pterygoid bone and jugal arch, the pterygoid–palatine complex slides at the articulation with the parasphenoid bone, thereby transmitting rostral forces to the maxilla through the palate and palatomaxillary syndesmosis. (*Courtesy of Hugues Beaufrére, DVM, PhD, DABVP (Avian Practice), DECZM (Avian), DACZM, Department of Clinical Studies, Ontario Veterinary College, University of Guelph, Guelph, Canada.*)

and stabilization (discussed elsewhere in this article) should be always prioritized in every traumatized bird.

Airway patency should be confirmed before undertaking any other evaluation. Blood frequently obstruct the nares and, although they are not essential in avian respiration, they must be cleaned to maximize comfort. Air sac cannulation may be recommended

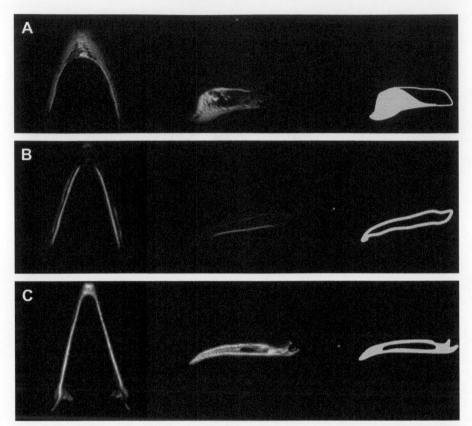

Fig. 6. Comparative aspect of the mandibula in various bird in a 3-dimensional reconstruction from computed tomography scans in ventral view, lateral view and a schematic drawing of bony part (*gray*) and pneumatic part (*black*). (*A*) *Psittacus erithacus*. The mandible is very large and thick in its rostral aspect, (*B*) *Accipiter melanoleucus*. The mandibula is long narrow and highly pneumatized. (*C*) *Gallus gallus*. The mandible is moderately pneumatized. (*Courtesy of* Minh Huynh, DVM, DECZM (Avian), DACZM, Centre Hospitalier Vétérinaire Frégis, Arcueil, France.)

if severe mandibular or hyoid trauma impairs the opening of the glottis or when the endotracheal tube may interfere with the required head manipulation during surgery.

Concurrent traumatic brain injuries are expected and may result in various neurologic signs (eg, partial or total loss of consciousness, head tilt, circling and cranial nerve deficits). A complete neurologic examination may be performed once the patient is stable enough to tolerate restraint.

Ophthalmic lesions are common in cases of trauma. The incidence of ophthalmic lesions may vary from 10% to 28% in raptors presented to wildlife rescue centers.[15,16] Some studies demonstrated a high prevalence (approximatively 80%) of ocular lesions in tawny owls affected by road traffic accidents.[17] A thorough ophthalmic evaluation is recommended in case of trauma, especially because most lesions are located in the posterior chamber.[17,18]

The clinical assessment of the skull includes a visual evaluation of the external beak, external palpation of the mandible and jugal arch, and mobilization of the jaws; intraoral, otic, and ophthalmic examinations should be also performed.

Stabilization

The bird should be placed in a quiet, dark, and temperature-controlled environment. Oxygen therapy is beneficial because hypercapnia can have a significant effect on intracranial pressure.

Head injuries and especially beak trauma, are known to be extremely painful; therefore, providing analgesia is a therapeutic priority. Species specific analgesic doses in birds are constantly reviewed and are beyond the scope of this article. The use of multimodal analgesia, parenteral when possible to avoid further manipulation of the head, is recommended.

If the beak is unstable, initial immobilization in most birds other than parrots can be achieved with tape (**Fig. 7**).

In cases of agitation and hyperventilation, sedation (eg, 0.2–0.5 mg/kg of intramuscular midazolam) may be beneficial to decrease stress levels, avoid further trauma on the beak, and avoid hypocapnia, which may cause cerebral vasoconstriction. As in every case of shock, intravenous or intraosseous fluid therapy is beneficial in enhancing tissue perfusion. Antimicrobials may be provided in case of skin infections or bite wounds.

Esophagostomy Tube

Esophagostomy tubes are useful to facilitate feeding and drug administration in cases of severe facial trauma (**Fig. 8**). The main limitation is the requirement of general anesthesia for its placement. Extreme care must be taken during the manipulation of the oral cavity. Curved forceps of an appropriate size are introduced in the oral cavity, advanced to the esophagus, and the tip is pushed against its lateral (normally left) wall in the midcervical region. The skin is incised over the forceps tip and the tip of the esophagostomy tube is grasped with the forceps and advanced directly into the distal esophagus. Retrograde insertion, the standard technique in which the tube is first advanced in cranially and then retroflexed into the esophagus, should be avoided because it may cause further damage to the maxillofacial area. Gentle manipulation of the tube allows bypassing the crop (not mandatory) and limits the risk of regurgitation. This procedure is relatively easy in raptors, but more difficult in parrots because of the shape of their crops.

Diagnostic Evaluation

Four radiographic projections (lateral, ventrodorsal, and right and left oblique) are classically required to evaluate the skull. Higher quality may be obtained under sedation or general anesthesia. Reverse contrast mode radiographs may help to visualize

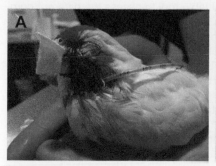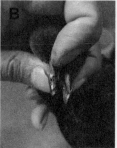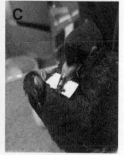

Fig. 7. Temporary stabilization in various birds after head trauma. (*A*) Stabilization of the mandible with tape in a Kakariki (*Cyanoramphus novezelandiae*). (*B*) Beak fracture in a rock piegon (*Columba livia*). (*C*) Stabilization of the distal mandible with tape in a rock pigeon (*Columba livia*). (*Courtesy of* Minh Huynh, DVM, DECZM (Avian), DACZM, Centre Hospitalier Vétérinaire Frégis, Arcueil, France.)

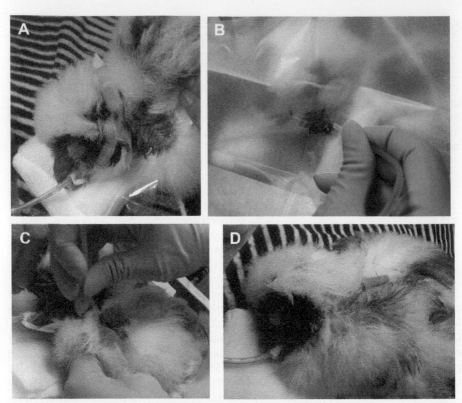

Fig. 8. Insertion of an esophagostomy tube in a spectacled owl chick *(Pulsatrix perspicillata)*. (*A*) The lateral side of the neck is prepared aseptically. (*B*) A clamp is inserted in the oral cavity and pushed against the esophagus. The skin is incised and the feeding tube grasped through the ostium created. (*C*) The feeding tube is inserted in a normograde fashion. (*D*) The tube is sutured and secured on the back of the bird. (*Courtesy of* Minh Huynh, DVM, DECZM (Avian), DACZM, Centre Hospitalier Vétérinaire Frégis, Arcueil, France.)

osseous structures (**Fig. 9**). Most anatomic structures are best evaluated in the lateral projection.[19] Nevertheless, structure superimposition and the presence of pneumatized bones can make the interpretation challenging.

Computed tomography scanning is an invaluable tool to assess the different complex elements of the avian skull and has been used in many case reports.[20–23] Reference images have been described in psittacines.[24] Examples of the anatomy including different articulations are provided (**Fig. 10**). Two major limitations are the potential small size of the patient and the presence of pneumatic bones composing the avian skull, which are difficult to distinguish from soft tissue by the routine diagnostic image algorithm used for bone examination in mammals. Optimal visibility of the 2 cortices of the avian skull bones may be achieved via a standard tissue filter and pulmonary window because most bones are pneumatized.[24] Deformities of the skull bone segment and complex fractures are best visualized with computed tomography scan and 3-dimensional reconstruction (**Figs. 11** and **12**).

ORTHOPEDIC PROCEDURES

The avian literature has focused on beak deviation and fracture, but limited information is available on precise clinical management. Most information comes from reviews or

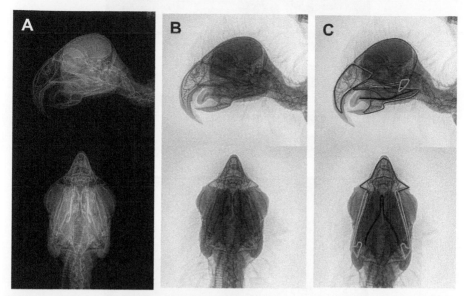

Fig. 9. Lateral and ventrodorsal views of the skull of a sun conure (*Aratinga solstitialis*). (*A*) Standard view. (*B*) Reverse contrast view. (*C*) Reverse contrast view annotated. Maxillary bone (*red*), palate (*blue*) composed of the jugal bars (*light blue*), quadrate (*light blue*), the palatovomeral complex and the pterygoid bones (*deep blue*), the mandible (*brown*), and the hyoid apparatus (*black*). (*Courtesy of* Minh Huynh, DVM, DECZM (Avian), DACZM, Centre Hospitalier Vétérinaire Frégis, Arcueil, France.)

book chapters describing the surgical techniques.[7,25–27] However, there are very limited data in the peer-reviewed literature on case series describing complications, outcomes, and expectations related with those surgeries. A summary of cases reported is presented in **Table 1**. It is noteworthy that 2 cases of mandibular fractures were managed successfully with conservative treatment and an esophagostomy tube.[22–28]

Only 7 papers covering 15 cases are published in the indexed peer-reviewed literature; the rest of the cases were presented as proceeding abstracts. Including peer-reviewed and not peer-reviewed reports, psittacines are the group of birds most represented (11 cases) followed by cranes (4 cases). Mandibular fractures and maxillary fractures are nearly equally represented (8 and 9 cases, respectively). Given the paucity of information, it is difficult to extrapolate the treatment of choice, the length of treatment (which may range from 6 days to 12 months), or the outcome (ranging from full recovery to misalignment) to new cases.

Overview of Dental Acrylics and Resin-Based Composites Used in Beak Disorders

Dental acrylics and resin-based composites such as polymethylmethacrylate (PMMA), bis-acrylic composite (Protemp Plus, 3M ESPE, St. Paul, MN; or Maxi-Temp, Henry Schein Inc., Melville, NY), urethane dimethacrylate-based material not containing methyl methacrylate (Triad Transheet, Dentsply International Inc., York, PA), methyl metacrylate (Technovit, Jorgensen Laboratories, Loveland, CO), or poly ethyl methacrylate plus isobutyl methacrylate (Koollner GC, America Inc, Alsip, IL) have proven useful for beak repair. Because both types of products produce an exothermic reaction during the polymerization process that may damage living tissues, the specific physicochemical properties of the product should be checked before using them. Resin-based composites generally reach lower temperatures than acrylics during

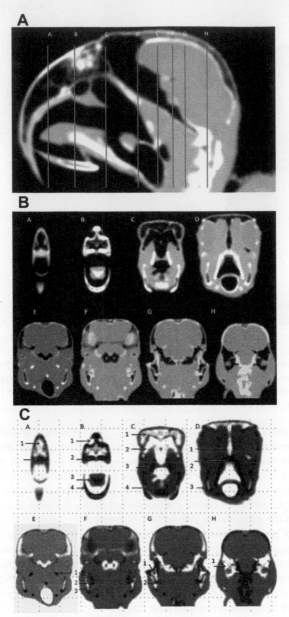

Fig. 10. Computed tomography scan multiplanar imaging of the skull of an African gray parrot (*Psittacus erithacus*) using a bone window. (*A*) Sagittal view. (*B*) Axial view corresponding to the slice mentioned on the sagittal view. (*C*) Same axial view with negative contrast annotated: Section A: (1) nasal diverticulum of the infraorbital sinus; (2) *Rostrum maxillare*. Section B: (1) nasal cavity; (2) palatine bone (junction of the palatine bone with the upper jaw); (3) hyoid bone; (4) mandible. Section C: (1) frontal bone; (2) infraorbital sinus; (3) palatine bone; (4) mandible. Section D: (1) Interorbital septum; (2) palatine bone (junction of the palatine bone-pterygoid bone and junction of the pterygoid bone–parasphenoid bone); (3) mandible. Section E: (1) pterygoid bone. Section F: (1) pterygoid bone (junction of the pterygoid bone and the quadrate); (2) quadrate bone; (3) mandible. Section G: (1) quadrate bone (junction of the quadrate and the mandible); (2) mandible. Section H: (1) otic bone. (*Courtesy of* Minh Huynh, DVM, DECZM (Avian), DACZM, Centre Hospitalier Vétérinaire Frégis, Arcueil, France.)

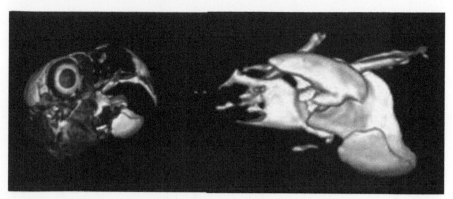

Fig. 11. Three-dimensional reconstruction from computed tomography (CT) scan in an eclectus parrot (*Eclectus* sp.) presented for acute trauma. The CT scan allows for the visualization of the comminuted fracture of the right mandible. (*Courtesy of* Minh Huynh, DVM, DECZM (Avian), DACZM, Centre Hospitalier Vétérinaire Frégis, Arcueil, France.)

polymerization.[29] Visible light curing composites are light-sensitive synthetic materials that can be molded and used to fill large defects or create beak prostheses. The use of a curing light may speed composite polymerization but, depending on the product, may not be mandatory. Methyl methacrylate (eg, Technovit) can be used as a light but strong binding adhesive material in the construction of external fixators. Once polymerization is completed, both resin-based composites and acrylics can be reshaped and/or polished with a drill, although some can be extremely hard and difficult to reshape. A review about bone cements and their potential use in mandibular endoprosthesis in humans concluded that plain PMMA is the default choice for the initial development phase of this procedure but modified PMMA cements, composite resin

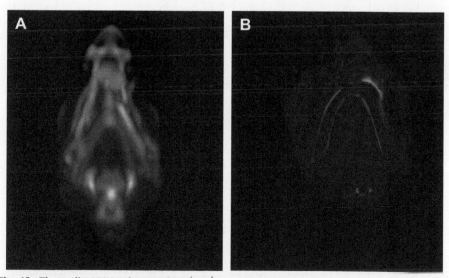

Fig. 12. Three-dimensional reconstruction from a computed tomography scan various birds presented for trauma. (*A*) Double fracture of the mandibula in a kakariki (*Cyanorhamphus novaezelandiae*). (*B*) The left mandibula is shorter than the right mandibula causing deviation of the gnathotheca in a cockatiel (*Nymphicus hollandicus*). (*Courtesy of* Minh Huynh, DVM, DECZM (Avian), DACZM, Centre Hospitalier Vétérinaire Frégis, Arcueil, France.)

Table 1
Clinical cases of beak deviation and mandibular or maxillary bone fracture surgically corrected reported in avian literature[a]

Reference	Species	Beak Disorder	Technique	Duration	Outcome
Lothamer et al,[36] 2014[a]	African gray parrot	Acute symphyseal mandibular fracture	Wire and acrylic to appose the mandible	47 d	Successful
	Red crowned Crane	Seven-week-old symphyseal fracture of the mandibular beak	Wire and acrylic to appose the mandible	21 wk	Successful
Lejnieks,[37] 2004	Sulfur-crested cockatoo	One-month-old mandibular symphyseal fracture	Steel plate and acrylic to appose the mandible	10 wk	Lateral deviation of the rhinotheca
Calvo Carrasco et al,[49]	Yellow billed kite	Mandibular fracture	External fixation and acrylic	6 d	Correct alignment
Morris and Weigel,[45] 1990	Marabout stork	Mandibular fracture and amputation of the beak	Pin and dental acrylic used as prothesis	9 mo	The prosthesis fell off
Fletcher,[46] 1979	Shoebill stork	Bilateral mandibular fracture	Steinmann pin, wire, and aluminum plate	Not mentioned	Successful
Speer and Powers,[7] 2016[a]	Cockatiel	Mandibular symphyseal diastasis/fracture	Transmandibular hypodermic needle looped with polypropylene suture and covered with liquid acrylic	Not mentioned	Successful
Calvo Carrasco et al,[47] 2016[a]	Swan	Deviated mandible	Osteogenesis distraction and esophagostomy tube	First surgery 2 wk Second surgery 3 wk	Moderate misalignment
Anderson et al,[48] 2018	Chicken	Deviated mandible	Osteogenesis distraction	3 wk	Requires occasional beak trim of the rhamphotheca

Reference	Species	Condition	Treatment	Duration	Outcome
Speer and Powers,[7] 2016[a]	Indian ring-necked parakeet	Mandibular prognathism	A 22G spinal needle stylet was placed dorsal to ventral through the rostral premaxilla and covered with liquid acrylic	6 wk	Successful
Beaufrere et al,[20] 2018	Hawk-headed parrot	Palatine bone and pterygoid luxation, fracture pterygoid, jugal bar, and palatine bone	Wire and dental acrylic	2 wk	Successful
Foerster et al,[51] 2000[a]	Blue-and-gold macaw	Palatine bone luxation	Stabilization with suture around the suborbital arch and jugal bone after reduction	—	Died shortly after the surgery
Schnellbacher et al,[34] 2010[a]	Blue-and-gold macaw	Scissor beak	Wire and dental acrylic for ramp prosthesis	6 wk	Prosthesis fell off
Fecchio et al,[35] 2010	Striped owl	Scissor beak	Wire and acrylic for ramp prosthesis	30 d	Successful
Speer and Powers,[7] 2016[a]	Blue-and-gold macaw	Scissor beak	Transfrontal pin and tension band	Not mentioned	Functional recovery in 3 d
Crosta,[41] 2002[a]	Black-necked aracari	Fractured rhinotheca	Alloplastic bill	3 mo	Died 3 mo later from an unrelated cause
	Channel-billed toucan	Fractured rhinotheca	Heteroplastic bill	2 mo	Lost to follow-up
Wade,[39] 2015	Senegal parrot	Fractured rhinotheca	Dental acrylic	1 mo	Successful
	Eclectus parrot	Fractured rhinotheca	Dental acrylic	3 mo	Successful
Speer and Powers,[7] 2016[a]	Blue-and-gold macaw	Fractured rhinotheca and premaxillary bone	Liquid acrylic around the rostral maxillary beak	Not mentioned	Not mentioned
Chitty,[50] 2004	Red-crowned crane	Maxillary beak fracture	Type 2 external fixator and cerclage wire	Wire removal after 2 wk; Pin removal after 3 wk	Deviation of the beak; Regular trimming of the gnathotheca was required every 8 wk

(continued on next page)

Table 1
(continued)

Reference	Species	Beak Disorder	Technique	Duration	Outcome
Lothamer et al,[36] 2014[a]	White-napped Crane	Maxillary beak fracture	Wire and acrylic to appose the mandible	Not mentioned	Successful
	Sandhill Crane	Maxillary beak fracture	Wire and acrylic to appose the mandible	Not mentioned	Successful
Speer and Powers,[7] 2016[a]	Pekin duck	Maxillary and mandibular avulsion	Prosthetic constructed from positive profile threaded external skeletal fixation pins, cerclage wire and epoxy	12 mo	12 mo of functional recovery before needing prosthetic replacement

[a] Case reports published in an indexed peer-reviewed journal.

cements, osteoinductive calcium phosphate compounds, and cementless fixation are options that offer advantages over PMMA cements, and, therefore, further research should be conducted to study their suitability.[30] PMMA can be supplemented with antibiotics if there is a significant risk of infection. Calcium hydroxide (Ca(OH)(2)) is a basic salt that has been widely used intralesionally in avian bone fractures repair owing to its antimicrobial effects and its capability of inducing hard tissue formation.

Overview of Pin Fixation

External pin fixation has been described in the management of mandibular fracture or in transfrontal pinning. No specific studies were performed on the avian mandible. Holding power studies of various pin designs in avian long bones suggest the use of threaded pins (preferably positive) with the smallest pitch possible.[31] Because mandibular bones are often pneumatic, they provide less pull-out strength compared with medullary bone.[32] Predrilling pilot holes of a smaller diameter than the threaded pin to be used improves its stability.[33] Air sac anesthesia may be beneficial in beak orthopedic procedures because it may allow for a better visualization and a greater range of movement of the structures involved.

BEAK DISORDERS
Scissor Beak

Scissor beak is a lateral deviation of the rhinotheca leading to beak malocclusion. Although scissor beak may occur in any species of psittacines, it seems to be more common in macaws and cockatoos.[26] It has been also reported in other species (eg, doves, raptors, and chickens).[7,26] Severe cases may prevent the prehension of food and cause abnormal wear on both sides of the gnathotheca. On the deviation side, the gnathotheca wears excessively, whereas the rhinotheca overgrows. In the contralateral side, the gnathotheca may overgrow and the rhinotheca may wear excessively. Any change in the normal rate of keratin migration (normally rostrally along the surface of the beak and laterally from the vascular bed), any change in the orientation of the premaxilla, or a malformation of the frontal bone or nasofrontal hinge could cause the beak to deviate laterally[25,26] (**Fig. 13**).

Scissor beak correction is easier in young individuals because the bones and rhinotheca are actively remodeling.[26] Radiography has been recommended as a prognostic aid before correction.[25] The objective of the correction procedures is to change the forces that direct the anterior growth of the rhinotheca. Multiple corrective alternatives have been reported.

a. If recognized early, scissor beak could be corrected by applying gentle manual pressure to the beak for 10 minutes 6 to eight times daily.[25]
b. Mild forms of scissor beak may be corrected with periodic corrective beak trimming.[25]
c. A ramp prosthesis may be applied in the lateral aspect of the gnathotheca ipsilateral to the lateral rhinothecal deviation to redirect it medially through keratin and bony remodeling[25,26,34] (**Fig. 14**). The keratin of the gnathotheca on the affected side can be grooved deep enough to increase the surface area for prosthetic attachment without inducing hemorrhage. The gnathotheca is disinfected and a prosthesis made of dental acrylic or stainless steel or nylon dental screen mesh covered with cyanoacrylate or dental acrylic is fixed to it. The prosthesis should be long enough to prevent the bird from slipping the rhinotheca over the prosthesis. Correction may take several weeks to several months, and normal keratin exfoliation may require reapplication of the prosthesis every 10 to 14 days until the

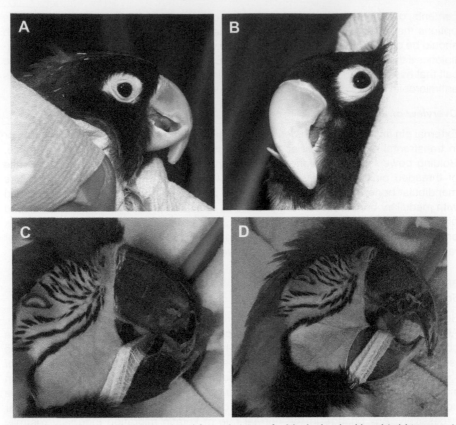

Fig. 13. Scissor beak. (*A, B*) Lateral and frontal views of a black-cheeked lovebird (*Agapornis nigrigenis*). (*C, D*) Lateral view of a blue-and-gold macaw (*Ara ararauna*) before and during beak trim. (*Courtesy of* Mikel Sabater, LV, CertZooMed, DECZM (Avian), MRCVS, Exoticsvet, Valencia, Spain.)

deviation is corrected and the prosthesis can be removed.[25] In most cases, 5 to 6 weeks of treatment are required.[34] A case of lateral maxillary beak deviation was successfully treated with a ramp orthosis in a striped owl (*Rhinoptynx clamator*).[35]

d. Contralateral constant lateral tension may be applied to the deviated maxilla using a tension band anchored to the skull by a transfrontal pin[7,21] (**Fig. 15**). A Kirshner or small Steinmann pin is placed perpendicular to the skull, through the frontal bones just caudal to the craniofacial hinge joint on a line between the lateral canthus of the eye and the cere. In macaws, a small bony protuberance marks the point where the pin is introduced on one side and exits on the other. On the side of beak contralateral to the direction of the deviation, the pin is cranially bent 90° as it leaves the skin and laterally bent at the level of the beak tip. The other end of the pin is trimmed and curled over on itself, preventing it from being pulled through the skull. A tension band is created by using a rubber band or wire (sometimes passing through a hole created in the distal rhinotheca) between the cranial aspect of the transfrontal pin and the distal rhinotheca. The tension can be adjusted by loosening or tightening the wire/rubber band and is maintained until the beak deviation is corrected. In young birds this can be as soon as 10 to 14 days. Once the beak deviation is

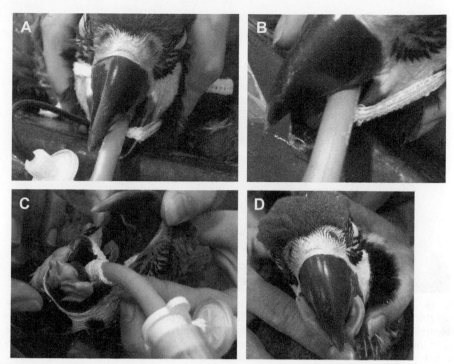

Fig. 14. Scissor beak in a blue-and-gold macaw (*Ara ararauna*) treated with a dental acrylic ramp prosthesis. (*Courtesy of* Minh Huynh, DVM, DECZM (Avian), DACZM, Centre Hospitalier Vétérinaire Frégis, Arcueil, France.)

corrected, the tension band is removed. The pin can be removed if the beak maintains a normal position for several days.

Scissor beak associated with prefrontal bone collapse is not yet amenable to treatment. These birds usually adapt to their disability and do well provided regular beak trimmings are performed to maintain a functionally normal occlusion.[27]

Mandibular Prognathism

Mandibular prognathism, also known as maxillary brachygnathism, is the anteroposterior discrepancy between the upper and the lower beaks in which the lower beak is rostrally displaced in relation to the upper beak. This malformation can vary from the tip of the rhinotheca resting on or just inside the gnathotheca, to severe cases in which the upper beak curls inside the oral cavity preventing normal food prehension. Cockatoos are the most common species reported and this may be related with the presence of cartilaginous lateral extensions on the tip of the maxilla in hatchings that, when contracted, may contribute to inward deviation of the maxillary tip.[7,27] Correction techniques are based on forcing the tip of the upper beak upward and outward so that it rests over the edge of the lower beak in the most natural position. In very young chicks, gentle manual pressure applied outward to the maxillary tip placing it over the mandible for 10 minutes 6 to 8 times daily may be enough to correct the malformation. Once the beak hardens, surgical correction is preferred.

Dental acrylic may be applied over the rhinotheca extending it until the gnathotheca fits inside (**Fig. 16**). Careful placement of a sterile pin dorsal to ventral through the tip of

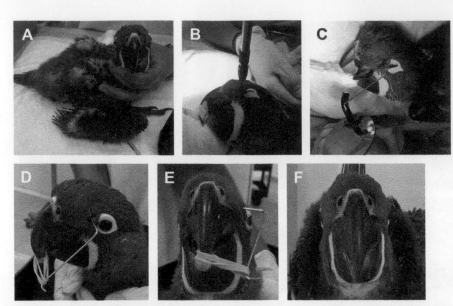

Fig. 15. Surgical correction of scissors beak in a hyacinth macaw (*Anodorhynchus hyacinthinus*) chick. (*A*) Frontal view before surgery. (*B*) Transsinus pin placement. (*C*) Use of a photopolymerizer light (Dent-Sply) to speed the polymerization of the dental acrylic placed in the tip of the rhinotheca. (*D*, *E*) Lateral and frontal views of the corrective device. (*F*) Postoperative frontal view. (*Courtesy of* Mikel Sabater, LV, CertZooMed, DECZM (Avian), MRCVS, Exoticsvet, Valencia, Spain.)

the premaxilla may help to stabilize the device. However, pins placed through the bone of growing birds may result in trauma to the softer and pliable tissues.[7] The prosthesis can be manually removed or using a rotating burr once the upper beak has is wider and more cranial than the lower beak, which may occur between 2 weeks and 6 months later, depending on the age of the chick.[25]

An alternative way to correct mandibular prognathism can be the use of a pin in the frontal bone, a pin in the maxilla, and 2 tension bands connecting their ipsilateral tips. After passing a Kirshner or small Steinmann transsinus pin through the frontal bones, the pin tips are bended in a hook shape close to the skin. A second pin is placed in the maxilla midway down the beak at the point at which the internal rotation of the maxilla is most severe and the tips should be also bent in a hook shape. The position of the pin can be reinforced with dental acrylic. Then, a tension band is created with a rubber band connecting the ipsilateral tips of the pins. The rubber band can be removed once the rhinotheca is properly positioned on the outer surface of the gnathotheca. The pins and the dental acrylic can be removed after several days not observing the recurrence of mandibular prognathism.[26]

Both surgical techniques apply tension to the *pterygoideus* and *pseudotemporalis profundus* muscles, often contracted in affected birds, resulting in abnormal flexion of the upper jaw and temporary discomfort.[7]

Beak Traumatic Injuries

The objectives of beak repair are providing reduction and stability to the beak structures, allowing normal function and restoring a protective barrier against microorganisms. Sequelae to serious beak trauma may include infection of the surrounding soft tissues and permanent beak deformities.[25]

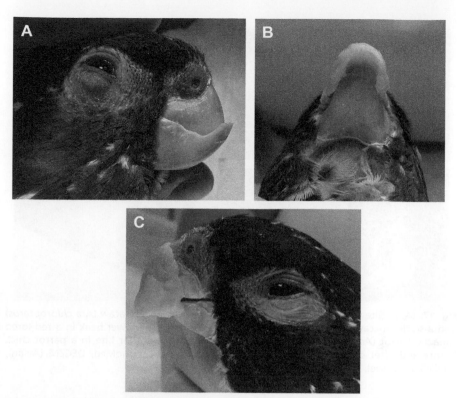

Fig. 16. Mandibular prognathism in 2 bronze-winged parrots (*Pionus chalcopterus*). (*A*) Lateral view. (*B*) Ventral view after dental acrylic placement on the upper beak. Note the lower beak fits within the prosthesis. (*C*) Both birds after acrylic resin placement. (*Courtesy of* Mikel Sabater, LV, CertZooMed, DECZM (Avian), MRCVS, Exoticsvet, Valencia, Spain.)

Abrasions, cracks, and fissures of the beak

Abrasions, cracks, and minor fissures should be disinfected and, sometimes, surgically debrided to prevent infection of the underlying dermis and nasal sinuses (**Fig. 17**). Any injury to the beak involving the germinal keratin layer is more likely to cause permanent keratin defects. Longitudinal fissures into the germinal epithelium do not heal well because the defect remains as the new beak grows. In these cases, the beak should be filed or trimmed to the full extent of the crack. Extensive cracks may benefit from the use of a tension band wire across the defect to prevent further cracking and to promote growth.[25]

Beak splits

Short anterior splits may be ground down to eliminate most or all the fracture, and the remaining defect can be covered with acrylic. Longer splits may require overlapping layers of mesh splinting in addition to the acrylic covering. The treatment is aimed at creating a functional lower beak edge that allows subsequent keratin growth to develop as a uniform sheet and prevents further splitting of the fracture. Complete recovery may take weeks to months.[26] Several cases (an African gray parrot and 3 cranes) were treated with interfragmentary wiring and acrylic composite.[36] The main principle of the therapy was to stabilize both fragment of the mandibula with a series of orthopedic wire, which were drilled through both sides of the mandibula or maxilla, twisted to achieve apposition, and reinforced with a bis-acryl composite splint. All

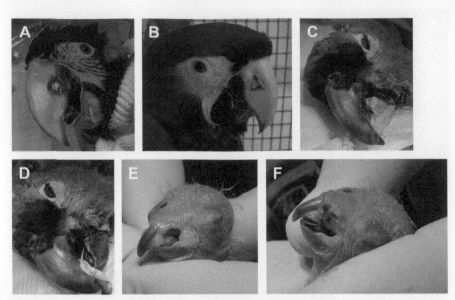

Fig. 17. (*A, B*) Bite wound in the rhinotheca of a red-and-green macaw (*Ara chloropterus*) and a scarlet macaw (*Ara macao*). (*C, D*) Partial avulsion of the lower beak in a red-lored Amazon parrot (*Amazona autumnalis*). (*E, F*) Chronic wound after bite in a parrot chick before and after surgery. (*Courtesy of* Mikel Sabater, LV, CertZooMed, DECZM (Avian), MRCVS, Exoticsvet, Valencia, Spain.)

cases were successful and allowed functional recovery[36] (**Fig. 18**). One case of mandibular disjunction that failed to heal after 1 month of cerclage wire was successfully treated with a steel plate in a lesser sulfur-crested cockatoo.[37] The steel plate was used to apply strong pressure against both mandibles to minimize the split. The plate fell off after 10 weeks and the bird recovered eventually.[37]

Beak punctures
The presentation of puncture wounds varies from slight irregularities to depressed or missing sections of the keratin surface. Superficial puncture wounds can be treated with local disinfectants and, if required, local or systemic antimicrobials and analgesics. Deeper wounds that may affect the structural integrity of the beak should be debrided carefully.[25] The prognosis is generally good, but punctures involving the germinal keratin layer are more prone to result in permanent keratin defects. Although resin-based composites to cover large beak defects have been widely reported in literature, these authors prefer the use of hydrogel dressings because resin composites delay beak tissues healing and may trap infection. Hydrogel dressings display greater wound contraction compared with hydrocolloid and polyethylene dressings.[38]

Partial beak tip fractures
Fractures of the beak tip are common in pet birds. Minimal fractures of the tip in which the germinal tissues are not exposed do not require treatment, but may benefit from edge polishing. If the beak tip is intact and partially attached to the rest of the beak, it can be cleaned gently and fixed back into place with dental acrylic. Dental acrylic has been used successfully to stabilize proximal rhinothecal fractures in a Senegal parrot and an eclectus parrot.[39] The acrylic was applied on the culmen, and the lateral

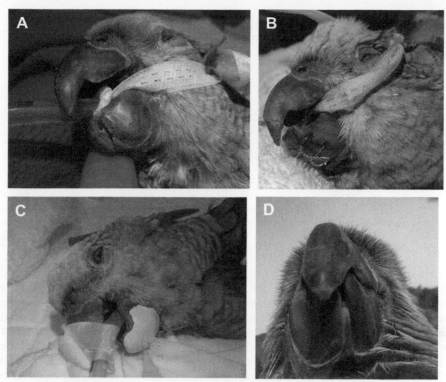

Fig. 18. (*A*) Mandibular beak fracture in a blue fronted Amazon parrot (*Amazona aestiva*). (*B*) The edge of the beak is thoroughly disinfected and 2 cerclage wires are placed to stabilize the fracture site. (*C*) Acrylic is apposed to reinforce the stability of the device. (*D*) Postoperative aspect 2 months after injury. The stabilization device was removed 1 month after the surgery. (*Courtesy of* Minh Huynh, DVM, DECZM (Avian), DACZM, Centre Hospitalier Vétérinaire Frégis, Arcueil, France.)

and proximal transverse aspect of the rhinotheca. Both birds recovered after 1 and 3 months.[39] Dental acrylic has also been used to stabilize fractured beaks in kiwis.[40]

Beak avulsions

Avulsions can be partial or complete (**Fig. 19**). Damage to the germinal epithelium in selected or entire beak regions generally does not allow for beak regeneration.[25] Hemorrhage, if present, should be controlled immediately. The stump should be disinfected carefully, preventing further damage of the exposed tissues. Analgesia, antimicrobials, and supportive care (including supportive feeding) should be provided until the wound has healed and the bird has adapted to eating with the abnormal beak. The rhamphotheca may require repeated beak trimming if the rhinotheca and gnathotheca do not appose anymore. Reattachment is generally unsuccessful and generally provokes further trauma to the exposed tissues[25] (**Fig. 20**). The use of alloplastic and heteroplastic bill prostheses in 2 ramphastids has been described, although long-term monitoring was not performed.[41]

In general, avulsions shorter than the rostral third of the maxilla will usually result in regrowth of the avulsed portion, whereas larger losses will usually result in permanent deformity.[27] Regrowth rates may be increased by oral administration of biotin (50 μg/kg daily for 2–3 months).[25] According to 1 case series, 9 of 10 psittacine birds with amputation of the beak survived, and all the survivors were able to self-feed within

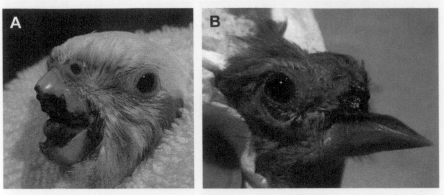

Fig. 19. (*A*) Upper beak avulsion in a cockatiel (*Nymphicus hollandicus*). (*B*) Upper beak avulsion in a European greenfinch (*Chloris chloris*). Both birds recovered well from the injury and were able to feed after the trauma. (*Courtesy of* Minh Huynh, DVM, DECZM (Avian), DACZM, Centre Hospitalier Vétérinaire Frégis, Arcueil, France.)

20 days[42] (**Fig. 21**). Avulsion of the maxillary beak can result in difficulty prehending food and exposure of the tongue in waterfowl and can also result in difficulty with self-feeding in other avian species, such as ramphastids and storks.[7] These birds may benefit from surgical placement of a beak prosthesis. However, cosmetic appearance should never be the only factor to consider in deciding whether to place a beak prosthesis, particularly in psittacine birds.[7] Prosthetic beaks can be constructed from epoxy or acrylic structural adhesive resins applied to intramedullary pins, Kirschner wires, or cerclage wire secured to the trabecular bony structures of the remaining beak. Prosthetic beaks designed and constructed using 3-dimensional printing have been reported in a bald eagle (*Haliaeetus leucocephalus*) and a green-billed toucan (*Ramphastos dicolorus*).[7] Unfortunately, beak prostheses are always temporary because the beak is composed of light trabecular bone and a dermal layer under permanent remodeling, and the

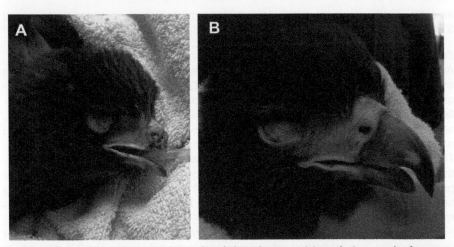

Fig. 20. Upper beak avulsion in a Harris hawk (*Parabuteo unicinctus*). One week after reattachment, the beak fell. However, the bird tolerated hand feeding very well by this time and, therefore, no further treatment was necessary until the beak regrew. (*Courtesy of* Mikel Sabater, LV, CertZooMed, DECZM (Avian), MRCVS, Exoticsvet, Valencia, Spain.)

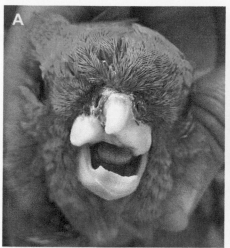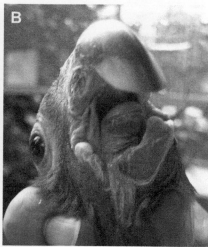

Fig. 21. (A) Healed nonunion fracture and partial avulsion of the premaxillary bone in a green parakeet (*Aratinga holochlora*). (B) Healed nonunion fracture of the mandible in a greater vasa parrot (*Coracopsis vasa*). (*Courtesy of* Mikel Sabater, LV, CertZooMed, DECZM (Avian), MRCVS, Exoticsvet, Valencia, Spain.)

prosthesis is exposed to strong kinetic forces during normal beak function. Diving birds and seed-cracking birds have limited success with prosthetic beaks owing to the high stresses applied to them.[25] Prosthetic beaks must be monitored closely for complications, such as failure and infection, and repaired and managed accordingly.[7] Prostheses implanted into bone by using screws or threaded pins remain in place longer, but eventually fail owing to bone resorption, implant infection, or both.[43] No long-term beak prosthesis has been reported in the peer-reviewed literature in parrots and birds of prey; however, longer durations seem to occur in toucans owing to their very slow keratin growth rate. If there is bone resorption, subsequent attempts to apply a prosthesis will generally fail more quickly because there is less bone available to fix them.[43] Kirschner pins inserted in the remaining osseous structures can be used as a frame for a prosthesis made of mesh, wire, bone cement, and dental acrylic, or some combination thereof.[25] The use of this technique in an ibis allowed the prosthesis to remain in place longer than 2 years.[44] Weakening and atrophy of the beak was suspected in a marabou stork (*Leptoptilos crumeniferus*) treated with this technique requiring removal of the maxillary prosthesis 9 months after placement.[45]

Maxillary fractures and nonsymphyseal mandibular fractures
Maxillary fractures and mandibular fractures are prone to nonunion because of the excessive motility of the area.[25] Fracture management requires adequate disinfection and debridement of the bone fragments, stabilization of the fracture, and the reapposition of the soft tissues overlying the fracture. To allow correct healing, the forces encountered by the beak from biting or muscular tension should be neutralized.[26] Depending on the size of the patient, pins, wires, screws, plates, hypodermic needles, cerclage wires, nylon or stainless steel mesh, and various dental acrylics may be used for fracture repair.[25] An original device using hooks attached to keratin with superglue and rubber bands bridging the fracture site has been used successfully on the maxilla of a kiwi.[40]

Simple unilateral mandibular fractures may be repaired by enveloping the fracture on 3 planes with multiple layers of dental acrylic, with or without nylon or stainless steel mesh for added stability. Fractures of the mandible, which is pneumatized and narrow

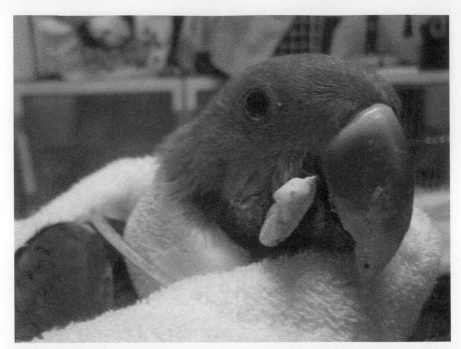

Fig. 22. Stabilization of a mandibular fracture with a cerclage wire and a dental acrylic in an eclectus parrot (*Eclectus roratus*). (*Courtesy of* Minh Huynh, DVM, DECZM (Avian), DACZM, Centre Hospitalier Vétérinaire Frégis, Arcueil, France.)

in most pet birds, are best stabilized with wires and acrylic (**Fig. 22**). When surgical fixation is attempted, it is important to debride the fractured ends of the bone and remove overlying keratin to have bone-to-bone contact. In large birds, surgical repair of mandibular fractures with bone defects is possible using external fixators and bone grafts.[25] A bilateral mandibular ramus open fracture in a shoebill stork (*Balaeniceps rex*) was successfully treated with a combination of Steinmann pins, cerclage wire, and a conformed external aluminum plate.[46]

A high rate of failure for nonsymphyseal mandibular fractures, especially at the junction with the skin, should be anticipated. In some or most of these cases, partial amputation of the overlapping fragments is recommended and there is an associated good outcome for the patient, who usually adapts quickly.

The use of an osteogenic distractor has been reported as a successful surgical option for the management of a unilateral mandibular rami fracture in a juvenile mute swan (*Cygnus olor*) and in a chicken.[47,48] Infected, multiple, and/or bilateral fractures carry a poor prognosis because of a high incidence of osteomyelitis, avascular necrosis, nonunion, and tissue avulsion.[25] Once the fracture is repaired, soft tissue injuries must be treated.[26] A rare case of congenital fracture of the lower mandible was suspected in a yellow billed kite.[49] The fracture was reduced with an osteotomy and an external fixation reinforced with dental acrylic.

Symphyseal fractures may be corrected with cerclage wires passed through predrilled holes in the mandible with transmandibular pins. The pins can be secured to each other externally by using elastic bands or with loops of polypropylene or stainless steel suture or wire. Covering the pin or wire with adhesive resin may provide additional support and protection to the external fixator.[7] The prognosis for successful

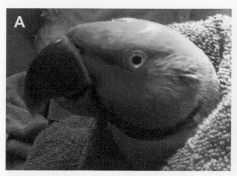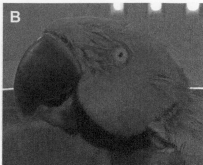

Fig. 23. (*A, B*) Luxation of the palatine-pterygoid complex bones after correction in an Alexandrine parakeet (*Psittacula eupatria*). (*Courtesy of* Mikel Sabater, LV, CertZooMed, DECZM (Avian), MRCVS, Exoticsvet, Valencia, Spain.)

repair is considered guarded to poor owing to the thin nature of vascular dermis and bone in this region.[7]

Fractures of the upper beak are generally more difficult to manage owing to involvement of small bones (eg, the quadrate and jugal bones) and prokinetic mobility, especially in parrots. Fractures involving the nasofrontal hinge carry a poor prognosis and severe trauma to the dermis may result in beak deformities.[25,26] A fracture of the quadrate bone managed conservatively in an Amazon parrot resulted in the bird being able to eat but unable to open the beak wider than 50% of the normal aperture.[22] Plastic or nylon mesh strips embedded in an acrylic cast, or the use of hypodermic needles, may be useful in fractures of premaxillae too small to hold wires or pins.[25,26] A maxillary fracture in a red-crowned crane (*Grus japonensis*) was treated by creating a type II external fixator by connecting with an epoxy resin a transfrontal pin and a pin transversally passed through the rostrum maxillare, and applying a cerclage wire placed across the fracture site of the dorsal nasal bone.[50]

A case of multiple fractures and luxation of palatofacial bones has been described in a hawk-headed parrot (*Deroptyus accipitrinus*). The left palatine bone was luxated as well as the pterygoid and the palatine complex. Fracture of the pterygoid bone, jugal bar, and palatine bone was also diagnosed. An interfragmentary wire was placed through the palatine bone, the maxilla and the rhinotheca to achieve stabilization of the palate–maxillary syndesmosis. No specific stabilization was performed on the bone fracture. The bird recovered 3 months after surgery.[20]

Luxation of the palatine–pterygoid complex (palatine bone luxation)
Traumatic palatine bone luxation has been reported in 2 blue-and-gold macaws (*Ara ararauna*). It happens in parrots biting hard a solid object and forcefully hyperextending the maxilla. The palatine–parasphenoid complex moves rostrally and then luxates dorsally beyond its normal endpoint on the parasphenoid–mesethmoid bones (interorbital septum) at the ventral base of the braincase. Because the interorbital septum is large in parrots and fused to the parasphenoid bone, it is unclear whether the palate gets hooked onto the parasphenoid or mesethmoid. Regardless, the luxation can be surgically reduced by introducing an intramedullary pin transversely across the infraorbital sinus dorsal to the palatine bones. Then, the maxillary beak is hyperextended while the pterygoid–parasphenoid–palatine complex is ventrally replaced into its anatomic position. Additional stabilization can be accomplished by passing absorbable suture around the suborbital arch and jugal bones bilaterally, but may not be necessary[26,51] (**Fig. 23**).

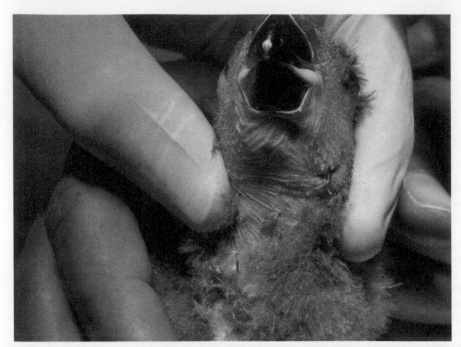

Fig. 24. Circumferential suture around the epibranchial bone and the ipsilateral maxillary bone to stabilize the luxation of the hyoid apparatus in a chick of purple-bellied lory (*Lorius hypoinochrous*). (*Courtesy of* Mikel Sabater, LV, CertZooMed, DECZM (Avian), MRCVS, Exoticsvet, Valencia, Spain.)

Luxation of the hyoid apparatus

Unilateral luxation of the hyoid apparatus was observed by the authors in a chick of purple-bellied lory (*Lorius hypoinochrous*; Video 1). Under general anesthesia, the luxated epibranchial bone was blindly anchored to the surface of the connective tissue that envelopes the jaw muscles as epimysia. Additional stability was provided by placing a circumferential absorbable suture around the epibranchial bone and the ipsilateral maxillary bone (**Fig. 24**). The chick completely recovered the normal function of the hyoid apparatus.

ACKNOWLEDGMENTS

The authors thank the Ménagerie du Jardin des plantes (Paris, France) for providing birds for computed tomography examinations.

SUPPLEMENTARY DATA

Supplementary data related to this article can be found online at https://doi.org/10.1016/j.cvex.2019.01.006.

REFERENCES

1. King AS, McLelland M. Skeletomuscular system. In: King AS, McLelland M, editors. Bird: their structure and function. Eastbourne (United Kingdom): Baillière Tindall; 1984. p. 9–22.

2. King AS, McLelland M. Integument. In: King AS, McLelland M, editors. Bird: their structure and function. Eastbourne (United Kingdom): Baillière Tindall; 1984. p. 24–52.
3. Coles B. Diversity in anatomy and physiology: clinical significance. In: Coles B, editor. Essentials of avian medicine and surgery. Oxford: Blackwell Publishing Ltd.; 2007. p. 1–21.
4. Buhler P. The functional anatomy of the avian jaw apparatus. In: King AS, McLelland M, editors. Form and function in birds, vol. 2. London: Academic Press; 1981. p. 439–68.
5. Zusi RL. Patterns of diversity in the avian skull. In: Hanken J, Hall BK, editors. The skull, volume 2: patterns of structural and systematic diversity, vol. 2. Chicago: University of Chicago Press; 1993. p. 391–437.
6. Hall BK. Variations outside the norm: neomorphs and atavism. In: Hall BK, editor. Bones and cartilage. Developmental and evolutionary skeletal biology. 2nd edition. San Diego (CA): Elsevier Academic press; 2015. p. 693–710.
7. Speer B, Powers LV. Anatomy and disorders of the beak and oral cavity of birds. Vet Clin North Am Exot Anim Pract 2016;19(3):707–36.
8. King AS, McLelland M. Respiratory system. In: King AS, McLelland M, editors. Bird: their structure and function. Eastbourne (United Kingdom): Baillière Tindall; 1984. p. 110–44.
9. Hertel F. Ecomorphological indicators of feeding behavior in recent and fossil raptors. Auk 1995;112(4):890–903.
10. Guangdi SI, Dong Y, Ma Y, et al. Shape similarities and differences in the skulls of scavenging raptors. Zoolog Sci 2015;32(2):171–7.
11. Tokita M. The skull development of parrots with special reference to the emergence of a morphologically unique cranio-facial hinge. Zoolog Sci 2003;20(6): 749–58.
12. Hall B. The distribution and fate of the adventitious cartilage in the skull of the eastern rosella, *Platycerus eximius* (Aves: Psittaciformes). Aust J Zool 1967; 15(4):685–98.
13. Maierl J, Liebich HG, Konig HE, et al. Head and trunk. In: Konig HE, Korbel RT, Liebich HG, editors. Avian anatomy: textbook and colour atlas. Sheffield (United Kingdom: 5M Publishing; 2009. p. 24–45.
14. Carril J, Degrange FJ, Tambussi CP. Jaw myology and bite force of the monk parakeet (Aves, Psittaciformes). J Anat 2015;227(1):34–44.
15. Murphy CJ, Kern TJ, McKeever K, et al. Ocular lesions in free-living raptors. J Am Vet Med Assoc 1982;181(11):1302–4.
16. Korbel RT. Disorders of the posterior eye segment in raptors - examination procedures and findings. In: Lumeij JT, Remple D, Redig P, editors. Raptor biomedicine III. Lake Worth (FL): Zoological Education Network; 2000. p. 179–93.
17. Cousquer G. Ophthalmological findings in free-living tawny owls (*Strix aluco*) examined at a wildlife veterinary hospital. Vet Rec 2005;156(23):734–9.
18. Buyukmihci NC. Lesions in the ocular posterior segment of raptors. J Am Vet Med Assoc 1985;187(11):1121–4.
19. Krautwald-Junghanns M-E, Kostka VM, Dorsch B. Comparative studies on the diagnostic value of conventional radiography and computed tomography in evaluating the heads of psittacine and raptorial birds. J Avian Med Surg 1998,12(3). 149–57.
20. Beaufrére H, Laniesse D, Kabachiev C, et al. Multiple fractures and luxations of palatofacial bones in a hawk-headed parrot (*Deroptyus accipitrinus*). J Am Vet Med Assoc 2019;254(2):251–6.

21. Duvall A, Greenacre C, Jones M. Use of computed tomography in the diagnosis of complicated skull fractures in two parrots. Paper presented at: Exoticscon, September 23–26, 2018; Atlanta, GA.

22. Ashe CC, Morandi F, Greenacre C, et al. What is your diagnosis? J Am Vet Med Assoc 2009;234(4):455–6.

23. Echols MS, Speer B. Diagnosis and treatment of nasal-frontal hinge joint arthrodesis in a hybrid macaw (*Ara macao x Ara ararauna*). Paper presented at: ICARE, April 20–26, 2013; Wiesbaden.

24. Veladiano IA, Banzato T, Bellini L, et al. Computed tomographic anatomy of the heads of blue-and-gold macaws (*Ara ararauna*), African grey parrots (*Psittacus erithacus*), and monk parakeets (*Myiopsitta monachus*). Am J Vet Res 2016; 77(12):1346–56.

25. Wheler CL. Orthopedic conditions of the avian head. Vet Clin North Am Exot Anim Pract 2002;5(1):83–95, vi.

26. Martin H, Ritchie BW. Orthopedic surgical techniques. In: Ritchie BW, Harrison GJ, Harrison LR, editors. Avian medicine: principles and application. Lake Worth (FL): Wingers Publishing; 1994. p. 1138–69.

27. Doneley B. Disorders of the beak and cere. In: Doneley B, editor. Avian medicine and surgery in practice: companion and aviary birds. 2nd edition. Boca Raton (FL): CRC Press; 2016. p. 187–96.

28. Monks D, Miles S, Sciacca E, et al. Treatment of bilateral mandibular fractures in a goose (Anser anser domesticus). Paper presented at: AAVAC, December 1–6, 2017; Auckland.

29. Rice CA, Riehl J, Broman K, et al. Comparing the degree of exothermic polymerization in commonly used acrylic and provisional composite resins for intraoral appliances. J Vet Dent 2012;29(2):78–83.

30. Lye KW, Tideman H, Merkx MA, et al. Bone cements and their potential use in a mandibular endoprosthesis. Tissue Eng Part B Rev 2009;15(4):485–96.

31. Castineiras Perez E, Segade Seoane M, Villanueva Santamarina B, et al. Comparison of holding power of three different pin designs for external skeletal fixation in avian bone: a study in common buzzard (*Buteo buteo*). Vet Surg 2008;37(7):702–5.

32. López Garcia M, Lopez Beceiro AM, Valcarcel Juarez V, et al. Holding power of three different pin designs in the femur and ulna of the common buzzard (*Buteo buteo*). J Zoo Wildl Med 2011;42(4):552–7.

33. Clary EM, Roe SC. In vitrobiomechanical and histological assessment of pilot hole diameter for positive-profile external skeletal fixation pins in canine tibiae. Vet Surg 1996;25(6):453–62.

34. Schnellbacher RW, Stevens AG, Mitchell MA, et al. Use of a dental composite to correct beak deviation in psittacine species. J Exot Pet Med 2010;19(4):290–7.

35. Fecchio RS, Petri BSS, Fitorra LA. Beak correction in a striped owl. Exotic DVM 2010;12(2):7–9.

36. Lothamer C, Snyder CJ, Mans C, et al. Treatment and stabilization of beak symphyseal separation using interfragmentary wiring and provisional bis-acryl composite. J Vet Dentistry 2014;31(4):255–62.

37. Lejnieks D. Treatment of a mandibular fracture using a steel plate in a lesser sulfur-crested cockatoo. Exot DVM 2004;6(4):15–7.

38. Pavletic MM. Dressings, bandages, external support and protective devices. In: Pavletic MM, editor. Atlas of small animal wound management and reconstructive surgery. 4th edition. Hoboken (NJ): Wiley Blackwell; 2018. p. 95–143.

39. Wade L. Acrylic stabilization for psittacine rhinothecal fractures (the "beak helmet"). Paper presented at: Proc Ann Assoc Avian Vet August 29 – September 2, 2015; San Antonio. p. 127–9.

40. Jolly M, Gartrell B. Bill injuries of the North island brown kiwi (*Apteryx mantelli*). Paper presented at: AAVAC, December 1–6, 2017; Auckland.

41. Crosta L. Alloplastic and heteroplastic bill prostheses in 2 ramphastidae birds. J Avian Med Surg 2002;16(3):218–22.

42. Ardisana R, Welle KR. Outcomes of beak amputation in psittacine birds. Proc Assoc Avian Veterinarian August 4–7, 2013; Jacksonville.

43. Bennett RA. Avian respiratory and thoracic surgery. Paper presented at: Proceeding CVC, October 1, 2009; San Diego.

44. Olsen GH. Oral biology and beak disorders of birds. Vet Clin North Am Exot Anim Pract 2003;6(3):505–21, vi.

45. Morris PJ, Weigel JP. Methacrylate beak prosthesis in a marabou stork (*Leptoptilos crumeniferus*). J Assoc Avian Vet 1990;10(2):103–6.

46. Fletcher KC. Repair of bilateral mandibular fractures in a shoebill stork (*Balaeniceps rex*). Journal of Zoo Animal Medicine 1979;10(2):69–72.

47. Calvo Carrasco D, Dutton TA, Shimizu N, et al. Distraction osteogenesis correction of mandibular ramis fracture malunion in a juvenile mute swan (*Cygnus olor*). J Avian Med Surg 2016;30(1):30–8.

48. Anderson K, Arango J, Dugat D, et al. Distraction osteogenesis for correction of scissor beak in a chicken (*Gallus gallus domesticus*). Paper presented at: Exoticscon September 23–26, 2018; Atlanta. p. 451.

49. Calvo Carrasco D, Abou-Zahr T, Shimizu N, et al. Correction of congenital rostrum mandibulare deformity in a yellow-billed kite chick (*Milvus aegyptius*). Paper presented at: ICARE2017; Venice.

50. Chitty J. Beak repair in a red-crowned crane grus (*Grus japonensis*). Paper presented at: Proc Annu Assoc Avian Vet August 16–20, 2004. New Orleans, LA, USA. p. 430.

51. Foerster SH, Gilson SD, Bennett RA, et al. Surgical correction of palatine bone luxation in a blue-and-gold macaw (*Ara ararauna*). J Avian Med Surg 2000; 14(2):118–21.

Orthopedics in Reptiles and Amphibians

Peter M. DiGeronimo, VMD, MSc[a],*, João Brandão, LMV, MS, DECZM (Avian)[b]

KEYWORDS

- Secondary hyperparathyroidism • Osteomyelitis • Snake • Lizard • Chelonian
- Anuran • Urodele • External coaptation

KEY POINTS

- The clinical approach to orthopedic cases in reptiles and amphibians starts with a thorough history and review of husbandry, and any underlying disease processes should be diagnosed and addressed.
- Local and systemic analgesia and general anesthesia should be provided as indicated, and diagnostic imaging and ancillary tests (eg, hematology and blood biochemistry panels) should be considered to further characterize the patient's condition.
- Medical management is indicated for pathologic fractures and for the treatment of underlying disease and may include antimicrobials, appropriate nutritional support, bandaging, and/or external coaptation.
- In cases of traumatic fractures, surgical stabilization may include external coaptation and/ or internal fixation and, in the case of chelonians, shell repair.
- Many techniques used in mammalian practice can be applied to reptiles and amphibians, although these species may require prolonged healing times by comparison.

INTRODUCTION

The clinical approach to any orthopedic presentation in a reptile patient begins with a thorough history and review of husbandry. Signalment and inappropriate husbandry may predispose some patients to orthopedic disease, including pathologic fractures, or make them particularly susceptible to traumatic injury. In cases for which surgery is considered, underlying medical problems should be identified and may need to be addressed before surgical intervention.

Reviews of the impacts of husbandry on the health of captive reptiles and amphibians are available.[1–3] However, significant knowledge gaps in species-specific natural

The authors have nothing to disclose.
[a] Department of Clinical Science and Advanced Medicine, School of Veterinary Medicine, University of Pennsylvania, 3900 Delancey Street, Philadelphia, PA 19140, USA; [b] Department of Veterinary Clinical Sciences, Center for Veterinary Health Sciences, Oklahoma State University, 2065 West Farm Road, Stillwater, OK 74078, USA
* Corresponding author. Adventure Aquarium, 1 Riverside Drive, Camden, NJ 08103.
E-mail address: pmdigeronimo@gmail.com

history still inhibit evidence-based husbandry recommendations, especially for amphibian species.[4,5] Husbandry recommendations should attempt to mimic the natural history and environment for each species as far as possible, with attention to microclimates and gradients.

UNDERLYING AND CONCOMITANT CONDITIONS

Hyperparathyroidism is a common condition of captive reptiles and amphibians and is often secondary to inappropriate diets, nutritional deficiencies, lack of exposure to ultraviolet B (UVB) radiation, or primary renal disease. Secondary nutritional hyperparathyroidism (SNHP) should be suspected in reptiles and amphibians fed diets deficient in calcium, vitamin A, and cholecalciferol, and those with inadequate or no UVB exposure.[2,5–8] Physical examination findings in reptiles and amphibians consistent with SNHP may include skeletal deformities (eg, scoliosis or kyphosis of the spine, rounded skull, or shortened mandible), inappropriate posture, nonspecific signs of weakness, and swollen long bones or mandible, including signs of "rubber jaw," resulting from fibrous osteodystrophy.[9,10] (**Fig. 1**) Reptile owners may report muscle fasciculation or tremors that are presumed to be secondary to hypocalcemia.[10] The episodic nature of these events may correlate with periods of growth in juveniles or with periods of reproductive activity in adult females. Reproductive physiology of egg-laying reptiles requires females to mobilize calcium stores in response to ovulation to form shells around their eggs. Therefore, gravid females may be more susceptible to osteomalacia, osteoporosis, and pathologic fractures than males kept under similar husbandry conditions.[11] Pathologic fractures and orthopedic disease should be considered in female reptiles presented for signs of dystocia.

Because of the chronic nature of SNHP, orthopedic disease may be occult and many patients may be presented for concomitant problems. Therefore, diseases of captivity, including SNHP and associated orthopedic disease, should be considered for all patients. In a retrospective study of captive bearded dragons (inland bearded dragon [*Pogona vitticeps*] and black-soil bearded dragon [*Pogona henrylawsoni*]), a majority of patients for which a blood biochemistry profile was performed had a reverse calcium/phosphorus (Ca:P) ratio regardless of the presenting complaint.[12] More than one-third of animals presented for constipation also had evidence of metabolic bone disease.[12] Chronic stress may predispose young growing reptiles to skeletal disease. Elevated plasma corticosterone concentrations have been associated with osteoporosis in juvenile growing American alligators (*Alligator mississippiensis*).[13]

Other than SNHP, reptiles may present for an orthopedic manifestation of other systemic diseases, particularly infection and neoplasia. Hematogenous spread is often

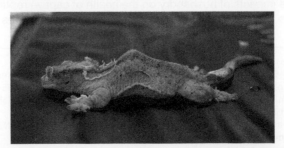

Fig. 1. Crested gecko (*Rhacodactylus ciliatus*) with marked kyphosis consistent with secondary hyperparathyroidism. (*Courtesy of* Mikel Sabater, LV, Dipl. ECZM [Avian], Exoticsvet, Valencia, Spain.)

suspected in cases of osteomyelitis and infectious osteoarthritis in reptiles. Bony lesions were the most common clinical sign associated with detection of Salmonella sp. by fecal cultures in reptiles in a zoologic collection.[14] Although most of these animals were subclinical, snakes were the most common taxa to exhibit signs of illness when testing positive for Salmonella.[14] Necrotizing osteomyelitis, granulomatous inflammation, osteomalacia, and fractures of vertebral bodies and intervertebral spaces caused by systemic infection (most commonly Salmonella sp., but also Pseudomonas sp. and Streptococcus sp.) have been well documented in a variety of captive snakes.[15–19] Blood samples may be used as a proxy for direct sampling of spinal lesions for culture and sensitivity testing to support the diagnosis and direct antimicrobial therapy.[19] An abscess of the epipterygoid bone caused by Salmonella enterica serovar Kintambo infection was described in a savannah monitor (Varanus exanthematicus) that was treated using local antibiotic instillation without aggressive surgical debridement.[20] Disseminated infection with Mycobacterium chelonae was diagnosed in a free-ranging Kemp's ridley sea turtle (Lepidochelys kempii) with a swollen elbow joint and osteolytic lesions on the proximal radius and ulna.[21] Progressive destruction of both humeroscapular joints, associated with Nocardia sp., Corynebacterium sp., α-hemolytic Streptococcus sp., and gram-negative nonfermenters was described in a stranded green sea turtle (Chelonia mydas).[22] Because there was a lack of external wounds, septic arthritis secondary to hematogenous spread was suspected.[22] Systemic mycoplasmosis has been associated with polyarthritis characterized by erosion of articular cartilage and bone and osteophyte formation in Nile crocodiles (Crocodylus niloticus).[23] Paravertebral boney masses believed to be secondary to soft-tissue infection were identified in a blue-tailed monitor (Varanus dorianus) with no lesions of the associated vertebral bodies themselves.[24]

For amphibians, water quality is also paramount to systemic and musculoskeletal health. Metabolic bone disease was documented in captive colonies of New Zealand frogs (Archey's frog [Leiopelma archeyi] and Hochstetter's New Zealand frog [Leiopelma hochstetteri]) as a result of excessive fluoride in water from municipal water sources.[25] Dietary calcium supplementation, UVB exposure, and use of defluorinated water reduced the morbidity, incidence of bone fractures, and mortality rates in these colonies.[25] Other musculoskeletal abnormalities of amphibians, such as limb deformities, are caused by trematode cysts (Ribeiroia sp.) that disrupt the cellular organization of limb buds and have been well documented in free-ranging anurans.[26]

Neoplasia has been well documented in snakes and other squamates.[27] Neoplasia may directly affect the skull and jaw or the axial skeleton. In a retrospective study of 358 tumor samples, 13 were bone neoplasias. In lizards, benign proliferations of the bone (ossifying fibroma [n = 2], fibrous dysplasia [n = 1]) as well as malignant cartilage (chondrosarcoma [n = 2]) and bone tumors (fibroblastic osteosarcoma [n = 2], small cell osteosarcoma [n = 1]) on the head (n = 5) and limbs (n = 3) were reported.[28] In snakes, only malignant cartilage neoplasms (chondrosarcoma [n = 2], undifferentiated chondrosarcoma [n = 3]) of the spine were diagnosed.[28] An ameloblastoma was documented to cause mandibular osteolysis in a free-ranging black rat snake (Pantherophis alleghaniensis).[29] An osteosarcoma originating from the ribs of an 18-month-old captive-bred woma python (Aspidites ramsayi) has been reported.[30] Chondroblastic osteosarcoma associated with the pelvic girdle was diagnosed in 2 related spiny-tailed monitor lizards (Varanus acanthurus).[31] An oral fibrosarcoma was diagnosed in a geriatric black iguana (Ctenosaura pectinata).[32] These cases suggest that advanced age and genetic predisposition may play roles in neoplasia of reptiles as they do for mammals.

When approaching reptile orthopedic cases, other disease processes to consider include osteitis deformans (Paget's disease) and congenital and developmental abnormalities. Osteitis deformans is a chronic focal disorder of bone remodeling that results in a disorganized mosaic of woven and lamellar bone.[33] The condition was documented in a Burmese python (*Python molurus bivittatus*) with impaired mobility and boney masses of the vertebral column similar to those documented in snakes with infectious vertebral osteomyelitis.[33] Exposure to inappropriate temperatures and humidity gradients has been documented to cause skeletal deformities developmentally in various reptile species. Besides developmental abnormalities from improper incubation, hereditary skeletal abnormalities have also been documented in reptiles. Congenital kyphosis that was present from hatching and progressively worsened with age has been reported in a Brazilian rainbow boa (*Epicrates cenchria crassus*).[34] The deformity was characterized by multiple dorsal deviations of the spinal column without the presence of osteoarthrosis, and was believed to be congenital because no other individuals in the clutch were affected despite the eggs having been incubated in an identical manner. Other congenital abnormalities of the axial skeleton, including kyphosis and scoliosis, have been documented in free-ranging viperids, jararaca (*Bothrops jararaca*), and cascabel rattlesnake (*Crotalus durissus terrificus*).[35]

TRIAGE AND DIAGNOSTICS

The clinician's intent should be to provide the same standard of care for reptile patients as for mammals. As such, analgesia is imperative for all patients with orthopedic problems. Although a discussion of analgesia in reptile and amphibian medicine is beyond the scope of this article, thorough evidence-based reviews may be found elsewhere.[36–39] Signs of pain in reptiles may be subtler than those in mammalian patients. Changes in feeding behavior may be the only indication of pain in some patients. In a study of ball pythons (*Python regius*), animals subjected to noxious chemical or surgical stimuli showed delays in striking prey items or would skip meals altogether relative to control animals.[40] Therefore, a thorough history should include detailed information on the patient's food consumption and feeding behavior. Fractures and open wounds should be assumed to be painful and treated accordingly with systemic analgesics, and general and/or local anesthesia. As in other species, manipulation and treatment of fractures should be performed under general anesthesia.

Consider administration of analgesics or induction of anesthesia before a physical examination. Findings on orthopedic examination may include lameness, swelling, necrosis of extremities, joint luxation, and impaired or inappropriate range of motion.[12] Obvious wounds should be further characterized by severity (open versus closed; clean versus contaminated versus infected), chronicity, and anatomic location. Open wounds should be thoroughly lavaged and debrided, and systemic and/or local antimicrobial therapy instituted before surgical closure.

Diagnostic imaging is often necessary to characterize orthopedic disease and institute appropriate treatment. Grossly apparently skeletal lesions and a history of trauma were cited as the most common indications for radiographic evaluation of lizards in one referral hospital.[41] Radiography is indicated in all cases where orthopedic disease is suspected. In addition to identifying traumatic and pathologic fractures, clinical radiography and computed tomography (CT) have been used to subjectively evaluate and to quantify bone density in amphibians, respectively.[7,42] Radiographic techniques for reptiles and amphibians follow similar principles to those applied for mammals and have been reviewed elsewhere.[43] Orthogonal views are indicated as in other species.

Additionally, in chelonians an anterior-posterior projection is recommended for evaluation of the lung fields and the carapace.

CT may not be readily available in most practices, but can be used to identify skeletal lesions not apparent radiographically. For chelonians, it is particularly useful for evaluation of proximal joints of the thoracic and pelvic limbs (shoulder and coxofemoral joints, respectively) and shell lesions. CT has been used to diagnose shoulder luxation in a radiated tortoise (Geochelone radiata) and scapular fracture and coxofemoral luxation in a common snapping turtle (Chelydra serpentina).[44] Because the bones of the shell do not align with the external scutes, CT is particularly useful in evaluating the axial skeleton of chelonians to aid clinical decision-making, especially when evidence of trauma is not externally apparent.[44,45] In boa constrictors (Boa constrictor imperator), CT has been used to guide biopsies of proliferative bone lesions observed radiographically on vertebral bodies.[17] Reviews of the application of CT in reptile practice are available.[46]

Ancillary diagnostics, including blood biochemistry profiles, low total serum calcium concentrations, low ionized calcium, inverse Ca:P ratios, high parathyroid hormone, and low serum calcidiol (25-hydroxycholecalciferol) concentrations, may be used to support a diagnosis of secondary hyperparathyroidism. Elevated alkaline phosphatase may reflect bone remodeling, and elevated creatinine kinase may reflect recent tissue damage.[33] Renal disease may lead to azotemia and, when severe, is one of the causes of secondary hyperparathyroidism. In a study of juvenile veiled chameleons (Chamaeleo calyptratus), total serum calcium concentrations lower than 2.3 mmol/L (9.2 mg/dL) were consistent with nutritional metabolic bone disease, and serum calcidiol concentrations greater than 100 μg/L (>250 nmol/L) were considered ideal.[8] Underlying and concomitant problems should be addressed.

Joint disease of the shoulder joint (eg, septic arthritis or degenerative osteoarthritis) is occasionally described in reptiles and is usually diagnosed by imaging. Arthroscopy is a surgical procedure used to visualize, diagnose, and potentially treat problems within a joint. Although this diagnostic tool has not been well investigated in reptiles, it may be of use for cases of osteoarthritis and potential joint infections. Fluoroscopic-guided arthroscopy was used in a yellow-headed snapping turtle (Elseya irwini) with focal degenerative joint disease of the left glenohumeral joint.[47] Arthroscopy allowed the assessment of the joint and collection of samples for aerobic bacterial, fungal, and mycobacterial cultures.[47] The investigators suggest that arthroscopy can provide a minimally invasive surgical technique to evaluate joint disorders in turtles.[47]

FRACTURE STABILIZATION

Once a fracture has been identified, the site should be immobilized promptly to promote healing and avoid complications associated with osseous nonunion. Urodeles, specifically axolotls (Ambystoma mexicanum), have been used in experimental models of bone healing and tissue regeneration.[48,49] These models are capable of successful healing of nonstabilized fractures if the fragments are within close proximity.[49] Therefore, in these species stabilization may be recommended for displaced fractures. Cage rest in small enclosures may also be a good option for small-sized patients or species in which the placement of bandage material may damage the skin.

External Coaptation

External coaptation is indicated for immediate stabilization of fracture sites on triage, for patients that are poor surgical or anesthetic candidates owing to concomitant disease, and for patients too small for internal or external surgical fixation. External coaptation may be the only treatment option for some patients, as surgical fixation of fractures should not be pursued in cases where the strength of the bone is compromised because of SNHP or other metabolic bone diseases. To stabilize the fracture site, the joints immediately proximal and distal to the fractured bone must be immobilized.

Ball bandages may be used to stabilize digit luxations and fractures by taping the digits to a ball of cotton or rolled gauze placed in the center of the palmar or plantar aspect of the manus or pes, respectively.[50,51] Nonadhesive dressing is used to incorporate the digits and the entire foot proximal to the carpal or tarsal joint into the bandage. In some cases, these fractures may be stabilized by taping the affected digit to an adjacent digit. In smaller lizards and crocodilians, fractures of the radius and/or ulna of the thoracic limb and of the tibia and/or fibula of the pelvic limb may be stabilized by extending the limb and binding it to the body wall or tail base, respectively, with adhesive medical tape or nonadhesive bandaging.[50–52] (**Fig. 2**) The use of custom-made foam material between the limb and the body may improve fracture alignment (**Fig. 3**), and stabilization may be improved by including a splint in the bandage. Because the risk of malunion is greater for humeral and femoral fractures using this technique, casting the thoracic or pelvic girdles, respectively, is recommended.[50,51] (**Fig. 4**) Care must be taken not to occlude the vent when including the pelvic girdle in bandaging or casting. In chelonians, the limb maybe taped or bandaged into place within the shell to restrict movement.[50] Scapulohumeral luxation and scapular fracture have been successfully treated in chelonians using this technique.[44] Only one thoracic or one pelvic limb should be restricted at a time because chelonians may experience breathing difficulties if all limbs are restricted simultaneously.

In reptiles, some skull and jaw fractures may be successfully treated by a restrictive bandage around the head and mouth. Prior placement of an esophagostomy tube allows for nutritional support and enteral medication administration during the convalescent period.[51] A 1.5-year-old male blue-tongued skink with an open, bilateral mandibular fracture and multiple rib fractures as a result of malnutrition and trauma was managed with a nonsurgical approach.[53–56] An intraoral U-shaped 2-mm plastic plate was placed, and two bands of tape were applied to minimize movement of the mouth.[53] The first tape was placed around the mandible and maxilla just caudal to the nares and in front of the eyes while the second tape was placed on the ventrorostral part of the mandible ascending in an angle behind both eyes.[53] Experimentally

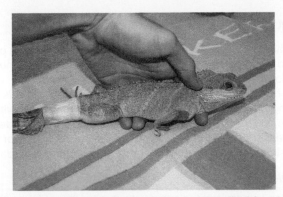

Fig. 2. Chinese water dragon (*Physignathus cocincinus*) with a tibial fracture stabilized using external coaptation by taping the length of the affected bone to the tail base. (*Courtesy of* Mikel Sabater, LV, Dipl. ECZM [Avian], Exoticsvet, Valencia, Spain.)

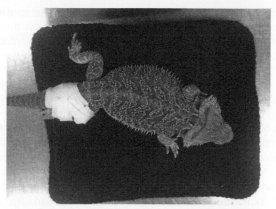

Fig. 3. Inland bearded dragon (*Pogona vitticeps*) with a femoral fracture stabilized using external coaptation. Foam was placed to improve limb placement. (*Courtesy of* Kailey Anderson, DVM, Oklahoma State University, Stillwater, Oklahoma, USA.)

induced unilateral mandibular fractures in adult spotted salamanders (*Ambystoma maculatum*) healed without treatment, with osseous union noted by 21 weeks after fracture.[57]

Amputation

In one retrospective study of captive bearded dragons, limb or tail amputation was the most common orthopedic surgery reported.[12] Digits should be amputated at the level of the metacarpus or metatarsus.[50] In smaller lizards, partial limb amputation may leave a stump to aid in locomotion, although there is risk of dehiscence, infection, and recurrent trauma at the site.[50,51] When possible, surgical incisions should be closed such that the incision is not in direct contact with the ground. In larger reptiles, complete amputation through the scapulohumeral or coxofemoral joints may be indicated.[50] A rolling prosthetic or wheel can be affixed to the plastron of chelonians to allow for walking.[50,51] Surgical excision of the femoral head and neck has been described to successfully treat an adult leopard tortoise (*Stigmochelys pardalis*) with

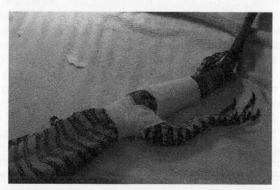

Fig. 4. Juvenile monitor lizard (*Varanus varius*) with a femoral and a hip fracture stabilized using external coaptation that incorporates both the coxofemoral joints and the stifle of the affected limb. Note that the vent is not occluded by the tape. (*Courtesy of* Mikel Sabater, LV, Dipl. ECZM [Avian], Exoticsvet, Valencia, Spain.)

chronic, non–weight-bearing lameness resulting from a coxofemoral luxation.[58] A cranial approach through the prefemoral fossa was used to access the joint.

Tail amputation follows the same surgical principles as in mammals. In male squamates, care must be taken not to damage the hemipenes should amputation at the proximal end of the tail be indicated. Some lizard species of the iguana (Iguanidae), skink (Scincidae), and gecko (Gekkonidae and Phyllodacylidae) families are capable of caudal (tail) autotomy. In these species, the skin may be incised caudal to the site of amputation and the tail snapped and slightly twisted at the intended site of amputation so as to break the tail through the natural fracture plane of a coccygeal vertebra.[50] This approach does not negate the need for general anesthesia, analgesia, and aseptic technique. If amputated as such, iguanids may regenerate their tail, although primary closure is indicated for all other taxa.

Limb amputation is often indicated for comminuted fractures of the long bones of amphibians.[59] Axolotls are capable of regenerating cartilage at articular surfaces, digits, and entire limbs, and may do so following surgical amputation.[48] In anurans, amputation of the hind limb at the coxofemoral joint is recommended.[59] Because male anurans require use of their forelimbs to achieve amplexus during mating, partial forelimb amputation is recommended especially for animals intended for breeding or release into the wild.[59] In Eastern newts (Notophthalmus viridescens), the skeletal elements of an amputated limb were restored in a proximal-to-distal direction, reiterating the developmental pattern; however, the portion of the humerus distal to the amputation site failed to ossify in synchrony with the regenerating radius and ulna.[60] By 270 days, most regenerated skeletal parts were undergoing ossification, but those of the wrist remained entirely cartilaginous.[61]

External Fixation

External fixation cannot be applied to the limbs of chelonians because the devices are prone to damage and failure when the patient attempts to withdraw the limb into the shell.[50] External skeletal fixation (ESF) devices can be fashioned using materials readily available in most practices. Bone pins or hypodermic needles are inserted through each fragment of the affected bone at various angles. A connecting bar is fashioned across the needles parallel to the bone by using an intravenous fluid line tubing or a Penrose drain filled with dental acrylic or polymethylmethacrylate (PMMA). ESF devices may be used for fractures of long bones and the mandible[62] (**Fig. 5**). In some cases, stabilization may be improved with the use of cerclage or Kirschner wires. In a captive Fly River turtle (Carettochelys insculpta), rostral mandibular, left mandibular, left maxillary, and bilateral orbital fractures were repaired using external skeletal fixators and cerclage wire.[63] Hypodermic needles may be inserted through the bone on each side of the fracture site and used to guide the passage of the wire through the bone. The needles are removed before twisting the ends of the wire to create an interfragmentary loop. Bilateral tibial fractures in an American bullfrog (Lithobates catesbeianus) were repaired using a type-I external fixator with 0.45 Kirschner wires.[64] Although pins were left in place until radiographic evidence of bone union was well established (69–85 days), earlier removal may have been possible based on palpation of the fracture and the presence of callus.[64] Osteomyelitis was suspected in multiple areas of the bone but seemed to improve with different antibiotic treatments, and at 1 year after surgery appeared to have healed appropriately on radiographic examination.[64] The animal was ultimately euthanized approximately 2 years later for suspected osteomyelitis, but necropsy was not performed.[64]

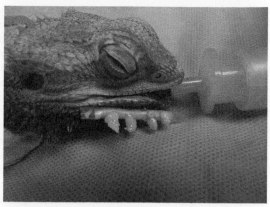

Fig. 5. External fixation of a mandibular fracture in an inland bearded dragon (*Pogona vitticeps*). (*Courtesy of* David Eshar, DVM, Dipl. ABVP (Exotic Companion Mammals), Dipl. ECZM [Small Mammal & Zoo Health Management], Kansas State University, Manhattan, Kansas, USA.)

Internal Fixation

In general, internal fixation techniques include intramedullary pins and bone plates, and follow the same principles in reptiles and amphibians as in other species.[51,59]

The successful treatment of a complete fracture of the ramus of the mandible of a boa constrictor with a plate and compression screws has been described.[65] A mandibular fracture in an Eastern bluetongue skink (*Tiliqua scincoides scincoides*) was repaired using a combination of an intramedullary pin and suture material.[66] A closed comminuted fracture of the femur of an American bullfrog was successfully treated with internal fixation by use of interfragmentary Kirschner wires and securing a positive profile pin along the femur with encircling sutures and modeling PMMA around the apparatus.[67] A common chameleon (*Chamaeleo chamaeleon*) with an oblique fracture of the metaphysis of the left humerus was treated by internal fixation using a 22-gauge needle placed in a retrograde approach.[68] The implant was removed after 3 months when a cartilaginous callus was noted.[68] A right femoral fracture was repaired with 1-mm Kirschner wire placed intramedullary in a 6-month-old green iguana (*Iguana iguana*).[69] During the postoperative period, the animal developed severe metabolic bone disease and died at approximately 4.5 months.[69]

Other Procedures

Joint injury and intervertebral disease may be diagnosed and treated similarly as in mammals. The successful stabilization of a stifle joint using an extra-articular surgical approach has been described in an American bullfrog with presumptive cruciate rupture.[70] A dorsal laminectomy successfully resolved clinical signs associated with proliferative boney lesions and kyphosis of the spine in a two-toed amphiuma (*Amphiuma means*), although the animal required subsequent euthanasia because of recurrence of an unidentified, underlying problem causing ongoing vertebral disorder.[71]

Shell Fracture Repair

Chelonians have their internal organs protected by the shell, which is composed of the carapace dorsally and plastron ventrally connected by the lateral bridges. The origin of the carapace has remained unclear for many years, and several hypotheses regarding the incorporation of the exoskeletal components into the costal and neural plates have been suggested.[72] It has recently been proposed that the major part of the carapace evolved solely by modification of the endoskeleton.[72] The shell structure protects the reptile from predator attacks by sustaining impact loads and dissipating energy.[73] A central longitudinal row of neural plates caps the neural spines of the dorsal vertebrae and a lateral row of costal plates is closely associated with the dorsal ribs. A marginal row of marginal plates, an anterior nuchal plate, and 1 or 2 posterior pygal plate(s) complete the carapace.[74] Because the shell is made of bone, the management of a shell fracture should follow the same principles as for any other bone repair.

Traumatic shell fracture is a common presenting complaint of chelonians, especially free-ranging individuals. Sea turtles are often presented with traumatic shell fracture or erosion resulting from a boat or propeller strike.[75] Terrestrial turtles are prone to lawn mowers and terrestrial and aquatic turtles are prone to vehicular trauma, especially during nesting seasons when the search for appropriate nesting sites leads gravid females across roadways.[52,76]

Wounds should be thoroughly cleaned by lavage and surgical debridement under general anesthesia before primary closure. In all cases, the wound should be lavaged with warm antiseptic solution (eg, dilute iodine) followed by sterile saline.[50] Standard wet-to-dry bandaging may be indicated to decontaminate infected wounds. Wounds that communicate with the coelom carry a poorer prognosis.

Vacuum-assisted closure (VAC) has been described as an alternative method for wound management in chelonians. VAC may lead to improvement of wound perfusion, reduction of interstitial edema and inflammatory or inhibitory cytokines, stimulation of the production of biochemical mediators, or changes in cellular function that may result in the enhancement of granulation tissue formation, reduction in bacterial contamination, and enhanced removal of exudative material from a wound.[77] Comparison of VAC and traditional bandages has not been reported in chelonians.

For partial-thickness, ulcerative shell lesions, photopolymerizable nanohybrid dental composite can be used to close the wounds in addition to local and systemic antibiotics and analgesics as needed.[78] Healing may be expected within 3 months.[78] For shell wounds in aquatic turtles that require recurrent dressing or topical treatment, the bottom may be removed from a resealable plastic container and affixed directly to the shell with epoxy or dental acrylic to provide a waterproof but accessible environment.[79]

Reduction and stabilization of shell fractures may be achieved using screws and wire or plates mounted through the shell itself (**Fig. 6**). Alternatively, a top-closure system may be used by affixing mounts for cable ties or wires to the outer surface of the shell using epoxy or dental acrylic.[80] This allows for reduction of central and marginal shell fractures without having to drill holes through the tissue to secure interfragmentary wires. Larger defects can be bridged with sterilized fiberglass patches or aluminum mesh.[50] Chelonians require appropriate care postoperatively including analgesics, antibiotics, and nutritional support. Repeat diagnostic imaging may be used to confirm osseous union of the bony plates below the visible scutes. Closely apposed fractures may heal within 12 to 18 weeks, whereas larger defects may require significantly longer healing times.[50] For free-ranging animals, all medical devices should be removed following rehabilitation before release to the wild.

It important to consider that covering infected wounds or fractures may provide an environment that allows bacteria to proliferate and lead to infections later in life. The use of bacterial cultures and cytology may provide clinicians with information regarding the presence of contamination before the application of such material (eg, fiberglass). Ideally the wound bed or fracture site should not be infected; however,

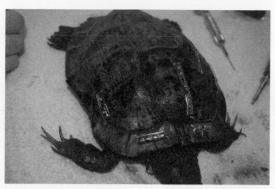

Fig. 6. Bone plates used to repair a shell fracture in a red-eared slider (*Trachemys scripta elegans*). (*Courtesy of* João Brandão, LMV, MS, Dipl. ECZM [Avian], Oklahoma State University, Stillwater, Oklahoma, USA.)

this may be difficult to determine and there will always be an inherent risk associated with it. Alternatively, the use of stabilization devices that do not directly cover the wounds allows for fracture healing and application of treatments (**Fig. 7**). Anecdotally, protective devices such as plastic food containers have been attached to the shell of chelonians, providing protection to the wound while allowing for the application of treatments (**Fig. 8**).

CONVALESCENCE

Appropriate nutritional support, maintenance within species-specific preferred optimal temperature zones and humidity levels, and local and systemic analgesia and antimicrobial therapy as indicated are essential during the convalescent period for healing to occur.[81] Gavage feeding and esophagostomy tubes should be considered in anorectic animals. Feeding tubes, as previously mentioned, may be of use for cases of skull fractures so as to minimize manipulation of the affected area during the healing process.

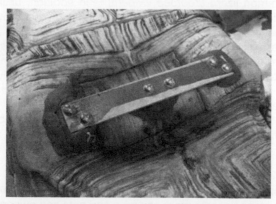

Fig. 7. A customized surgical osteotomy repair in an African spurred tortoise (*Geochelone sulcata*). Note that the metal bar is elevated from the plastron and not covering the surgical cut surface. (*Courtesy of* João Brandão, LMV, MS, Dipl. ECZM [Avian], Oklahoma State University, Stillwater, Oklahoma, USA.)

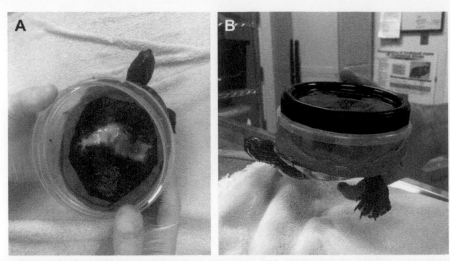

Fig. 8. A captive river cooter (*Pseudemys concinna*) with lesions of the carapace caused by infection with *Pseudomonas aeruginosa*. (*A*) Application of a plastic food storage container using a low exothermic coral reef epoxy to protect the wound but still allow access for the application of topical treatments. (*B*) Plastic food storage container secured to the carapace. The animal, after a period of habituation, was able to be kept in its regular aquatic enclosure. (*Courtesy of* João Brandão, LMV, MS, Dipl. ECZM [Avian], Oklahoma State University, Stillwater, Oklahoma, USA.)

In general, wounds and bone fractures in reptiles take longer to heal than in mammals of similar sizes.[81] In some cases of complete bone fractures, it can take up to 3 months until there is radiographic evidence of bony callus and more than 5 months until radiographic confirmation of osseous union.[62] Following stabilization, reptiles generally form a larger cartilaginous callus than may be expected in mammals.[81] Radiographically this may cause the ends of the fractures to appear further apart in the weeks following stabilization than at the time of initial presentation. In an experimental model, endochondral ossification was first apparent radiographically at 3 weeks in a common lizard (*Zootoca vivipara*).[81] In addition, unlike in mammals, experimental models of Italian wall lizards (*Podarcis muralis*) have shown that the articular cartilage of reptiles has high regenerative potential.[82]

Unlike other Classes, amphibians achieve fracture healing by subsequent ossification of a callus formed by periosteal hyperplasia rather than by secondary cartilage.[57] In untreated spotted salamanders with mandibular fractures, the callus was apparent by 5 weeks after fracture, and calcified bony tissue was observed between 7 and 11 weeks after fracture with complete osseous union by 21 weeks.[57]

ESF devices, interfragmentary wires, and intramedullary pins may be removed after radiographic confirmation of bony callus and osseous union.

SUMMARY

Orthopedics in reptiles and amphibians has evolved significantly over the years. As reptiles and amphibians become more common and pets and owners demand higher quality of care, veterinarians need to develop and improve new techniques and new management options. Nonetheless, some species have anatomic characteristics that limit or impair the veterinarian's ability to completely resolve some of the conditions, such as a limb fracture in a chelonian. New equipment that can be adapted to reptiles and amphibians will likely be developed and become available in the future. The use of an evidence-based approach to reptile and amphibian orthopedics is recommended, and additional research is warranted.

REFERENCES

1. Chinnadurai SK, Kane LP. Advances in amphibian clinical therapeutics. J Exot Pet Med 2014;23:50–5.
2. Watson MK, Mitchell MA. Vitamin D and ultraviolet B radiation considerations for exotic pets. J Exot Pet Med 2014;23:369–79.
3. Antwis R, Browne R. Ultraviolet radiation and vitamin D 3 in amphibian health, behaviour, diet and conservation. Comp Biochem Physiol A Mol Integr Physiol 2009;154:184–90.
4. Michaels CJ, Gini BF, Preziosi RF. The importance of natural history and species-specific approaches in amphibian ex-situ conservation. Herpetol J 2014;24: 135–45.
5. Pessier AP, Baitchman EJ, Crump P, et al. Causes of mortality in anuran amphibians from an ex situ survival assurance colony in Panama. Zoo Biol 2014;33: 516–26.
6. Michaels C, Antwis R, Preziosi R. Impacts of UVB provision and dietary calcium content on serum vitamin D3, growth rates, skeletal structure and coloration in captive oriental fire-bellied toads (*Bombina orientalis*). J Anim Physiol Anim Nutr (Berl) 2015;99:391–403.
7. Tapley B, Rendle M, Baines FM, et al. Meeting ultraviolet B radiation requirements of amphibians in captivity: a case study with mountain chicken frogs (*Leptodactylus fallax*) and general recommendations for pre-release health screening. Zoo Biol 2015;34:46–52.
8. Hoby S, Wenker C, Robert N, et al. Nutritional metabolic bone disease in juvenile veiled chameleons (*Chamaeleo calyptratus*) and its prevention. J Nutr 2010;140: 1923–31.
9. Liu N, Niu J, Wang D, et al. Spinal pathomorphological changes in the breeding giant salamander juveniles. Zoomorphology 2016;135:115–20.
10. Wright K. Two common disorders of captive bearded dragons (*Pogona vitticeps*): nutritional secondary hyperparathyroidism and constipation. J Exot Pet Med 2008;17:267–72.
11. Raiti P, Haramati N. Magnetic resonance imaging and computerized tomography of a gravid leopard tortoise (*Geochelone pardalis pardalis*) with metabolic bone disease. J Zoo Wildl Med 1997;28:189–97.
12. Schmidt-Ukaj S, Hochleithner M, Richter B, et al. A survey of diseases in captive bearded dragons: a retrospective study of 529 patients. Vet Med (Praha) 2017; 62:508–15.
13. Elsey RM, Joanen T, McNease L, et al. Stress and plasma corticosterone levels in the American alligator—relationships with stocking density and nesting success. Comp Biochem Physiol A Physiol 1990;95:55–63.
14. Clancy MM, Davis M, Valitutto MT, et al. Salmonella infection and carriage in reptiles in a zoological collection. J Am Vet Med Assoc 2016;248:1050–9.
15. Hardt I, Gava MG, Paz JS, et al. Inclusion body disease and spondylitis by *Salmonella* sp. in a *Boa constrictor constrictor*. Pesqui Vet Bras 2017;37:984–90.
16. de Souza SO, Casagrande RA, Guerra PR, et al. Osteomyelitis caused by *Salmonella enterica* serovar Derby in boa constrictor. J Zoo Wildl Med 2014;45:642–4.

17. Di Girolamo N, Selleri P, Nardini G, et al. Computed tomography-guided bone biopsies for evaluation of proliferative vertebral lesions in two boa constrictors (*Boa constrictor imperator*). J Zoo Wildl Med 2014;45:973–8.

18. Ramsay EC, Daniel GB, Tryon BW, et al. Osteomyelitis associated with Salmonella enterica SS arizonae in a colony of ridgenose rattlesnakes (*Crotalus willardi*). J Zoo Wildl Med 2002;33:301–10.

19. Isaza R, Garner M, Jacobson E. Proliferative osteoarthritis and osteoarthrosis in 15 snakes. J Zoo Wildl Med 2000;31:20–7.

20. Barboza T, Beaufrère H, Chalmers H. Epipterygoid bone Salmonella abscess in a Savannah monitor (*Varanus exanthematicus*). J Herpetol Med Surg 2018;28: 29–33.

21. Greer LL, Strandberg JD, Whitaker BR. *Mycobacterium chelonae* osteoarthritis in a Kemp's Ridley sea turtle (*Lepidochelys kempii*). J Wildl Dis 2003;39:736–41.

22. Guthrie A, George J, deMaar TW. Bilateral chronic shoulder infections in an adult green sea turtle (*Chelonia mydas*). J Herpetol Med Surg 2010;20:105–8.

23. Huchzermeyer FW, Groenewald HB, Myburgh JG, et al. Osteoarthropathy of unknown aetiology in the long bones of farmed and wild Nile crocodiles (*Crocodylus niloticus*). J S Afr Vet Assoc 2013;84:1–5.

24. Rothschild BM. Paravertebral masses in blue-tailed monitor, *Varanus dorianus*, indicative of soft-tissue infection with associated osteomyelitis. J Zoo Wildl Med 2014;45:47–52.

25. Shaw SD, Bishop PJ, Harvey C, et al. Fluorosis as a probable factor in metabolic bone disease in captive New Zealand native frogs (*Leiopelma species*). J Zoo Wildl Med 2012;43:549–65.

26. Stopper GF, Hecker L, Franssen RA, et al. How trematodes cause limb deformities in amphibians. J Exp Zool 2002;294:252–63.

27. Page-Karjian A, Hahne M, Leach K, et al. Neoplasia in snakes at Zoo Atlanta during 1992–2012. J Zoo Wildl Med 2017;48:521–4.

28. Dietz J, Heckers K, Pees M, et al. Bone tumours in lizards and snakes. A rare clinical finding. Tierarztl Prax Ausg K Kleintiere Heimtiere 2015;43:31–9.

29. Comolli JR, Olsen HM, Seguel M, et al. Ameloblastoma in a wild black rat snake (*Pantherophis alleghaniensis*). J Vet Diagn Invest 2015;27:536–9.

30. Cowan M, Monks D, Raidal S. Osteosarcoma in a woma python (*Aspidites ramsayi*). Aust Vet J 2011;89:520–3.

31. Needle D, McKnight CA, Kiupel M. Chondroblastic osteosarcoma in two related spiny-tailed monitor lizards (*Varanus acanthurus*). J Exot Pet Med 2013;22:265–9.

32. Salinas EM, Arriaga BOA, Lezama JR, et al. Oral fibrosarcoma in a black iguana (*Ctenosaura pectinata*). J Zoo Wildl Med 2013;44:513–6.

33. Preziosi R, Diana A, Florio D, et al. Osteitis deformans (Paget's disease) in a Burmese python (*Python molurus bivittatus*)—a case report. Vet J 2007;174:669–72.

34. Sesoko NF, Bortolini Z, Miranda BS, et al. Congenital bone malformation in a rainbow boa *Epicrates cenchria crassus*—case report. Medicina Veterinaria-Recife 2011;5:281–4.

35. de Carvalho MPN, Sant'Anna SS, Grego KF, et al. Microcomputed tomographic, morphometric, and histopathologic assessment of congenital bone malformations in two neotropical viperids. J Wildl Dis 2017;53:804–15.

36. Perry SM, Nevarez JG. Pain and its control in reptiles. Vet Clin North Am Exot Anim Pract 2018;21:1–16.

37. Stevens CW. Analgesia in amphibians: preclinical studies and clinical applications. Vet Clin North Am Exot Anim Pract 2011;14:33–44.

38. Mosley C. Pain and nociception in reptiles. Vet Clin North Am Exot Anim Pract 2011;14:45–60.
39. Balko JA, Chinnadurai SK. Advancements in evidence-based analgesia in exotic animals. Vet Clin North Am Exot Anim Pract 2017;20:899–915.
40. James LE, Williams CJ, Bertelsen MF, et al. Evaluation of feeding behavior as an indicator of pain in snakes. J Zoo Wildl Med 2017;48:196–9.
41. Lojszczyk-Szczepaniak A, Szczepaniak KO, Grzybek M, et al. Causes of consultations and results of radiological and ultrasound methods in lizard diseases (2006-2014). Medycyna Weterynaryjna 2018;74:65–9.
42. van Zijll Langhout M, Struijk RP, Könning T, et al. Evaluation of bone mineralization by computed tomography in wild and captive European common spadefoots (*Pelobates fuscus*), in relation to exposure to ultraviolet B radiation and dietary supplements. J Zoo Wildl Med 2017;48:748–56.
43. Schumacher J, Toal RL. Advanced radiography and ultrasonography in reptiles. Semin Avian Exot Pet Med 2001;10:162–8.
44. Abou-Madi N, Scrivani PV, Kollias GV, et al. Diagnosis of skeletal injuries in chelonians using computed tomography. J Zoo Wildl Med 2004;35:226–31.
45. Spadola F, Barillaro G, Morici M, et al. The practical use of computed tomography in evaluation of shell lesions in six loggerhead turtles (*Caretta caretta*). Vet Med (Praha) 2016;61:394–8.
46. Gumpenberger M, Henninger W. The use of computed tomography in avian and reptile medicine. Sem Avian Exot Pet Med 2001;174–80.
47. Hadfield CA, Canapp SO Jr, Clayton LA, et al. Fluoroscopic-guided shoulder arthroscopy in a yellow-headed snapping turtle (*Elseya irwini*) with focal degenerative joint disease. J Herpetol Med Surg 2011;21:45–9.
48. Cosden R, Lattermann C, Romine S, et al. Intrinsic repair of full-thickness articular cartilage defects in the axolotl salamander. Osteoarthritis Cartilage 2011;19:200–5.
49. Hutchison C, Pilote M, Roy S. The axolotl limb: a model for bone development, regeneration and fracture healing. Bone 2007;40:45–56.
50. Alworth LC, Hernandez SM, Divers SJ. Laboratory reptile surgery: principles and techniques. J Am Assoc Lab Anim Sci 2011;50:11–26.
51. Raftery A. Reptile orthopedic medicine and surgery. J Exot Pet Med 2011;20:107–16.
52. Mitchell MA. Diagnosis and management of reptile orthopedic injuries. Vet Clin North Am Exot Anim Pract 2002;5:97–114.
53. Köchli B, Schmid N, Hatt J, et al. Nonsurgical treatment of a bilateral mandibular fracture in a blue-tongued skink. Exot DVM 2008;10:25–8.
54. Naganobu K, Ogawa H, Oyadomari N, et al. Surgical repair of a depressed fracture in a green sea turtle, *Chelonia mydas*. J Vet Med Sci 2000;62:103–4.
55. Goldberg DW, Adeodato A, de Almeida DT, et al. Green turtle head trauma with intracerebral hemorrhage: image diagnosis and treatment. Ciência Rural 2010;40:2402–5.
56. Franchini D, Cavaliere L, Valastro C, et al. Management of severe head injury with brain exposure in three loggerhead sea turtles *Caretta caretta*. Dis Aquat Organ 2016;119:145–52.
57. Hall BK, Hanken J. Repair of fractured lower jaws in the spotted salamander: do amphibians form secondary cartilage? J Exp Zool 1985;233:359–68.
58. Naylor AD. Femoral head and neck excision arthroplasty in a leopard tortoise (*Stigmochelys pardalis*). J Zoo Wildl Med 2013;44:982–9.
59. Gentz EJ. Medicine and surgery of amphibians. ILAR J 2007;48:255–9.

60. Stock SR, Blackburn D, Gradassi M, et al. Bone formation during forelimb regeneration: a microtomography (microCT) analysis. Dev Dyn 2003;226:410–7.
61. Libbin RM, Singh IJ, Hirschman A, et al. A prolonged cartilaginous phase in newt forelimb skeletal regeneration. J Exp Zool 1988;248:238–42.
62. Nau MR, Eshar D. Rostral mandibular fracture repair in a pet bearded dragon (*Pogona vitticeps*). J Amer Vet Med Assoc 2018;252:982–8.
63. Tuxbury KA, Clayton LA, Snakard EP, et al. Multiple skull fractures in a captive fly river turtle (*Carretochelys insculpta*): diagnosis, surgical repair, and medical management. J Herpetol Med Surg 2010;20:11–9.
64. Johnson D. External fixation of bilateral tibial fractures in an American bullfrog. Exotic DVM 2003;5:27–30.
65. Castro JLC, Santalucia S, Pachaly JR, et al. Mandibular osteosynthesis in a *Boa constrictor* snake. Semin Cienc Agrar 2014;35:911–8.
66. Scheelings TF. Surgical management of maxillary and mandibular fractures in an eastern bluetongue skink, *Tiliqua scincoides scincoides*. J Herpetol Med Surg 2007;17:136–40.
67. Royal LW, Grafinger MS, Lascelles BDX, et al. Internal fixation of a femur fracture in an American bullfrog. J Amer Vet Med Assoc 2007;230:1201–4.
68. Di Giuseppe M, Faraci L, Luparello M. Use of intramedullary pin for humeral fracture repair in a *Chamaeleo chamaeleon*. Natura Rerum 2013;3:63–9.
69. Matičić D, Stejskal M, Vnuk D, et al. Internal fixation of a femoral fracture in a green iguana developing metabolic bone disease—a case report. Vet Arh 2007;77:81–6.
70. Van Bonn W. Clinical technique: extra-articular surgical stifle stabilization of an American bullfrog (*Rana catesbeiana*). J Exot Pet Med 2009;18:36–9.
71. Waffa BJ, Montgerard AC, Grafinger MS, et al. Dorsal laminectomy in a two-toed amphiuma (*Amphiuma means*). J Zoo Wildl Med 2012;43:927–30.
72. Hirasawa T, Nagashima H, Kuratani S. The endoskeletal origin of the turtle carapace. Nat Commun 2013;4:2107.
73. Achrai B, Wagner HD. Micro-structure and mechanical properties of the turtle carapace as a biological composite shield. Acta Biomater 2013;9:5890–902.
74. Rieppel O. Turtles as hopeful monsters. Bioessays 2001;23:987–91.
75. Orós J, Torrent A, Calabuig P, et al. Diseases and causes of mortality among sea turtles stranded in the Canary Islands, Spain (1998-2001). Dis Aquat Org 2005; 63:13–24.
76. Sack A, Butler E, Cowen P, et al. Morbidity and mortality of wild turtles at a North Carolina wildlife clinic: a 10-year retrospective. J Zoo Wildl Med 2017;48:716–24.
77. Knapp-Hoch H, de Matos R. Clinical technique: negative pressure wound therapy-general principles and use in avian species. J Exot Pet Med 2014;23: 56–66.
78. Spadola F, Morici M. Treatment of turtle shell ulcerations using photopolymerizable nano-hybrid dental composite. J Exot Pet Med 2016;25:288–94.
79. Sypniewski LA, Hahn A, Murray JK, et al. Novel shell wound care in the aquatic turtle. J Exot Pet Med 2016;25:110–4.
80. Horowitz IH, Yanco E, Topaz M. Top closure system adapted to chelonian shell repair. J Exot Pet Med 2015;24:65–70.
81. Pritchard J, Ruzicka A. Comparison of fracture repair in the frog, lizard and rat. J Anat 1950;84:236.
82. Alibardi L. Regeneration of the epiphysis including the articular cartilage in the injured knees of the lizard *Podarcis muralis*. J Dev Biol 2015;3:71–89.

Locoregional Anesthesia in Exotic Pets

Dario d'Ovidio, DMV, MSc, SPACS, DECZM (Small Mammal), PhD[a],*,
Chiara Adami, DMV, MRCVS, RCVS, EBVS European Specialist in Veterinary Anaesthesia and Analgesia, DECVAA, DACVAA, PhD[b]

KEYWORDS

- Exotic pets • Locoregional anesthesia • Analgesia • Nerve stimulator
- Ultrasonography

KEY POINTS

- Locoregional anesthesia is widely used in exotic pets.
- The effectiveness of the techniques that have been described is anecdotally reported.
- Nerve stimulators and ultrasonographic guidance increase the success rate of nerve blocks and help decrease the risk of iatrogenic complications.

INTRODUCTION

In human and canine patients, locoregional anesthesia helps decrease the perioperative requirement of systemic analgesics and improve the quality of recovery after invasive procedures. The use of locoregional techniques is becoming more and more popular in exotic pet practice and, within the past decade, the number of published reports describing the use of blocks to provide analgesia during various surgical procedures has significantly increased.

Locoregional anesthesia is accomplished with local anesthetics (LAs). These agents interrupt the nerve conduction by blocking the sodium channels along the neuronal axons and, therefore, interfering with the axonal depolarization caused by the intracellular current of positively charged ions. None of the modern LAs, namely bupivacaine, levobupivacaine, and ropivacaine, has a marketing authorization for animals in either Europe or the United States; nonetheless, the extralabel use of these molecules for clinical purposes is widely described in veterinary medicine. The lack of published work investigating the pharmacodynamics and pharmacokinetics of LAs in exotic animal species implies that, in most cases, the dosages used in the clinical setting are extrapolated from studies conducted in species that share biological and evolutional

Disclosure Statement: The authors have nothing to disclose.
[a] Private Practitioner, Via Cristoforo Colombo 118, Arzano, NA 80022, Italy; [b] Clinical Sciences and Services, Royal Veterinary College, University of London, Hawkshead Campus, Hatfield AL97TA, United Kingdom
* Corresponding author.
E-mail address: dariodovidio@yahoo.it

similarities or are based on observational studies that include a small number of subjects.

To increase the success rate and decrease the incidence of iatrogenic complications, nerve stimulator–guided and, more recently, ultrasound-guided techniques became popular.

EQUIPMENT AND PATIENT PREPARATION

For most ultrasound-guided nerve blocks, the ultrasound machine should be equipped with a 10-MHz to 12-MHz linear probe.

For the nerve stimulator–guided technique, a 23-gauge, 35-mm insulated needle and an electrical stimulator, capable of delivering a current of 0.2 Hz to 1 Hz and 1 mA to 2 mA, should be prepared. The skin electrode is usually placed at 3 cm to 5 cm from the needle entry point. The current, initially set at 2 mA, is used to locate, by means of the target motor response, the motor component of the nerve. Once the motor response is evoked, the current should be decreased to 0.2 mA. If the motor response is still present with a current between 0.5 mA and 0.2 mA, the needle is close to the nerve and the LA should be injected. If the motor response is still elicited by a current as low as 0.2 mA or less, however, inadvertent intraneural injection is possible.

Most locoregional techniques are performed under anesthesia, ideally after intravenous catheter placement and while monitoring the physiologic variables of the patient. The area to be blocked should be clipped and aseptically prepared. Volumes of LA of 0.05 mL to 0.1 mL per nerve are commonly used in the clinical setting. An aspiration test should precede the LA injection to avoid inadvertent intravascular administration.

SMALL MAMMALS
Anesthesia of the Eye Globe

Anesthesia of the eye globe is performed as an aid to general anesthesia during ophthalmic surgeries, with the purpose of achieving both analgesia and akinesia of the eye.

Neuroanatomy
In the rabbit, the oculomotor nerve contains efferent motor fibers and parasympathetic fibers. The former innervate the extrinsic striated muscles of the eye, whereas the latter provides innervation to the ciliary and sphincter pupillae intrinsic muscles, which control the lens curvature and the pupillary constriction/dilation, respectively. The oculomotor nerve also innervates the elevator palpebrae muscle of the dorsal eyelid.[1]

Technique
Two variations of the ultrasound-guided eye block, the intraconal and the periconal approaches, have been described in rabbits.[2] In both cases, the needle is inserted within the orbital cavity, inside and outside the muscular cone, respectively. To perform the periconal block, the ultrasound probe is positioned at the supraorbital rim, 90° opposite to the needle that is inserted at the lateral aspect of the inferior orbital rim (**Fig. 1**). The tip of the needle should be forwarded until it reaches the area behind the eye globe, in the periconal space outside the muscular cone, where the LA should be injected.

Cranial Nerve Blocks

The distal branches of various cranial nerves can be blocked to provide analgesia during surgeries involving the oral cavity. Blind techniques have been described for rabbits, rodents, and ferrets.[3–5]

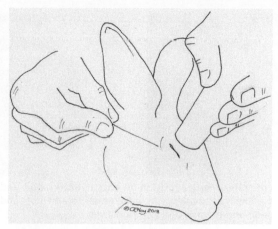

Fig. 1. Positioning in sternal recumbency for ultrasound-guided periconal block in a rabbit. The needle is inserted perpendicularly to the ultrasound transducer (out-of-plane technique). (*Courtesy of* Caroline Hoy, RVNVTS (Anes/Analgesia) NCert (A&CC).)

Neuroanatomy

The mandibular and the maxillary nerves are branches of the trigeminal nerve. The mandibular nerve is both sensory and motor, whereas the maxillary has solely sensory function. The mandibular nerve emerges the skull through the oval foramen and provides motor innervation to the lower jaw and sensory innervation to lower teeth and adjacent soft tissues.[1] The maxillary nerve exits the skull through the round foramen and, its extensions, the infraorbital and the palatine nerves, provide sensory innervation to the upper teeth and the adjacent soft tissues.

Technique

The rostral maxillary nerve block, also called infraorbital, provides analgesia during surgical procedures involving the maxilla and its components, including the upper teeth.[3,4] The anatomic landmark to perform the block is the infraorbital foramen, identified by palpation on the lateral aspect of the maxilla, at midway and slightly rostral to an imaginary line running from the lacrimal process to the facial tuber. The needle should be inserted toward the nerve as it exits the maxilla, in the immediate proximity of the first maxillary cheek tooth[4] (**Fig. 2**A).

The block of the cranial mandibular nerve, also called mental block, provides analgesia during surgeries involving the rostral component of the mandible. The anatomic landmark to perform the block is the mental foramen, located in the upper third of the lateral aspect of the mandible, just rostral to the first mandibular cheek tooth[4] (see **Fig. 2**B).

The block of the caudal mandibular nerve, also called inferior alveolar nerve, is preferred over the mental nerve block when a large area of desensitization, including bone and lower teeth, is desirable. The anatomic landmark is the mandibular foramen, located on the medial aspect of the mandible.[4] In rabbits, the narrow oral cavity makes the intraoral approach technically difficult; as a result, an extraoral insertion of the needle through the medial pterygoid muscle is preferred.

The infraorbital block and the pulp injection technique also have been described in ferrets.[6]

Brachial Plexus Block

A combined ultrasound–nerve stimulator–guided technique for axillary brachial plexus nerve block has been described in rabbits.[7]

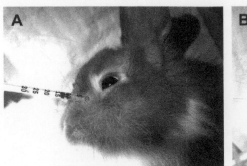
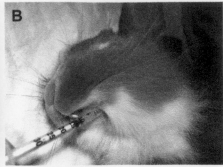

Fig. 2. Performance of cranial nerve blocks in an anesthetized rabbit undergoing a dental surgical procedure. Needle insertion into the infraorbital foramen (A) and mental foramen (B) for infraorbital and mental nerve blocks, respectively.

Neuroanatomy

The brachial plexus of the rabbit is composed of the ventral branches of the last 4 cervical spinal nerves, combined with the first thoracic spinal nerve.[1,8] The plexus is located within the connective tissue of the axillary space, medial to the scapula, near the axillary artery and vein. It gives origin to the suprascapular, the subscapular, the axillary, the musculocutaneous, and the radial nerves as well as the common trunk of the median and ulnar nerves.[8]

Technique

The rabbit should be placed in lateral recumbency, with the limb to be blocked abducted and uppermost. The plexus appears as a complex of hyperechoic structures, dorsal to the axillary artery and vein.[7] The needle is inserted with an in-plane technique, parallel to the transducer (ultrasound beam) plane, and advanced, while being visualized as a hyperechoic line, toward the brachial plexus (**Fig. 3**). The LA should be injected so that each nerve trunk is surrounded by a pocket of fluid visible with the ultrasound.

Sciatic-Femoral Nerve Block

A nerve stimulator–guided sciatic-femoral nerve block has been described in pet rabbits for surgeries involving the hind limb distal to the stifle joint.[9]

Neuroanatomy

In rabbits, as well as in other animal species, the sciatic and the femoral nerves arise from the lumbosacral plexus. The femoral nerve originates from the fourth, fifth, and sixth lumbar nerves. It courses along the medial surface of the thigh, in close proximity to the femoral artery and vein, where it innervates the adjacent muscles, and then continues toward the foot as the saphenous nerve.[10,11] The sciatic nerve forms mainly from the seventh lumbar and the first sacral nerves, with little contribution of the sixth lumbar and the second sacral nerves. Its trunk courses dorsally, between the ilium and the vertebral column, and then it continues ventrally toward the thigh. Proximal to the stifle, it branches into the peroneal and the tibial nerves.[10,11]

Technique

The rabbits should be positioned in lateral recumbency. For the femoral nerve block, the limb to be blocked is abducted 90° and extended caudally. The anatomic landmarks described by Mahler and Adogwa for dogs are used to locate the nerves.[9]

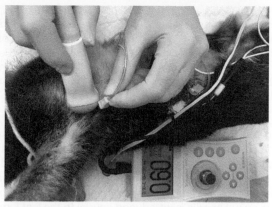

Fig. 3. Combined nerve locator and ultrasound-guided technique (dual guidance) for brachial plexus block in a pet rabbit. The stimulating needle is advanced toward the brachial plexus roots under ultrasound guidance.

For the femoral nerve, the needle is inserted cranial to the femoral artery, identified by palpation, and toward the femur (**Fig. 4**A). The target motor response consists of the contraction of the quadriceps femoris and the extension of the stifle.

Regarding the sciatic nerve block, the rabbit should remain in lateral recumbency, with the limb to be blocked uppermost. The greater trochanter (GT) of the femur and the ischiatic tuberosity (IT) are identified by palpation and the needle inserted at 60° to the skin, at approximately one-third (the closest to the GT) of the distance between the GT and IT (see **Fig. 4**B). Successful nerve location is confirmed by plantar extension and contraction of both the semitendinosus and the semimembranosus muscles.

Neuroaxial Anesthesia

Neuroaxial anesthesia has been described in ferrets, rabbits, and guinea pigs undergoing surgery involving reproductive tract, hind limbs, pelvis, perineum, vertebral column, and tail.[5,12–14]

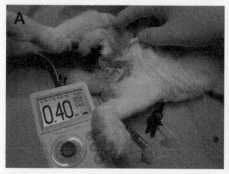
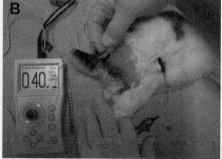

Fig. 4. Performance of a sciatic-femoral nerve block under nerve locator guidance in a pet rabbit prior to hind limb surgery. Positioning in lateral recumbency and stimulating needle insertion for femoral nerve (A) and sciatic nerve (B) locations.

Neuroanatomy

Rabbits have 6 to 7 lumbar vertebrae and 4 sacral vertebrae. The first 3 sacral vertebrae are fused whereas the fourth may be fused or not.[1] The spinal cord may terminate
within the first, most commonly second, or third sacral vertebra.[11] Ferrets have 5 to 7
lumbar vertebrae and 3 fused sacral vertebrae. The spinal cord of most often termi-
nates cranial to the lumbosacral space.[13,15] Guinea pigs have 6 lumbar and 2 to 3
sacral vertebrae.[16]

Technique

The animal should be positioned in sternal recumbency, with the hind limbs flexed
cranially under the abdomen. A 22-gauge, 38 mm (1.5 in) spinal needle may be
used to perform single epidural injections. Rigorous asepsis should be encouraged.
The lumbosacral junction is identified by palpation using as landmarks the spinous
processes of the last lumbar vertebra, the sacrum, and the ileum wings.[5,13] Thereafter,
an appropriate-size spinal needle is introduced caudal to the last lumbar vertebra and
advanced through the skin and subcutaneous layers. At this point, the stylet is
removed from the needle and the latter is advanced, with a drop of sterile saline
applied onto the hub of the needle, until a pop sensation, indicative of intervertebral
ligaments crossing, is felt, and the saline drop is aspirated. LAs alone or in combination with opioids are injected over 30 seconds to 60 seconds.[5] The loss of motor and
sensory functions confirms the successful block.[12]

Topical Applications

LAs can be applied as topical eye drops, to anesthetize the cornea during minor procedures. A eutectic mixture of lidocaine and prilocaine (EMLA Cream, AstraZeneca,
Karlskoga, Sweden) can be applied to the skin 30 minutes to 60 minutes before veni-
puncture or intravenous catheterization.[17] Hair clipping and application of a bandage
help to optimize absorption of the cream through the skin and subcutaneous layers in
the area of interest.[14]

Intratesticular Injections

Intratesticular injections are commonly performed in exotic pets undergoing castra-
tion. The LA is injected into the testicle and the spermatic cord in volumes up to
1 mL per testicle, depending on the size of the animal.[5,14,18–20]

BIRDS
Brachial Plexus Block

The brachial plexus block has been described in anesthetized or sedated individuals
belonging to multiple avian species (**Fig. 5**).[21–29]

The clinical effects of the brachial plexus block in birds were reported to be variable,
and it was suggested that the sensory block may be concentration dependent and/or
volume of LA dependent.[25] In chickens, blind brachial plexus block performed with
lidocaine, ropivacaine, or bupivacaine, at a volume of 1 mL/kg, was found technically
easy. The success rate of this technique, however, was less than 70%.[22,23]

Neuroanatomy

The anatomy of the brachial plexus varies greatly among avian species. This implies
that techniques described for 1 species are not necessarily valid for other species.[28]
In 3 Hispaniolan Amazon parrot (*Amazona ventralis*), the brachial plexus is formed by
the last 3 cervical and the first thoracic nerves. These nerves merge from the lateral
edge of the corresponding vertebrae before branching into the dorsal and ventral

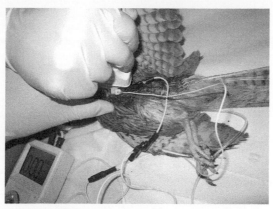

Fig. 5. Combined nerve stimulator and ultrasound-guided technique (dual guidance) for brachial plexus block in a common kestrel (*Falco tinnunculus*) prior to wing surgery.

fascicles. The eleventh and twelfth nerves give rise to the ventral fascicle of the brachial plexus that innervates the biceps brachii, the skin of the ventral aspect of the shoulder, and the large pectoralis muscle. The ventral fascicle continues then as the medioulnar nerve, which divides near the elbow into the ulnar and median nerves. The twelfth and thirteenth nerves form the dorsal fascicle, which gives origin to the radial nerve.[30]

Technique

In Hispaniolan Amazon parrots, both blind and ultrasound-guided techniques were described. Neither of them, however, resulted in muscle relaxation at the doses of lidocaine used by the authors (2 mg/kg in a total volume of 0.3 mL).[28]

Two nerve stimulator–guided approaches have been described in mallard ducks (*Anas platyrhynchos*): axillary and dorsal. The target motor response is a muscular twitch of the wing. Both techniques, however, resulted in clinically inadequate nerve block.[25]

Axillary technique

The duck should be positioned in lateral recumbency, with the wing extended to facilitate the access to its ventral aspect. The anatomic landmark is a triangular depression in the axillary region, delimited by the medial edge of the pectoralis muscle, the cranial edge of the biceps brachii muscle, and the dorsal aspect of the serratus ventralis (**Fig. 6**). The brachial plexus is subcutaneous and craniodorsal to this depression.[25]

Dorsal technique

The bird is positioned as for the axillary approach, and the dorsal spine is palpated to identify a depression between the last cervical vertebra and the first thoracic vertebra. The brachial plexus is located cranioventral to that depression, beneath the scapula.[25]

Sciatic-Femoral Nerve Block

A combined nerve stimulator–guided sciatic-femoral nerve block has been described in the peregrine falcon (*Falco peregrinus*) undergoing surgical treatment of pododermatitis.[31]

Neuroanatomy

The organization of avian peripheral nerves is similar to that of mammals.[32,33] The lumbosacral plexus is formed by the union of 2 lumbar and 4 sacral nerves. In some

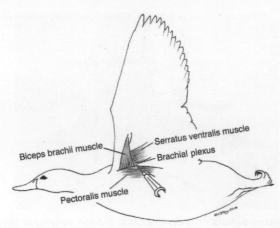

Fig. 6. Positioning in lateral recumbency for brachial plexus nerve block through the axillary approach in a duck. Needle entry is at the triangular depression in the axillary region formed by the intersection of the 3 depicted muscles. (*From* Brenner DJ, Larsen RS, Dickinson PJ, et al. Development of an avian brachial plexus nerve block technique for perioperative analgesia in mallard ducks (*Anas platyrhynchos*). J Avian Med Surg 2010;24(1):28; with permission.)

species (eg, fowl), 2 distinct portions of the plexus can be distinguished. The anterior portion gives origin to several branches, including the femoral, the internal saphenous and the obturator nerves, whereas the posterior portion gives rise to the sciatic nerve.[34]

Technique
For the femoral nerve block, the bird is placed in lateral recumbency, with the limb to be blocked abducted 90° and extended caudally. For the sciatic nerve block, lateral recumbency is preferred, with the limb to be blocked uppermost.

Femoral nerve block
The landmarks described for dogs also can be used for falcons.[35] After identifying the femoral artery by palpation, the needle is inserted in the quadriceps femoris muscle cranial to the vein, pointing toward the femur (**Fig. 7**A). The targeted motor response consists of the contraction of the quadriceps femoris and the extension of the stifle.

Sciatic nerve block
For the sciatic nerve block, the GT of the femur and the IT are the anatomic landmarks identified by palpation. The needle is inserted at approximately one-third of the distance along the GT-IT line, slightly nearer to the GT, with a 60° angle (see **Fig. 7**B). The targeted motor responses are the plantar extension and the contraction of the caudal thigh muscles.

Topical Application

The use of an LA (either lidocaine or bupivacaine at 2 mg/kg) for topical irrigation has been described in premedicated pet birds to provide analgesia during wound surgical curettage.[36]

Local Infiltration

A combination of lidocaine (2 mg/kg) and bupivacaine (2 mg/kg) has been successfully used in 2 species of psittacines, the blue-crowned conure (*Thectocercus*

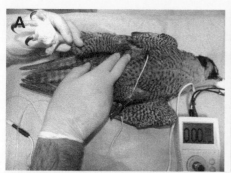
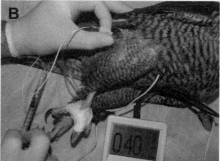

Fig. 7. Nerve stimulator–guided sciatic-femoral nerve block in a peregrine falcon (*Falco peregrinus*). The femoral artery is palpated and the puncture site for femoral block is selected, just cranial to it (*A*). The stimulating needle is inserted percutaneously with a 60° angle at approximately one-third of the distance along the GT-IT line for sciatic nerve block (*B*).

acuticaudatus) and the cockatiel (*Nymphicus hollandicus*), undergoing minor surgeries under sedation.[36]

REPTILES
Cranial Nerve Blocks

The mandibular nerve block has been performed in several species of crocodilians, the American alligator (*Alligator mississippiensis*), the yacare caiman (*Caiman yacare*), and the dwarf crocodile (*Osteolaemus tetraspis*), undergoing dental biopsy.[37]

Neuroanatomy
In crocodilian species, the mandibular nerve originates from the trigeminal nerve and runs ventral past the cranial aspect of the external mandibular foramen. It provides sensory innervation to the mandible and its components and motor innervation to the intermandibularis muscle, in the area between the mandibular rami[38] (**Fig. 8**).

Technique
The mandibular block has been performed in patients restrained on a board using nylon straps, with the mouth open and fixed around a padded polyvinyl chloride piping using electrical tape. Two nerve stimulator–guided approaches, lateral and intraoral, have been described.

For the lateral approach, the needle is inserted into the cranial aspect of the external mandibular foramen, which can be palpated on the lateral aspect of the mandible.

To perform the block with the intraoral technique, the needle is inserted ventrocaudal to the lateral commissure of the mouth, along the lingual surface of the mandibular ramus and toward the mandibular foramen (**Fig. 9**).

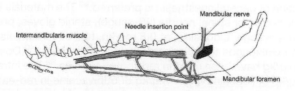

Fig. 8. Neuroanatomy of the mandibular branch of the trigeminal nerve in the American alligator (*Alligator mississippiensis*). (*Courtesy of* Caroline Hoy, RVNVTS (Anes/Analgesia) NCert (A&CC).)

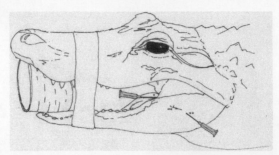

Fig. 9. Anatomic landmarks for mandibular nerve block techniques in crocodilians. Puncture sites for the lateral (*double asterisk*) or intraoral (*asterisk*) approach to the mandibular nerve. (*From* Wellehan JF, Gunkel CI, Kledzik D, et al. Use of a nerve locator to facilitate administration of mandibular nerve blocks in crocodilians. J Zoo Wildl Med 2006;37:406; with permission.)

The target motor response is a pulsatile contraction of the intermandibularis muscle; mepivacaine at 2 mg/kg divided into 2 injection sites has been used for this block.[37]

Neuroaxial Anesthesia

The use of intrathecal anesthesia has been reported in red-footed tortoise (*Chelonoidis carbonarius*), red-eared sliders (*Trachemys scripta elegans*), and Galápagos tortoise (*Geochelone nigra*), to provide analgesia during surgeries involving the cloaca, the urinary bladder, the genitalia, and the hind limbs.[39,40]

Neuroanatomy

In chelonians, the nerves originating from the caudal portion of the sacral plexus, in combination with the coccygeal nerves, provide innervation to the cloaca, the genitalia, and the hind limbs.[41,42] Chelonians lack a proper epidural space; however, they do have a well-developed intrathecal space. As a result, spinal anesthesia is preferred over the epidural technique.[43] Owing to the fusion of the vertebral column to the carapace, access to the intrathecal space is limited to the cervical and coccygeal vertebrae. The intrathecal spinal injection of LAs has been described in these species in the coccygeal area; at this level, there is only a thin skin layer above the neural arch, which makes the access to the intrathecal space technically easy (**Fig. 10**).

Technique

Despite that spinal anesthesia has been performed in conscious tortoises positioned in ventral recumbency without adverse effects, performing the procedure with the animal under sedation or general anesthesia is preferred.[43] The materials to be prepared consist of a hypodermic or spinal needle (28-gauge), sterile gloves, preservative-free opioids, LA, and a syringe. Lidocaine, at 0.8 mg/kg, has been administered intrathecally in 15 hybrid Galápagos tortoises undergoing phallectomy.[40] Dosages between 4 mg/kg and 8 mg/kg have been used in red-footed tortoise.[39] The intrathecal administration of 4 mg/kg of lidocaine and 1 mg/kg of bupivacaine in red-eared sliders has been reported to provide regional anesthesia of the tail, cloaca, and hind limbs with a duration of 1 hour and 2 hours, respectively. The addition of 0.1 mg/kg to 0.2 mg/kg of preservative-free morphine increased the duration of the sensory block up to 48 hours.[43]

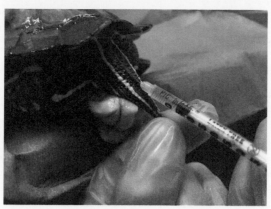

Fig. 10. Intrathecal lidocaine injection for induction of spinal anesthesia in a female river cooter turtle (*Pseudemys concinna*) undergoing cloacal surgery.

Topical Application

EMLA cream (1 g/10 cm²), applied on the penile mucosa and combined with systemic tramadol (10 mg/kg, orally), has been reported to provide successful analgesia during phallectomy in chelonians.[44]

Bilateral desensitization of infrared-detecting facial pits has been achieved in prairie rattlesnakes (*Crotalus viridis*) by injecting a drop of 2% lidocaine solution into each pit chamber.[45]

Local Infiltration

Local infiltration of lidocaine (5 mg/kg) has been successfully used as an aid to general anesthesia in an Argentine black and white tegu (*Tupinambis merianae*) undergoing humeral osteosynthesis, and in a Burmese python (*Python molurus*) undergoing surgical treatment of cloacal prolapse.[46,47] Additionally, local infiltration with 2 mg/kg of lidocaine can be used at the prefemoral incision site, in combination with intrathecal lidocaine, for sterilization of chelonians.[48]

Prevention of Block-related Complications

The main complications associated with nerve blocks are nerve damage and LA systemic toxicity, the latter more commonly associated with overdose and/or unintentional intravascular injection.[9] The most common signs of cardiovascular lidocaine toxicity reported in dogs are bradyarrhythmia and collapse, whereas neurotoxicity is characterized by muscle twitching, convulsions, unconsciousness, respiratory arrest, and coma.[14] At the time of this writing, the maximum lidocaine dose has been reported in few species (eg, broiler chickens [6 mg/kg] and rabbits [4 mg/kg]).[49,50]

Peripheral nerve injury is rare in human medicine, accounting for 0.5% to 1.0% of the cases.[51] Inadvertent globe perforation, damage to the optic nerve and persistent diplopia represent uncommon complications of the eye blocks, especially when blind techniques are used.[2] Ultrasonography has proved to reduce the occurrence of iatrogenic injury.[2]

SUMMARY

Locoregional anesthesia is widely used in exotic pets. In most cases, the available information about the effectiveness of the described techniques is anecdotally reported rather than evidence based. Nevertheless, their use, as well as the development of new nerve blocks, should be encouraged as a measure to alleviate pain and to promote a multimodal approach to analgesia.

ACKNOWLEDGMENTS

The authors gratefully acknowledge Caroline Hoy for supplying illustrations and granting permission for their use.

REFERENCES

1. Osofsky A, LeCouter RA, Vernau KM. Functional neuroanatomy of the domestic rabbit. Vet Clin Exot Anim 2007;10:713–30.
2. Najman IE, Ferreira JZ, Abimussi CJ, et al. Ultrasound-assisted periconal ocular blockade in rabbits. Vet Anaesth Analg 2015;42:433–41.
3. Lennox AM. Clinical technique: small exotic companion mammal dentistry-Anesthetic considerations. J Exot Pet Med 2008;17:102–6.
4. Böhmer E. Anesthesia and analgesia. In: Böhmer E, editor. Dentistry in rabbit and rodents. 1st edition. Chichester (United Kingdom): Wiley Blackwell; 2015. p. 90–106.
5. Hawkins MG, Pascoe PG. Anesthesia, analgesia and sedation of small mammals. In: Quesenberry KE, Carpenter JW, editors. Ferrets, rabbits and rodents clinical medicine and surgery. 3rd edition. St Louis (MO): Elsevier/Saunders; 2012. p. 429–51.
6. Johnson-Delaney CA. Disorders of the oral cavity. In: Ferret medicine and surgery. Boca Raton (FL): CRC Press; 2016. p. 1–514.
7. Fonseca C, Server A, Esteves M, et al. An ultrasound-guided technique for axillary brachial plexus nerve block in rabbits. Lab Anim (NY) 2015;44:179–84.
8. Mencalha R, dos Santos Sousa CA, Costa O, et al. Ultrasound and gross anatomy of the brachial plexus and major nerves of the forelimb. An anesthetic approach using the domestic rabbit (*Oyctolagus cuniculus*) as an experimental model. Acta Cir Bras 2016;3:218–26.
9. d'Ovidio D, Rota S, Noviello E, et al. Nerve stimulator-guided sciatic-femoral block in pet rabbits (*Oryctolagus cuniculus*) undergoing hind limb surgery: a case series. J Exot Pet Med 2014;23:91–5.
10. Hyman LH. The comparative anatomy at the nervous system and the sense organs. In: A laboratory manual for comparative vertebrate anatomy. Chicago: University of Chicago Press; 1922. p. 339–40.
11. Greenaway J, Partlow G, Gonsholt N, et al. Anatomy of the lumbosacral spinal cord in rabbits. J Am Anim Hosp Assoc 2001;37:27–34.
12. Kero P, Thomasson B, Soppi AM. Spinal anaesthesia in the rabbit. Lab Anim 1981;15:347–8.
13. Eshar D, Wilson J. Epidural anesthesia and analgesia in ferrets. Lab Anim 2010; 39:339–40.
14. Wenger S. Anesthesia and analgesia in rabbits and rodents. J Exot Pet Med 2012;21:7–16.
15. Lichtenberger M, Ko J. Anesthesia and analgesia for small mammals and birds. Vet Clin North Am Exot Anim Pract 2007;10:293–315.
16. Quesenberry KE, Donnelly TM, Mans C. Biology, husbandry and clinical techniques of Guinea pigs. In: Quesenberry KE, Carpenter JW, editors. Ferrets, rabbits and rodents clinical medicine and surgery. 3rd edition. St Louis (MO): Elsevier/Saunders; 2012. p. 279–94.

17. Lester PA, Moore RM, Shuster KA, et al. Anesthesia and analgesia. In: Suckow MA, Stevens KA, Wilson RP, editors. The laboratory rabbit, Guinea Pig, hamster, and other rodents. San Diego (CA): Academic press; 2012. p. 33–56.

18. Gleeson M, Hawkins MG, Howerton CL, et al. Evaluating postoperative parameters in Guinea pigs (Cavia porcellus) following routine orchiectomy. J Exot Pet Med 2016;25:242–52.

19. Kharbush RJ, Richmond RV, Steinberg H, et al. Surgical resection of a testicular seminoma in a Guinea Pig (Cavia porcellus). J Exot Pet Med 2016;2:53–6.

20. Malbrue RA, Arsuaga CB, Collins TA, et al. Scrotal stalk ablation and orchiectomy using electrosurgery in the male sugar glider (Petaurus breviceps) and histologic anatomy of the testes and associated scrotal structures. J Exot Pet Med 2018;27: 90–4.

21. Vilani RGDC, Montiani-Ferreira F, Lange R, et al. Brachial plexus blocks in birds. Exotic DVM 2006;8:86–91.

22. Figueireido JP, Cruz ML, Mendes GM, et al. Assessment of brachial plexus blockade in chickens by an axillary approach. Vet Anaesth Analg 2008;35:511–8.

23. Cardozo LB, Almeida RM, Fiúza LC, et al. Brachial plexus blockade in chickens with 0.75% ropivacaine. Vet Anaesth Analg 2009;36:396–400.

24. Shaver SL, Robinson NG, Wright BD, et al. A multimodal approach to management of suspected neuropathic pain in a prairie falcon (Falco mexicanus). J Avian Med Surg 2009;23:209–13.

25. Brenner DJ, Larsen RS, Dickinson PJ, et al. Development of an avian brachial plexus nerve block technique for perioperative analgesia in mallard ducks (Anas platyrhynchos). J Avian Med Surg 2010;24(1):24–34.

26. d'Ovidio D, Noviello E, Nocerino M. Combination of fentanyl and lidocaine for brachial plexus block in a peregrine falcon (Falco peregrinus). Proceedings of the 11th Conference of the European Committee of the Association of Avian Veterinarians (EAAV). Madrid, 26–30 April, 2011. p. 394–6.

27. d'Ovidio D, Noviello E, Nocerino M, et al. Application of brachial plexus block (BPB) in wild birds undergoing surgery of the wings. Proceedings of the International Conference on Diseases of Zoo and Wild Animals (EAZWV). Verona, 16–17 May, 2012. p. 23.

28. da Cunha AF, Strain GM, Rademacher N, et al. Palpation- and ultrasound-guided brachial plexus blockade in Hispaniolan Amazon parrots (Amazona ventralis). Vet Anaesth Analg 2013;40:96–102.

29. Machin KL. Avian analgesia. Semin Avian Exot Pet Med 2005;14:236–42.

30. Broussard KH, da Cunha AF, Beaufrere H, et al. Clinical neuroanatomy of the wing of the Hispaniolan Amazon parrot (Amazona ventralis). Proceedings of the 11th Conference of the European Committee of the Association of Avian Veterinarians (EAAV). Madrid, 26–30 April, 2011. p. 389–91.

31. d'Ovidio D, Noviello E, Adami C. Nerve stimulator-guided sciatic-femoral nerve block in raptors undergoing surgical treatment of pododermatitits. Vet Anaesth Analg 2015;42:449–53.

32. Bennett AR. Neurology. In: Ritchie BW, Harrison GJ, Harrison LR, editors. Avian medicine: principles and application. Lake Worth (FL): Wingers Publishing Inc; 1994. p. 723–45.

33. Harcourt-Brown NH. Birds of prey-Anatomy, radiology and clinical conditions of the pelvic limb. CD-ROM. Lake Worth (FL): Zoological Education Network Inc; 2000.

34. Chauveau A, Arloing S, Fleming G. The nervous system in birds. In: Chauveau A, Arloing S, Fleming G, editors. The comparative anatomy of the domesticated animals. 2nd edition. New York: Appleton & C; 1908. p. 790–1.
35. Mahler SP, Adogwa AO. Anatomical and experimental studies of brachial plexus, sciatic, and femoral nerve-location using peripheral nerve stimulation in the dog. Vet Anaesth Analg 2008;35:80–9.
36. Lee A, Lennox AM. Sedation and local anesthesia as an alternative to general anesthesia in 3 birds. J Exot Pet Med 2016;25:100–5.
37. Wellehan JF, Gunkel CI, Kledzik D, et al. Use of a nerve locator to facilitate administration of mandibular nerve blocks in crocodilians. J Zoo Wildl Med 2006;37: 405–8.
38. Schumacher GH. The head muscles and hyolaryngeal skeleton of turtles and crocodilians. In: Gans C, Parsons TS, editors. Biology of the reptilia, vol. 4. San Diego (CA): Academic Press; 1973. p. 101–99.
39. Fontenelle J, Carvalho do Nascimento C, Lozano Cruz M, et al. Epidural anesthesia of Amazonian tortoises (Geochelone carbonaria). Proccedings of the 4th Congress and 9th ABRAVAS Meeting, São Pedro, São Paulo, January 7, 2000.
40. Rivera S, Divers SJ, Knafo SE, et al. Sterilisation of hybrid Galapagos tortoises (*Geochelone nigra*) for island restoration. Part 2: phallectomy of males under intrathecal anaesthesia with lidocaine. Vet Rec 2011;168:78.
41. Bojanus LH. Anatome testudinis europaeae. An anatomy of the turtle. Indiana University, Society for the study of amphibians and reptiles; 1970. p. 178.
42. Wyneken J. Reptilian neurology: anatomy and function. Vet Clin North Am Exot Anim Pract 2007;10:837–53.
43. Mans C. Clinical technique: intrathecal drug administration in turtles and tortoises. J Exot Pet Med 2014;23:67–70.
44. Spadola F, Morici M, Knotek Z. Combination of lidocaine/prilocaine with tramadol for short time anaesthesia-analgesia in chelonians: 18 cases. Acta Vet Brno 2015; 84:71–5.
45. Chiszar D, Dickman D, Colton J. Sensitivity to thermal stimulation in prairie rattlesnakes (*Crotalus viridis*) after bilateral anesthetization of the facial pits. Behav Neural Biol 1986;45:143–9.
46. George PL, Joseph J. Prolapse of cloaca in a python (*Python molurus*). Indian Vet J 1989;66:648–9.
47. Guirro ECB, DP, Cunha OD, et al. Multimodal anesthesia in tegu lizard *Tupinambis merianae*: case report. Ciência animal brasileira 2010;11:458–60.
48. Knafo SE, Divers SJ, Rivera S, et al. Sterilisation of hybrid Galapagos tortoises (*Geochelone nigra*) for island restoration. Part 1: endoscopic oophorectomy of females under ketamine-medetomidine anaesthesia. Vet Rec 2011;168:47.
49. Brandao J, da Cunha AF, Pypendop B, et al. Cardiovascular tolerance of intravenous lidocaine in broiler chickens (*Gallus gallus domesticus*) anesthetized with isoflurane. Vet Anaesth Analg 2015;42:442–8.
50. Barter LS. Rabbit analgesia. Vet Clin North Am Exot Anim Pract 2011;14:93–104.
51. Jeng CL, Rosenblatt MA. Intraneural injections and regional anesthesia: the known and the unknown. Minerva Anestesiol 2011;77:54–8.

Exoskeleton Repair in Invertebrates

Sarah Pellett, BSc (Hons), MA, VetMB, CertAVP (ZM), DZooMed (Reptilian), MRCVS[a],*,
Michelle O'Brien, BVetMed, CertZooMed, DECZM (ZHM), MRCVS[b]

KEYWORDS

- Invertebrate • Exoskeleton • Arthropod • Mollusk • Trauma • Repair

KEY POINTS

- Pathologic conditions of the invertebrate integument include any disorders that weaken or disrupt the normal physiologic function of the skin.
- Invertebrates may present as an emergency because of trauma to the exoskeleton resulting in penetrating wounds to the soft tissue, shell, or cuticle. Arthropods may present with exoskeleton damage because of dysecdysis or may present with damaged appendages or setae.
- Hemolymph loss may occur from cuticular wounds and this must be dealt with immediately, because death can occur rapidly.
- Active hemorrhage must be controlled immediately.
- Emergency hemostasis may be achieved by applying a small amount of talcum powder, icing sugar, paraffin wax, plasticine or sticky tape over the area. A more permanent seal may be achieved using tissue adhesives, nonheating/minimally exothermic epoxy, or plaster of Paris depending on the species and the area.

INTRODUCTION

Invertebrates range from single-celled protozoa to multicellular mollusks, arthropods, worms, leeches, sponges, and corals.[1] Invertebrates can often evoke fear in people, especially spiders, because humans have a cognitive mechanism to perceive certain animals that may have been harmful throughout evolutionary history.[2] This apparent fear may be reinforced in children who may have learnt it from other people who are also scared of spiders.[3] However, there are also many invertebrate enthusiasts, and many different invertebrate species are gaining popularity as pets. Many species of invertebrates are also part of zoologic collections in which some species are used in demonstration and outreach sessions to educate members of the public. Invertebrate

The authors have nothing to disclose.
[a] Animates Veterinary Clinic, 2 The Green, Thurlby, Lincolnshire PE10 0EB, UK; [b] Wildfowl & Wetlands Trust, Slimbridge, Gloucestershire GL2 7BT, UK
* Corresponding author.
E-mail address: sarah_pellett@hotmail.com

Vet Clin Exot Anim 22 (2019) 315–330
https://doi.org/10.1016/j.cvex.2019.01.008
1094-9194/19/© 2019 Elsevier Inc. All rights reserved.

collections are frequently seen within animal care teaching colleges, schools, and research/scientific laboratories, as pets or study animals but also as a source of food both for animals in captivity or humans. Although invertebrate medicine is still in its infancy compared with other exotic pet species, there has been more of a demand from both owners and veterinarians seeking advice in treating these animals over the last few years.[4]

The invertebrates most likely to be relevant to the practitioner are members of the phylum Arthropoda and the phylum Mollusca, and emphasis on species within these phyla will be discussed in this article.

INVERTEBRATE INTEGUMENT

The structure of the invertebrate integument, in addition to its pathology, was described in the eighteenth century by John Hunter, and specimens of normal and pathologic invertebrate material are displayed in the Hunterian Museum at the Royal College of Surgeons of England in London.[1] The integument of invertebrates varies from a simple epithelial layer to highly specialized chitinous structures.[5] Cuticle varies amongst invertebrate species, including the amount and orientation of chitinous fibers, the extent of cross-linking of the protein matrix, the thickness of the exocuticle and endocuticle, and the shape of these structures.[6] In 1892, Metchnikoff developed the understanding of inflammation and immune processes by his work on amebocyte cells in invertebrates and explaining their response to insults.[7,8] For this article, a generalized description of the invertebrate exoskeleton will be given, but for more detailed comparative information on the anatomy of invertebrates, including their integument, please refer to more specific literature.[9–13]

Phylum Arthropoda

Arthropods have an exoskeleton made of chitin.[1] The main functions of a chitinous exoskeleton are to provide support and impede fluid loss. Amongst the phylum Arthropoda, there are several classes of invertebrates that are more commonly found within the pet trade or kept within zoologic collections and are more likely to present to veterinarians with cases of integument damage and/or disease. The classes Insecta, Arachnida, Diplopoda, Chilopoda and Crustacea include species seen within the pet trade. The class Insecta includes many species of stick insects, mantises, beetles, and cockroaches. The class Arachnida includes many species of tarantula (theraphosids) and scorpions. The class Diplopoda includes species of millipedes kept within collections. The class Chilopoda includes species of centipede kept by experienced enthusiasts and within collections. The class Crustacea includes species of hermit crab and crayfish seen amongst collections.

Arthropod exoskeleton consists of 3 layers: the epicuticle (which is generally 1–3 μm thick depending on species), the procuticle (1–100 μm), and the epidermal cell layer, which is often a monolayer.[5] In general, the arthropod chitinous exoskeleton is secreted by the epidermis and is divided into hard plates with flexible joints.[1] The epicuticle is not made of chitin but is a wax depot, responsible for waterproofing, pheromone functions and, in some cases, antimicrobial (mostly antimycotic) functions.[5]

The composition and thickness of the arthropod cuticle varies on the species. In some species, such as New World theraphosids, the integument is protected by hollow outgrowths of the cuticle referred to as setae or urticating hairs. In some species, there are invaginations of the cuticle, which form respiratory organs. In many species of Crustacea the integument is calcified. Arthropoda undergo ecdysis, requiring the cuticle to be shed at intervals depending on the species. Although the new cuticle is being formed and hardening, the animal exoskeleton is particularly vulnerable to trauma.[1]

Phylum Mollusca

Mollusks do not have an exoskeleton made of chitin.[1] The most common species seen within the pet trade belong to the class Gastropoda, which includes, among others, the terrestrial, pulmonate snails such as the giant African land snails, *Achatina* spp. Gastropod mollusks have a shell made of calcium carbonate crystals in the form of calcite, aragonite, or both, depending on species, to protect the soft tissues.[14] The mantle epithelium secretes the shell that is composed of inner and outer epithelial layers, with connective tissue between them.[5] The protective shell consists of an outer layer composed of sclerotized protein and the periostratum with inner calcified layers.[5]

Alongside the shell, the muscular foot and 2 pairs of retractable tentacles on the frontal surface of the head can be easily identified during external macroscopic examination. Mollusks do not undergo ecdysis but grow slowly and constantly.[1]

PATHOLOGIC CONDITIONS OF THE INVERTEBRATE INTEGUMENT

Pathologic conditions of the invertebrate integument include any disorders that weaken or disrupt the normal physiologic function of the skin. This may be due to infectious (viral, bacterial, fungal, or parasitic) and noninfectious (eg, trauma) causes. There is an overlap in this generalization because specific neoplastic conditions may be caused by living organisms.[1] Noninfectious diseases affecting the invertebrate integument are often referred to as noncommunicable diseases by invertebrate pathologists.[1]

This article focuses on exoskeleton repair in invertebrates presented due to physical trauma with impairment of the integument and often with hemolymph loss. Invertebrates, especially the larger-bodied arthropods, can severely damage their exoskeleton if dropped or if they are handled during ecdysis. Invertebrates have an open circulatory system and even a small defect can lead to a significant loss of hemolymph and death if hemostasis is not rapidly achieved.

In most arthropods, damage to the integument stimulates the release of factors, leading to an increase in RNA and DNA replication and consequently protein production.[15] Tissue healing in higher invertebrates involves inflammatory cells and their mediators; however, studies have shown that in lower invertebrates there is no such response but healing still occurs.[16] Methods to combat infection seem to depend on phagocytes within the hemolymph, agglutination, coagulation, and bactericidins in most invertebrate species.[17] An invertebrate's ability to manage integumentary compromise is assisted by factors such as free fatty acids on the surface of the body and lysozyme-like secretions.[18,19] Ecdysterone, a hormone that controls the ecdysis and metamorphosis of arthropods, is secreted by injured cells.[12] In the pearl oyster (*Pinctada fucata*), a marine bivalve mollusk, the bone morphogenetic protein (BMP) group is important in the biomineralization process and BMP7b may be vital in the process of shell formation and repair. This was deduced by an experiment in which BMP7b showed an increased expression level 24 hours after a shell notch was performed.[20]

Arthropods and mollusks are ectothermic but able to control their body temperature to a certain point by behavioral means. Growth, regeneration, and repair of the invertebrate integument are temperature dependent.[1,21] Similarly to other species of exotic animals kept in captivity, excellent husbandry must be provided because suboptimal conditions (eg, environmental temperatures being too high or low or an incorrect relative humidity) can significantly affect the animals' homeostasis.

EXOSKELETON DAMAGE

Trauma

Invertebrates may present as an emergency because of trauma to the exoskeleton resulting in penetrating wounds to the soft tissue, shell, or cuticle. Arthropods may present with exoskeleton damage because of dysecdysis or may present with damaged appendages or setae. The loss of setae in some arthropods, such as New World Tarantulas, is used as a defense mechanism and these setae are replaced in the next molt. Regeneration of limbs occurs in some arthropods such as theraphosids. Hemolymph loss may occur from cuticular wounds and this must be dealt with immediately. Crushing injuries can also occur, resulting in bruising to underlying tissue, which has been reported to be a common finding in wild-caught cephalopods.[22] Healed shell fractures in mollusks are also not an uncommon finding.[23] In mollusks subdermal muscular contraction occurs in parallel with amebocyte infiltration, which results in the formation of a cellular plug.[5] Some studies state that a fibrillar mesh occurs; however, other investigators do not believe this to be the case.[24] Amebocytes are responsible for removing devitalized material from the wound and for eliminating infectious organisms. A collagenous substratum is secreted by the amebocytes and fibrocytes. This enables the epithelial cells to migrate, although in some situations, the amebocytes form a permanent cover over the wound.[25]

Suboptimal Temperatures

Dysecdysis can result from thermal stress related to temperatures lower or higher than the animal's zone of thermal tolerance.[26] Suboptimal temperatures are often associated with deviations from the preferred range for relative humidity. High temperatures may result in skin wounds and necrosis, whereas low temperatures may cause sloughing of the epidermis, appendages, and underlying tissues.

Nutritional Deficiencies

Giant African land snails require calcium in the diet. A diet deficiency in calcium causes brittle and/or soft shells that predispose the snail to shell fractures. Calcium-deficient snails may also rasp the shells of other snails increasing the likelihood of traumatic injury. Other observations include irregular or slow shell growth[27] (**Fig. 1**).

Dietary calcium has an important role in shell calcification. A calcium-enriched diet may lead to thickening of the shell in a dose-response manner.[28] Studies have shown that 25-hydroxycholecalciferol (25(OH)D3) seems to be biologically active in invertebrates.[29] Nutrient and light restrictions have led to changes in vitamin D metabolism, resulting in an increase in the weight and mineral content of shells. The molluscan metabolite E was found to accelerate the transfer of calcium from the mantle to the shell.[30]

STABILIZATION AND TREATMENT

The animal must be accurately identified and whether it is a venomous or dangerous species determined. Active hemorrhage must be controlled immediately, often with the animal conscious or, if considered to be dangerous, then under anesthesia (see later discussion). Once the animal has been stabilized, a thorough history addressing environmental factors and husbandry must be taken.

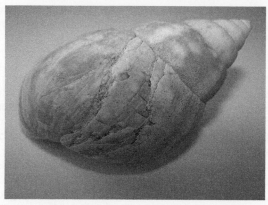

Fig. 1. Rasped shell due to a calcium-deficient snail within the same enclosure. (*Courtesy of* Michelle O' Brien, BVetMed, CertZooMed, DipECZM(ZHM), MRCVS, Wildfowl & Wetlands Trust, Slimbridge, Gloucestershire, UK.)

In general, to treat an invertebrate, the following points must be considered:

- Maintain the invertebrate at its preferred body temperature.
- Ensure the relative humidity is correct for the species. The relative humidity may be increased slightly to minimize fluid loss.
- Keep the invertebrate in a clinical environment that minimizes the risk of secondary bacterial or fungal infections. The author (SP) uses plastic Really Useful Boxes (RUBs) with paper towel as a substrate for most species. Caution must be taken to ensure that invertebrates are not put into any container that has housed an exotic species that has been treated for ectoparasites. It is vital that no flea sprays or insecticides are used in the room housing invertebrates. Hands must be thoroughly washed and gloves worn when handling invertebrates, especially if flea or deworming medication has been applied to any other animal. Clinical signs of insecticide toxicity in invertebrates include anorexia, incoordination, twitching, and death. Fatalities in theraphosids due to residual effects of fipronil (Frontline, Merial, UK) on a container, despite being thoroughly washed before use, have been described.[31]
- Topical antibiotics and antifungals may be necessary to minimize infection with triple-antibiotic ointment and clotrimazole, applied sparingly using a cotton-tipped applicator, having been reported to have been used with some success in terrestrial arthropods.[32] One author (SP) has used F10 germicide cream applied sparingly to a lesion on a giant millipede and the other author (MOB) has used fusidic acid (Isathal 10 mg/mL eye drops, Dechra, UK) topically on a theraphosid. Caution must be taken to prescribe products not containing insecticide (eg, F10 wound spray containing insecticide must be avoided).
- Fluid therapy, orally or parenterally administered, may be required for invertebrates having undergone hemolymph loss.
- If a client calls in for advice due to hemolymph loss after a traumatic incident, the animal may not survive the journey to the surgery; therefore, providing correct instructions to try to achieve hemostasis is vital. Emergency hemostasis can be achieved by applying a small amount of talcum powder, icing sugar, paraffin wax, plasticine, or sticky tape over the area.[33] The animal can be brought into the surgery afterward for assessment, stabilization, and placement of a more permanent seal to the wound, such as tissue adhesives, nonheating epoxy, or

plaster of Paris depending on the species and the traumatized area. For more information, please refer the following discussion for specific examples.

Fluid Therapy

Dampened paper towels can aid in increasing humidity and reducing evaporative fluid loss. Chlorinated tap water should be avoided in invertebrates and instead use dechlorinated water, reverse-osmosis water, or distilled water.[32] Rehydration in mildly dehydrated theraphosids is accomplished by placing the cephalothorax of the spider in a shallow dish of water. Caution must be taken as not to submerge the book lungs, which are situated on the ventral surface of the opisthosoma (**Fig. 2**). Most spiders will drink readily, and hydration will be achieved within a few hours. Theraphosids and other invertebrates may also be offered water from a syringe.[32,34] Snails can be placed in a shallow dish of tepid water, taking care not to cover the pneumostome, or by lightly spraying the enclosure and the food. The pneumostome is located beneath the shell rim in the mantle.

Severely dehydrated spiders will require parenteral fluids. Extension of appendages depends on hemolymph pressure; therefore, in extremely dehydrated spiders, movement is not possible.[35] Spiders are therefore often observed with their limbs pulled inwards toward the prosoma. Isotonic fluids are administered into the heart located on the dorsal midline of the opisthosoma via a 30-Gauge insulin needle and syringe. Tissue adhesive must be applied after fluid administration to ensure that the cuticle is closed to prevent iatrogenic hemorrhage. An alternative site for fluid administration is intracelomic, with the needle inserted from the lateral side of the opisthosoma.[34]

Analgesia and Anesthesia

Anesthesia may be necessary to allow physical examination and to facilitate treatment such as exoskeleton repair in some invertebrate species. A detailed description on anesthesia is beyond the scope of this article. Factors limiting successful anesthetic and analgesic use in invertebrates include subjectivity in pain assessment; inadequate knowledge of anesthetic and analgesic efficacy; safety, dosages, and dosing frequency across species; the inability to monitor anesthetic depth; pharmacokinetics of anesthetic and analgesic drugs; and the unknown relationship between risks and benefits for specific drugs.[36]

Volatile organic anesthetics are the method of choice for anesthetizing fractious theraphosids and scorpions to allow restraint and exoskeleton repair. Isoflurane and

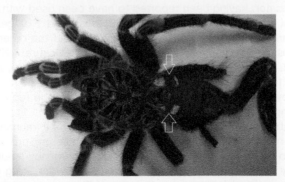

Fig. 2. A molt (exuvia) of a theraphosid to show the book lungs, which are situated on the ventral surface of the opisthosoma (*arrows*). (*Courtesy of* Sarah Pellett, BSc(Hons), MA, VetMB, CertAVP(ZM), DZooMed (Reptilian), MRCVS, Animates Veterinary Clinic, Thurlby, UK.)

sevoflurane are both effective and commonly used anesthetic gases in the clinical setting.[37–39] Induction takes place in an anesthetic chamber. Induction may be slow, taking as long as 20 minutes before there is a loss of righting reflex. Anesthesia is maintained in theraphosids by placing the opisthosoma within a facemask; the book lungs are located on the ventral abdomen of a tarantula. Injectable anesthesia, using alphaxalone, has been studied in *Grammostola rosea*, with 200 mg/kg administered into the heart provided a moderate anesthesia with a median duration of 28 minutes.[40] The authors prefer to use gaseous anesthesia if anesthesia is required for fractious theraphosids.

Anesthesia of giant African land snails is challenging and should be regarded as higher risk than that of arthropods. The use of anesthesia and risks associated with this must be discussed with owners.[31] For shell repair on land snails the authors do not induce anesthesia. Anesthesia of mollusks is covered in other texts.[37,41–50]

It is unknown whether invertebrates experience pain or they simply demonstrate a reflexive response to a painful stimulus.[51] There is a lack of published information relating to signs of pain in invertebrates, which may not be comparable to pain perception in other species. Arthropods and mollusks have nerve endings or similar sensory structures within internal tissues and the body wall.[52] In other taxa, such as cephalopods, there are well-developed nervous systems and brains together with demonstration of complex behaviors including the ability to respond to environmental cues.[53,54] Many invertebrate species have endogenous opioids and respond to noxious stimuli, and some species also respond to exogenous opioids.[55–63]

The clinician must view each case on an individual basis and base analgesia doses on publications (although most are anecdotal) from exotic animal formularies. In one study, administration of morphine at 50 to 100 mg/kg intracelomically or butorphanol at 20 mg/kg has been shown to decrease responses to noxious stimuli.[36] The paucity of information within the literature emphasizes the need for further research on analgesia use in invertebrates. Hypothermia is not considered a humane method of anesthesia or analgesia because there is no loss of sensation.

Euthanasia

Except for cephalopods, in the UK invertebrates are not governed by the same legislation and standards as are vertebrate species. Invertebrates are often not given the same ethical consideration. Further information on euthanasia for invertebrate taxa can be found in documents specifically produced to outline ethical and humane euthanasia techniques.[64]

Adequate analgesia and/or anesthesia must be provided before euthanasia. Carbon dioxide does not provide analgesia and therefore must not be used as the sole method of euthanasia.[65] The preferred method is to use an inhalant volatile anesthetic gas that can be administered to most invertebrate species. Once anesthetized, pentobarbitone can be injected into the hemocoel.[32] Death can be confirmed by the cessation of respiratory rate (observed at the cranial lateral side) and heart rate with a Doppler probe. An exception to inducing with gaseous anesthesia is for the giant African land snail. Gaseous anesthesia is not recommended for terrestrial snails because this may cause excess mucus production, and therefore be deemed as stressful.[64] Giant African land snails may be euthanized by using a bath of 100% phenoxyethanol (Aqua-Sed, VETARK Professional) to cover the muscular foot. Once nonresponsive, sodium pentobarbitone can be administered (R. Saunders, 2013, personal communication). An 8 MHz Doppler probe can be used to confirm cessation of a heartbeat.[66]

Other methods of euthanasia in invertebrates involve administration of potassium chloride, resulting in hyperkalosis and in theraphosids can be administered via the sternum into the prosoma ganglia or into the heart.[67]

Euthanasia may be an option for arthropods, spiders, and snails with severe traumatic injuries or for arthropods and spiders that have presented with unmanageable dysecdysis.

COMMON DISORDERS ACROSS TAXA
Theraphosids

Trauma
Hemolymph loss may result in fatalities, and therefore, tarantulas suffering traumatic injuries must be considered an emergency. Immediate first aid is essential, and instructions may have to be given to the client over the phone if the animal is housed a distance from the surgery. Cotton-tipped applicators may be used to apply gentle pressure over the area of cuticular damage to achieve hemostasis. If the wound is small, talcum powder with no added perfume or additive to it can be used to dry up the area. Wounds may also be sealed with tissue glue (in the surgery) or superglue (if at home). The animal should be placed in a small clean container on paper towel for 24 to 48 hours to monitor for further hemolymph loss. Hemolymph is clear and slightly blue in color but should be visible on paper towel. Fluid therapy may be necessary after hemolymph loss.[68]

Limbs may be damaged if they are caught on cloth fibers or mesh cage material; tarantulas have fine hairs on their feet. If the spider pulls away, complete autotomy may occur, or in some cases partial autotomy may occur, resulting in loss of hemolymph from the joints. It is a best practice to not perform autotomy under anesthesia because autotomy is an active process and anesthesia may prevent muscle spasms that aid in stopping hemolymph leakage. If the species is fractious or dangerous then anesthesia will have to be performed. The femur segment of the damaged limb is held with forceps and the limb is pulled rapidly upwards. If required, the area can be sealed with wax or cyanoacrylate glue.[68] Regeneration of the limb will take place, returning to normal size within the subsequent 2 to 3 molts.[31,68]

Dysecdysis
Theraphosids undergo ecdysis (molting), usually once a year. A new exoskeleton forms beneath the old cuticle from the living epidermal tissue. During ecdysis, the old exoskeleton splits to reveal the new cuticle. The new cuticle is soft to allow body expansion and then over a few hours to days, will harden. Tarantulas in dorsal recumbency are normally undergoing ecdysis and this may take up to 24 hours. They are very susceptible to trauma, and minimal interference is essential.[68]

Spiders may present because of dysecdysis and subsequent trauma to the exoskeleton. Owners have often tried to remove the old cuticle, and this often results in damage to the delicate exoskeleton underneath. It is not uncommon to have hemolymph loss. Attempts to free trapped limbs in retained exoskeleton cannot be made until the new cuticle has hardened. The old cuticle can be gently removed by wetting with mild detergents; the book lungs must be avoided to prevent drowning. The old cuticle may also be removed with iris scissors but there is a significant risk of iatrogenic exoskeleton damage resulting in loss of hemolymph.[32] If attempts to free the limbs are unsuccessful, autotomy can be performed and tissue glue adhesive applied at the site to prevent leakage of hemolymph. The authors have found that ligatures using fine suture material are inappropriate for spiders because this often results in cuticle damage.[68] Euthanasia must be considered for welfare reasons if too many limbs are damaged or deformed during dysecdysis and the spider is unable to move well enough to manage until the next molt.

Gastropods

Trauma

A fall or drop from a small distance can result in shell fracture or damage to soft tissues especially in calcium-deficient snails. This may result in hemolymph leakage, and death often occurs rapidly.[34] In giant African land snails, trauma usually results in damage to the calcareous shell with the consequences of dehydration due to exposure, desiccation to the underlying soft tissues, or hemorrhage if the soft tissues are penetrated. The snail should be placed in a shallow bowl of water or 0.9% saline pending shell repair. Shell fractures can be repaired by cleaning the fracture site with sterile saline, aligning the break and stabilizing the fracture sites with adhesive tape, adhesive plastic film, and then repairing using plaster of Paris or minimally exothermic epoxy resin (**Fig. 3**). Clear nail varnish can be applied over the repair once it has dried to make it water resistant. Damage to the tissues of the mantle can lead to shell growth deformities.[69–71] Dietary calcium supplementation with a natural chalk block or cuttlefish bone is advised for snails presented with shell damage.

If the tip of the shell is damaged it will not regrow. A repair may still be considered to enable a membrane to form over the area of injury (**Fig. 4**).

Lepidoptera

It is not uncommon to see collections with butterfly houses, and veterinarians may be asked to examine specimens. Lepidoptera may present with damaged wings that have torn or folded because of poor handling, becoming trapped, or from trauma in flight. A first-aid technique involving splinting the wing may be implemented. Gloves should be worn to prevent further damage to the Lepidoptera wing and the moth or butterfly should be placed upside down on a soft surface such as a towel. To gently restrain, a lightweight object (such as a wire coat hanger hook) can be placed over the animal (**Fig. 5**). The wings must be carefully straightened. A small splint can be made from cardboard and should be cut as small as possible to minimize the weight added to the wing. Apply a small amount of glue to the back of the cardboard using a toothpick or cocktail stick to avoid getting too much adhesive onto the cardboard. Using forceps place the cardboard across the break on the bridge of the wing and apply gentle pressure (see **Fig. 5**). Once secured, a small amount of unscented talcum

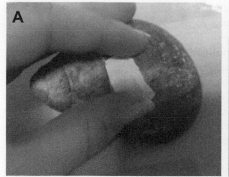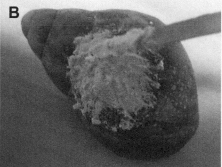

Fig. 3. Repair of shell in a giant African land snail using adhesive plastic film (*A*) and then applying plaster of Paris over the dressing (*B*). These images were taken during an invertebrate first-aid course using snail shells only. Gloves should be worn in practice. (*Courtesy of Lauren Lane, Paignton Zoo, Devon, UK.*)

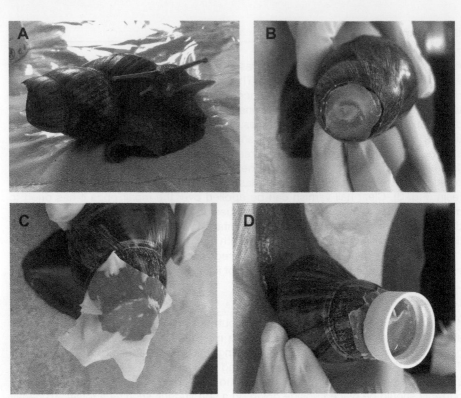

Fig. 4. (*A*) The tip of the damaged shell will not regrow, but a membrane may form over the area of injury. (*B*) The soft tissue is cleaned and an amorphous hydrogel (Intrasite gel, Smith and Nephew) is placed over the soft tissue. (*C*) A dressing is placed over the injury. (*D*) An adhesive is used to secure it. (*Courtesy of* Sonya Miles, BVSc, CertAVP(ZM), MRCVS, Highcroft Veterinary Group, Bristol, UK.)

powder is applied to ensure that the glue is covered and the adhesive dried to prevent the glue sticking to other parts of the animal.[71]

Fluid therapy can be challenging for Lepidoptera but may be essential. To provide fluids for butterflies and moths a shallow container such as a milk bottle top can be used. A sugar solution can be made using 2 teaspoons of sugar or honey to 100 mL of water. The solution is placed in the container, in addition to placing some on kitchen towel. The animal is held gently between the forefinger and thumb, with the wings held gently shut. The butterfly or moth's feet are placed on to the dampened kitchen towel and the animal is held in the natural sitting position, in front of the cap of sugar solution. A toothpick can be used to locate the proboscis and gently roll this into the sugar solution. This needs to be done with care, and multiple attempts may be needed before the animal settles and feeds. As the animal feeds, a pumping action of the proboscis can be seen. For debilitated animals the wings can be gently opened and closed repeatedly to attempt to stimulate feeding.[71] The animal can then be released back into the flight area.

Another technique that may be used to allow a butterfly or moth with a section of wing missing to fly, and to continue breeding, is to repair the wing using a wing from a deceased butterfly. Gloves are worn, and the animal is restrained as described earlier. The wings are straightened out to assess the severity of the damage. To repair the wing, a matching sized wing to the broken wing of the live animal must be found. It

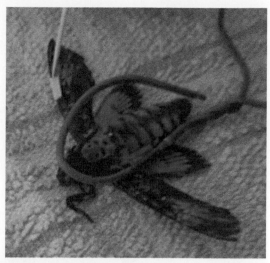

Fig. 5. Restraint of Lepidoptera may be achieved using a lightweight wire coat hanger. A small splint may be used across the break on the bridge of the wing. This image was taken on a postmortem specimen at an invertebrate first-aid course. (*Courtesy of* Lauren Lane, Paignton Zoo, Devon, UK.)

is not essential that the wing of the same species is used. Cut the broken side of the wing straight with sharp scissors and overlap the matching wing on to the broken one. A small amount of adhesive is applied using a toothpick and this is applied to the back of the new wing. This is then stuck to the broken wing. If the same species has been used attempt to match up the veins. Gentle pressure is applied using forceps until the adhesive is dry. Once the new wing is secured, unscented talcum powder is applied to the area and the animal is released.[71]

Other Arthropods

For smaller insects such as phasmids, beetles, or cockroaches damage to the exoskeleton may occur from incorrect handling, dysecdysis, or damage from cage furniture or browse such as bramble spikes. In phasmids, falling from a height from browse onto a hard surface can result in compression injuries. Repair to the exoskeleton can be achieved by applying gentle pressure with a cotton-tipped applicator and by applying a small amount of talcum powder or tissue adhesive as described earlier. An alternative approach is to make a drape using a piece of paper cutting out an area the size of the wound. The drape is placed over the invertebrate, protecting the rest of the exoskeleton and shielding respiratory openings such as the spiracles (**Fig. 6**). Excessive hemolymph is removed using a cotton-tipped applicator and then a liquid bandage or spray on plaster is applied covering the wound. Before placing the invertebrate into a darkened humid environment for recovery, ensure the liquid plaster has thoroughly dried.[71]

In general, placement of sutures in the exoskeleton is ineffective and may result in more injuries to the exoskeleton. Other approaches to sealing the exoskeleton, reported to be successful, include using an acrylic nail and cyanoacrylate glue to repair a fracture of the exoskeleton in a giant millipede.[32] Myriapods (millipedes and centipedes) are sensitive to desiccation, and ensuring adequate humidity when stabilizing any millipede or centipede after exoskeleton injury is paramount.[32,72]

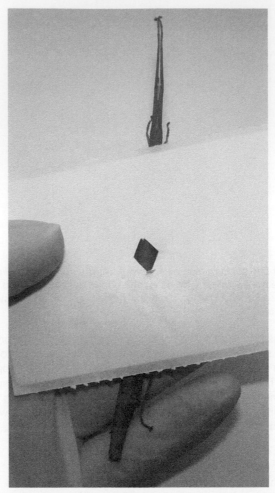

Fig. 6. A drape is made to allow the wound to be treated by applying talcum powder, tissue adhesive, or liquid plaster that can be sprayed on to the wound. The drape protects the respiratory openings. (*Courtesy of* Michelle O' Brien, BVetMed, CertZooMed, DipECZM (ZHM), MRCVS, Wildfowl & Wetlands Trust, Slimbridge, Gloucestershire, UK.)

Hermit crabs commonly present because of damage to the freshly molted exoskeleton and/or dysecdysis where the animals often lose legs and claws if there is inadequate provision of a deep substrate to burrow. Hermit crabs may also damage limbs or exoskeleton from fighting where crabs try and remove each other from their shells.[73,74] If there is no hemolymph loss, the animal should be separated from conspecifics and placed in a dark container with damp substrate and left undisturbed for 12 to 24 hours to allow the exoskeleton to harden. If hemolymph loss has occurred, the area must be dried and repaired using cyanoacrylate glue.[32]

SUMMARY

Invertebrates are becoming more popular within the pet trade and amongst teaching colleges, schools, and zoologic collections. It is not uncommon for these animals to be dropped or suffer from trauma where emergency treatment is essential to achieve hemostasis. Clinicians are encouraged to familiarize themselves with the basic first-aid techniques for invertebrate exoskeleton repair. With simple techniques and using items found in most homes, clients can be guided through basic first-aid procedures to prevent fatalities from hemolymph loss until the animal can be properly attended by a clinician.

ACKNOWLEDGMENTS

We would like to thank colleagues and organizations that have contributed in expanding invertebrate knowledge; colleagues at the British and Irish Association of Zoos and Aquariums (BIAZA) Terrestrial Invertebrate Working Group for their continued work on increasing awareness of invertebrate husbandry and welfare and developing the invertebrate first-aid workshop, which has been delivered to many organizations, and members of the Veterinary Invertebrate Society, an international association of veterinarians, veterinary nurses, scientists, and keepers interested in, and working with, invertebrates. We would like to acknowledge the Royal College of Veterinary Surgeons (RCVS) library for performing a literature review on this topic.

REFERENCES

1. Cooper JE. Skin disease in invertebrates. In: Locke PH, Harvey RG, Mason IS, editors. Manual of small animal dermatology. Cheltenham (United Kingdom): British Small Animal Veterinary Association (BSAVA); 1993. p. 198–212.
2. Rakison DH, Deringer J. Do infants possess an evolved spider-detection mechanism? Cognition 2008;107:381–93.
3. Lebowitz ER, Shic F, Campbell D, et al. Avoidance moderates the association between mothers' and children's fears: findings from a novel motion-tracking behaviour assessment. Depress Anxiety 2015;32:91–8.
4. Pellett S, Kubiak M. A review of invertebrate cases seen in practice. Proceedings Veterinary Invertebrate Society Summer Scientific Meeting. Cambridge (United Kingdom), July 12, 2017. p. 4.
5. Williams D. Integumental disease in invertebrates. Vet Clin North Am Exot Anim Pract 2001;4(2):309–20.
6. Parle E, Dirks JH, Taylor D. Damage, repair and regeneration in insect cuticle: the story so far, and possibilities for the future. Arthropod Struct Dev 2017;46(1): 49–55.
7. Metchnikoff E. Leçons sur la pathogie compare d'inflammation. Paris: Masson; 1893. p. 268.
8. Turk JL. Metchnikoff revisited. J R Soc Med 1991;84:579.
9. Fretten V, Graham A. A functional anatomy of invertebrates. London: Academic Press; 1976. p. 589.
10. Laverack MS, Dando J. Lecture notes on invertebrate zoology. 3rd edition. Oxford (United Kingdom): Blackwell; 1987. p. 212p.
11. Leake LD. Comparative histology. London: Academic Press; 1975. p. 738.
12. Wigglesworth VB. Insect physiology. 8th edition. London: Chapman and Hall; 1984. p. 191.
13. Bereiter-Hahn J, Matoltay AG, Richards KS, editors. Biology of the integument, vol 1. Invertebrates. Heidelberg (Germany). Springer-Verlag; 1984. p. 841.
14. Cusack M, DuJiao G, Chung P, et al. Biomineral repair of abalone shell apertures. J Struct Biol 2013;183(2):165–71.
15. Yeaton RW. Wound responses in insects. Am Zool 1983;23:195.

16. Silva JRMC, Mendes EG, Mariano M. Wound repair in the Amphioxus (*Branchiostoma plafae*): an animal deprived of inflammatory phagocytes. J Invertebr Pathol 1995;65:147–51.

17. Dales RP. Defense of invertebrates against bacterial infection. J R Soc Med 1979; 72:688.

18. Smith RJ, Grula EA. Toxic components on the larval surface of the corn earworm (*Heliothis zea*) and their effects on germination and growth of *Beauveria bassiana*. J Invertebr Pathol 1982;39:15.

19. Canicatti C, D'Ancona G. Biological protective substances in *Marthasterias glacialis* (Asteroidea) eoidermal secretion. J Zool 1990;222:373.

20. SiGang F, DaiZhi Z, BaoSuo L, et al. Molecular cloning and expression analysis of BMP7b from *Pinctada fucata* [Chinese]. South China Fisheries Science 2018; 14(1):121–6.

21. Sparks AK. Invertebrate Pathology: non-communicable diseases. New York: Academic Press; 1972. p. 387.

22. Boyle PR. The UFAW Handbook on the care and management of cephalopods in the laboratory. Potters Bar (United Kingdom): Universities Federation for Animal Welfare; 1991. p. 63.

23. Brandwood A, Jayes AS, Alexander RMCN. Incidence of healed fracture in the skeletons of birds, molluscs and primates. J Zool 1986;208:55.

24. Sminia RJ, Petersen K, Scheerboom JEM. Histochemical and ultrastructural observations on wound healing in the freshwater pulmonate *Lymnaea stagnalis*. Zeitung Zellschaft Mikroskopische Anatomie 1973;141:561–73.

25. Ruddell CL. Elucidation of the nature and function of the granular oyster amoebocyte through histochemical studies of normal and traumatized oyster tissues. Histochemie 1968;26:98–112.

26. Fry FEJ. Effects of the environment on animal activity. Ontario (Canada): University of Toronto Biology Services, Publication of Ontario Fisheries Research Laboratory; 1947. p. 5568.

27. O' Brien M. Dealing with giant African land snails. Veterinary Times 2009. Available at: http://www.vettimes.co.uk. Accessed August 8, 2017.

28. Ireland MP. The effect of dietary calcium on growth, shell thickness and tissue calcium distribution in the snail, *Achatina fulica*. Comp Biochem Physiol 1971; 98A(1):111–6.

29. Kriajev L, Otremski I, Edelstein S. Calcium cells from snails: response to vitamin D metabolites. Calcif Tissue Int 1994;55:204–7.

30. Kriajev L, Edelstein S. Effect of light and nutrient restriction on the metabolism of calcium and vitamin D in land snails. J Exp Zool 1995;272:153–8.

31. Pizzi R. Invertebrates. In: Meredith A, Johnson-Delaney CA, editors. BSAVA manual of exotic pets. 5th edition. Gloucester (United Kingdom): BSAVA Publications; 2010. p. 373–85.

32. Dombrowski D, De Voe R. Emergency care of invertebrates. Vet Clin North Am Exot Anim Pract 2007;10(2):621–45.

33. Cooper JE. A veterinary approach to spiders. Journal of Small Animal Practice 1987;28:229.

34. Braun ME, Heatley JJ, Chitty J. Clinical techniques of invertebrates. Vet Clin North Am Exot Anim Pract 2006;9:205–21.

35. Ellis CH. The mechanism of extension in the legs of spiders. Biol Bull 1944;86: 41–50.

36. Sladky KK. Current understanding of fish and invertebrate anaesthesia and analgesia. Proceedings Association of Reptilian and Amphibian Veterinarians. Orlando (FL), October 18–24, 2014. p. 122–4.

37. Zachariah TT, Mitchell MA, Guichard CM, et al. Isoflurane anaesthesia of wild-caught goliath birdeater spiders (*Theraphosa blondi*) and Chilean rose spiders (*Grammostola rosea*). J Zoo Wildl Med 2009;40:347–9.

38. Dombrowski DS, De Voe RS, Lewbart GA. Comparison of isoflurane and carbon dioxide anaesthesia in Chilean rose tarantulas (*Grammostola rosea*). Zoo Biol 2013;32:101–3.

39. Zachariah TT, Mitchell MA, Watson MK, et al. Effects of sevoflurane anaesthesia on righting reflex and haemolymph gas analysis variables for Chilean rose tarantulas (*Grammostola rosea*). Am J Vet Res 2014;75:521–6.

40. Gjeltema J, Posner LP, Stoskopf M. The use of injectable alphaxalone as a single agent and in combination with ketamine, xylazine, and morphine in the Chilean rose tarantula, *Grammostola rosea*. J Zoo Wildl Med 2014;45:792–801.

41. Clark TR, Nossov PC, Apland JR. Anaesthetic agents for use in the invertebrate sea snail, *Aplysia californica*. Contemp Top Lab Anim Sci 1996;35:75–9.

42. O'Brien M. Invertebrate anaesthesia. In: Longley L, editor. Anaesthesia of exotic pets. St Louis (MA): Elsevier Saunders; 2008. p. 279–95.

43. Runham NW, Isarankura K, Smith BJ. Methods for narcotizing and anaesthetising gastropods. Malacologia 1965;2:231–8.

44. Ross LG, Ross B. Anaesthesia of aquatic invertebrates. In: Ross LG, Ross B, editors. Anaesthetic and sedative techniques for aquatic animals. 2nd edition. Oxford (United Kingdom): Blackwell Science; 1999. p. 46–57.

45. Aquilina B, Roberts R. A method for inducing muscle relaxation in the abalone, *Haliotis iris*. Aquaculture 2000;190:403–8.

46. Edwards S, Burke C, Hindrum S. Recovery and growth effects of anaesthetic and mechanical removal on greenlips (*Haliotis laevigata*) and blacklip (*Haliotis rubra*) abalone. J Shellfish Res 2000;19:510.

47. White HI, Hecht T, Potgeiter B. The effect of four anaesthetics on *Haliotis midae* and their suitability for application in commercial abalone culture. Aquaculture 1996;140:145–51.

48. Gunkel C, Lewbart GA. Invertebrates. In: West G, Heard D, Caulkett N, editors. Zoo animal and wildlife immobilization and anesthesia. Ames (IA): Blackwell Publishing; 2007. p. 147–57.

49. Joosse J, Lever J. Techniques for narcotisation and operation for experiments with Lymnaea stagnalis (Gastropoda Pulmonata). Proceedings, Koninklijke Nederlandse Akademie van Wetenschappen. Amsterdam, 1959;2. p. 145–9.

50. Mutani A. A technique for anaesthetising pulmonate snails of medical and veterinary importance. Z Parasitenkd 1982;68:117–9.

51. Murray MJ. Euthanasia. In: Lewbart GA, editor. Invertebrate medicine. Oxford (United Kingdom): Blackwell Publishing; 2012. p. 441–3.

52. Cooper JE. Emergency care of invertebrates. Vet Clin North Am Exot Anim Pract 1998;1(1):251–64.

53. Tarsitano MS, Jackson RR. Araneophagic jumping spiders discriminate between detour routes that do and do not lead to prey. Anim Behav 1997;53:257–66.

54. Jackson RR, Carter CM, Tarsitano MS. Trial and orror solving of a confinement problem by a jumping spider, *Portia fibriata*. Behaviour 2001;138:1215–34.

55. Dyakonova VE. Role of opioid peptides in behaviour of invertebrates. J Evol Biochem Physiol 2001;37:335–47.

56. Kavaliers M, Hirst M, Teskey GC. A functional role for an opiate system in snail thermal behaviour. Science 1983;220:99–101.
57. Mather JA. Animal suffering: an invertebrate perspective. J Appl Anim Welfare Sci 2001;4:151–6.
58. Manev H, Dimitrijevic N. Fruit flies for anti-pain drug discovery. Life Sci 2005;76: 2403–7.
59. Elwood RW, Appel M. Pain experience in hermit crabs? Anim Behav 2009;77: 1243–6.
60. Nathaniela TI, Pankseppb J, Hubera R. Effects of a single and repeated morphine treatment on conditioned and unconditioned behavioural sensitisation in Crayfish. Behav Brain Res 2010;207:310–20.
61. Cooper JE. Anaesthesia, analgesia, and euthanasia of invertebrates. Inst Lab Anim Res J 2011;52:196–204.
62. Keller DL, Abbott AD, Sladky KK. Invertebrate antinociception: are opioids effective in tarantulas? Proc Am Assoc Zoo Vet. Oakland (CA), October 21–26, 2012. p. 97.
63. Lewbart GA. Clinical anaesthesia and analgesia in invertebrates. J Exot Pet Med 2012;21:59–70.
64. Pellett S, Kubiak M, Pizzi R, et al. BIAZA recommendations for ethical euthanasia of invertebrates. 2017 (Version 3.0 - April 2017). Available at: http://www.biaza. org.uk/In press. Accessed December 2, 2019.
65. Cooper JE, Knowler C. Snails and snail farming: an introduction for the veterinary profession. Vet Rec 1991;129:541–9.
66. Rees Davies R, Chitty JR, Saunders R. Cardiovascular monitoring of an Achatina snail using a Doppler ultrasound unit. Proceedings of the British Veterinary Zoological Society Autumn Meeting. RVC London, November 18–19, 2000. p. 101.
67. Bennie NAC, Loaring CD, Bennie MMG, et al. An effective method for terrestrial arthropod euthanasia. J Exp Biol 2012;215:4237–41.
68. Pizzi R. Spiders. In: Lewbart GA, editor. Invertebrate medicine. 2nd edition. Oxford (United Kingdom): Blackwell Publishing; 2012. p. 187–221.
69. Connolly C. Repair of the shell of a giant African landsnail (Achatina fulica), using Leucopor tape and Nexabond tissue adhesive. Veterinary Invertebrate Society Newsletter 2004;8–11.
70. Zwart P, Cooper JE. Shell deformities in the European edible snail (Cornu aspersum) and the giant African snail (Achatina achatina) In preparation for the Veterinary Invertebrate Society Journal, in press.
71. British and Irish Association of Zoos and Aquariums (BIAZA) Terrestrial Invertebrate Working Group First-aid Workshop. Twycross Zoo, 6th–8th December 2015.
72. Chiariello TM. Centipede care and husbandry. Journal of Exotic Pet Medicine 2015;24:326–32.
73. Marnell C. Tarantula and hermit crab emergency care. Vet Clin Exot Anim 2016; 19:627–46.
74. Elwood RW, Briffa M. Information gathering and communication during agnostic encounters: a case study of hermit crabs. Adv Stud Behav 2001;30:53–97.

Moving?

Make sure your subscription moves with you!

To notify us of your new address, find your **Clinics Account Number** (located on your mailing label above your name), and contact customer service at:

Email: journalscustomerservice-usa@elsevier.com

800-654-2452 (subscribers in the U.S. & Canada)
314-447-8871 (subscribers outside of the U.S. & Canada)

Fax number: 314-447-8029

Elsevier Health Sciences Division
Subscription Customer Service
3251 Riverport Lane
Maryland Heights, MO 63043

*To ensure uninterrupted delivery of your subscription, please notify us at least 4 weeks in advance of move.

ELSEVIER

Printed and bound by CPI Group (UK) Ltd, Croydon, CR0 4YY

03/10/2024

01040406-0003